GUA SHA 刮痧

An Ancient Therapy for Contemporary Illnesses

Other Related Titles from World Scientific

Acupuncture Understood: Rediscovering Traditional Five Element Healthcare
by Stuart Lightbody
ISBN: 978-981-4583-77-0
ISBN: 978-981-4583-78-7 (pbk)

Cancer Management with Chinese Medicine: Prevention and Complementary Treatments
Revised Edition
by Rencun Yu and Hong Hai
ISBN: 978-981-3203-88-4

The Healing Art of Tai Chi: Becoming One with Nature
by Martin J Lee, Emily Lee, Joyce Lee and Melinda Lee
ISBN: 978-981-3271-88-3
ISBN: 978-981-3273-08-5 (pbk)

Traditional Chinese Medicine, Western Science, and the Fight Against Allergic Disease
by Xiu-Min Li and Henry Ehrlich
ISBN: 978-981-4733-68-7
ISBN: 978-981-4733-69-4 (pbk)

Traditional, Complementary and Alternative Medicine: Policy and Public Health Perspectives
edited by Gerard Bodeker and Gemma Burford
ISBN: 978-1-86094-616-5
ISBN: 978-1-911299-69-1 (pbk)

GUA SHA 刮痧

An Ancient Therapy for Contemporary Illnesses

Kai Wen TANG

World Scientific

NEW JERSEY • LONDON • SINGAPORE • BEIJING • SHANGHAI • HONG KONG • TAIPEI • CHENNAI • TOKYO

Published by

World Scientific Publishing Co. Pte. Ltd.

5 Toh Tuck Link, Singapore 596224

USA office: 27 Warren Street, Suite 401-402, Hackensack, NJ 07601

UK office: 57 Shelton Street, Covent Garden, London WC2H 9HE

Library of Congress Cataloging-in-Publication Data
Names: Tang, Kai Wen, author.
Title: Gua sha : an ancient therapy for contemporary illnesses / Kai Wen Tang.
Description: Hackensack, NJ : World Scientific, [2020] |
Includes bibliographical references and index.
Identifiers: LCCN 2019047783 | ISBN 9789811209055 (hardcover)
Subjects: LCSH: Acupressure. | Medicine, Chinese.
Classification: LCC RM723.A27 T35 2020 | DDC 615.8/222--dc23
LC record available at https://lccn.loc.gov/2019047783

British Library Cataloguing-in-Publication Data
A catalogue record for this book is available from the British Library.

For any available supplementary material, please visit
https://www.worldscientific.com/worldscibooks/10.1142/11519#t=suppl

Typeset by Stallion Press
Email: enquiries@stallionpress.com

Preface

My earliest encounter with *Gua Sha* 刮痧 was a week before the National High School (GCE A Levels) Examination. As a martial-arts loving teenager from a modest family, I could only pursue my passion at the generosity of my friends who practiced with me after school during the hottest hours of the day.

On one occasion, I returned home perspiring heavily, feeling extremely exhausted and dozed off on the cement floor. I woke up in the evening with chills, teary eyes, splitting headache, severe muscular and joint pains and high temperature. I sensed I was in trouble and requested my mother to bring me to a hospital immediately.

Diagnosed with viral fever and admitted for symptomatic treatment, I was told to live the course of the illness that might take a fortnight. This obviously did not augur well with the timing of my impending national examination and knowing that there was no immediate threat to my life, asked my mum to arrange for my discharge against the orders of the doctors.

Reaching home, my mum applied *Gua Sha* on me that brought quick relief and I slept soundly through the night until the following afternoon. Fever subsided, *sans* body aches, a repaired body and a new-found respect for an effective traditional remedy I once scorned upon.

I subsequently learned that my mum's skill was inherited from her great grandmother who operated boarding houses for sea-faring traders from China. These travelers, when failed to adapt to the local climate, often succumbed to heat stroke and were saved by *Gua Sha.*

Decades later when I embarked on my journey to read Traditional Chinese Medicine (TCM), I resolved to demystify and rationalize *Gua Sha* by building a knowledge base of the topic from ancient as well as contemporary literature and connecting the dots to explore and discover the underlying concepts. In clinical practice, *Gua Sha* has also consistently produced favorable therapeutic outcomes for my patients. It is, therefore, time for me to share my understanding of this topic for the benefit of all.

This book is written in non-technical language and does not require the reader to have prior knowledge of the subject. For ease of reading, the subject is presented in bite-size topics with technical terms duly referenced and explained briefly in plain language within the same topic space. Dividing the subject into bite-size topics also permits the reader to selectively explore the subject from multiple points of entry.

Organized into three parts, the first section of the book helps build a theoretical framework for the reader by introducing TCM theories relevant to the subject. A reader without an understanding of TCM basics may, however, have to persevere in order to progress from theory to practice. Building on this foundation, the next segment on Treatment Protocols presents the practice aspects of the subject that lay further groundwork for the chapter on Applications. In this final part, the nature of disorders is deliberated from both contemporary medicine and TCM perspectives and with adequate depth before touching on the treatment protocol. The informed reader may, then on the premise of potential risks and benefit, make a judgment call if *Gua Sha* was indeed fitting for a situation encountered. For in any treatment, there shall be a therapeutic benefit only when the situation is correctly assessed but risks of delay and deterioration if otherwise.

This book is, however, not a forum for disease diagnosis. Knowledge in medical diagnosis, whether based on contemporary medical science or TCM, requires years of formal training to acquire and it is a conscious decision to exclude this aspect to ensure that the reader obtains a competent opinion of any condition before turning to *Gua Sha* as therapy.

As far as permissible, translations for TCM terminologies in this book are imported from the *WHO International Standard Terminologies on Traditional Medicine in the Western Pacific Region 2007*. Where necessary, reference is also made to WHO Standard Acupuncture Nomenclature 2nd Ed (1993).

Another feature of this book is that although written for the general public, it provides a comprehensive compilation of published findings from scientific journals that a practitioner may wish to review.

Gua Sha is an ancient therapy drawn from TCM. It is an extension of the Acupuncture discipline. It is however non-invasive in nature and leaves little permanent adverse effects on people without pre-existing conditions so that *Gua Sha* may be executed safely and without fear by an informed user. For this reason, unlike Acupuncture, the practice of *Gua Sha* is not regulated and there is no licensing requirement in Singapore.

As a healing technique, *Gua Sha* is effective in promptly relieving symptoms of many ailments and may be applied at various levels of proficiency that result in differing therapeutic effectiveness. It can also be deployed singularly or applied in conjunction with other treatment modalities.

Like any medical science, *Gua Sha* is a pragmatic skill. The author encourages anyone to put into practice what is shared in this book to fully appreciate the benefits of *Gua Sha* for therapeutic purpose or general health promotion.

But please do not stop here. The duration and distance of the learning journey are solely determined by the reader and what unfolds along the way shall prove that the art of *Gua Sha* is indeed a gem from the treasure trove of Traditional Chinese Medicine that may serve the reader a lifetime.

Tang Kai Wen PhD (Nanjing)
Registered Physician

A Note on Reading

Gua Sha, originally popularized as a folk treatment, shares the same theoretical framework as Acupuncture. Admittedly, its therapeutic range may not be as wide as Acupuncture but the training required for a student of *Gua Sha* to become productive is also correspondingly less demanding than that mandated for a professional acupuncturist. These are simple trade-offs in life.

Notwithstanding, *Gua Sha* can be used even today to treat or alleviate a fair range of contemporary ailments.

However, with the passage of time, Gua Sha has also advanced to include many of the acupuncture techniques especially in the adoption of Meridian Dredging and Acupoint *Gua Sha.*

This book makes considerable reference to meridians and their acupoints in an attempt to explain the rationale of *Gua Sha* applications and prescriptions. The author, therefore, recommends that the reader should avail himself to a convenient source of reference to acupoints in order to fully appreciate the discussion.

Aside from getting a hardcopy Acupuncture manual at a price, there are various free sources of acupoint references accessible online over the internet. These sites are usually hosted by professional acupuncturist bodies or schools to provide students of Acupuncture with convenient and credible sources of reference. Most of these sites have search facilities and many of them are platform-independent i.e. support multiple operating systems like Microsoft Windows, Apple iOS, Android, etc.

The reader may wish to visit https://tcmpoints.com for this purpose.

This book does not make any medical claims and no intention is therefore made for its content to substitute the advice of other healthcare professionals. It is always prudent for individuals to consult a licensed healthcare practitioner before adopting any integrative or complementary medical option.

Contents

Part 1

Theoretical Framework

Topic 1

Introduction to *Gua Sha* Therapy

Traditional Chinese Medicine (TCM) has more than 3000 years of history. Through its unique yet internally consistent theories and practices, it holds major influence over the lives of the Chinese population. Like contemporary medicine, TCM has two distinct but complementary branches of practice — herbal therapy and external interventions 外治法.

The commonly known of these external intervention techniques are acupuncture and fire-cupping 火罐. *Gua Sha* is another of the many external intervention techniques that are equally effective but somewhat less explored by modern society.

In a nutshell, *Gua Sha* is an ancient folk remedy in which the lubricated skin of the person seeking treatment is repeatedly "press-stroked" with a smooth-edged instrument in a methodical manner to produce a moderate bruising. This superficial bruising, however, is different from traumatic bruising that one sustained in accidents. In so doing, stagnated energy is dissipated, blood flow improved, lymphatic circulation stimulated, inflammation reduced and the body's physiological balance restored.

In fact, the word *Gua* 刮 literally means "scraping" while the word *Sha* 痧 carries several different connotations that may categorically be explained as metabolic waste or toxins the body failed to remove that resulted in an impeded flow of Qi or vital energy in the body.

Nobody really knows when *Gua Sha* was developed but it is fair to assume it evolved from some skin scraping/stabbing therapy originated during the Palaeolithic Age when scraping or stabbing certain parts of the body with hands, hard objects or stones offered relief to someone's symptoms or even loss of consciousness. Notwithstanding, the earliest glimpse of this therapeutic technique may be found among the records of emergency treatment from "Prescriptions for 52 Diseases 五十二病方". Prescriptions for 52 Diseases is a collection of medical manuscripts unearthed in 1973 during the excavation of the Ma Wang Dui Han tomb at Changsha in Hunan 湖南长沙马王堆三号汉墓. This manuscript is officially now the earliest known record of Chinese *materia medica* and is estimated to be compiled between 1065 BCE and 771 BCE or the Shang-Zhou era.

With the passage of time, the technique of *Gua Sha* became more refined and sophisticated. The most comprehensive work on *Sha* entitled "Diagnosis of *Sha* Distention 痧胀玉衡" was completed during Qing dynasty by Guo Zhizhen 郭志邃. In his manuscript, Guo elaborated on the choice of instruments and techniques of *Gua Sha* for appropriate application to various parts of the body.

Traders, explorers, and emigrants helped propagate the technique of *Gua Sha* beyond the shores of China. This was out of necessity as traveling to and residing in a foreign land made familiar medical treatment less accessible when the danger of contracting illness was greatest. And of course, the practical reason of choice to arm oneself with *Gua Sha* skills before a trip is that the technique is extremely effective in providing quick relief for a wide range of disorders, has a very short learning curve, does not require specialized instrument and relatively risk-free and error-prone in execution.

Gua Sha made its way to South Asia in early 15th Century along with the maritime expeditions of Admiral Zheng He 郑和 when the Ming naval fleet visited Champa (Vietnam), Siam (Thailand), Malacca (Malaysia), Java (Indonesia) and the Malabar Coast of India and Ceylon (Sri Lanka).

The technique retained its original name in Malaysia and Singapore but adopted the name *cạo gió* in Vietnam, a term that translates to “wind scraping” as TCM associates wind to be the carrier of many other exogenous pathogens. In Indonesia, it took on yet a different name *kerokan* or literarily “scraping technique” in the Indonesian language. Little is known about the prevalence of *Gua Sha* in India but suffice to say the deeply rooted Ayurvedic medicine may have limited *Gua Sha* to only sporadic practice and therefore its popularity.

Topic 2

How *Gua Sha*, Cupping and Acupuncture Differ From One Another

Gua Sha, Fire Cupping 火罐 and Acupuncture are different techniques of TCM external intervention 外治法 that are predicated on the Meridian Theory, the principles of which are detailed in the Book of Miraculous Pivot 灵枢, the second volume of HuangDi's Internal Classics 黄帝内经.

In addition, *Gua Sha* and Fire Cupping are also rooted in the Discourse on Skin 皮部论 enunciated in Chapter 56 of Plain Questions 素问, the first volume of HuangDi's Internal Classics. More of the Skin Theory shall be discussed under subsequent topics.

Simply put, these external interventions are not creations from trivial sources for HuangDi's Internal Classics, believed to be a compilation of medical manuscripts by eminent physicians during the Warring States period (475 BCE–221 BCE) and the Han dynasty (206 BCE–220 CE), is the most authoritative and influential source of reference in TCM even today.

It may also be of interest to note that the gap between 221 BCE and 206 BCE where no medical literary works were produced coincided with the Qin Dynasty period when literary works of all nature were massively destroyed by the ruling Emperor.

Though these three techniques share relatively similar theoretical foundation, they are markedly different in terms of execution as indicated in the tables below:

Equipment Used

Cupping	Cupping requires the administration of a vacuum within an airtight vessel over skin of the patient. This vacuum is created either by specialized equipment with a one-way air valve or traditionally by burning off the air in a glass or bamboo vessel before attaching it on the skin.
Acupuncture	Fine surgical quality steel needles of varying lengths for cutaneous needling, intradermal needles for subcutaneous insertion, knife needles, point catgut embedding, three-edge needles, fire needle, hypodermic needle and syringe and moxi.
Gua Sha	No specific equipment necessary so long as the instrument offers a smooth edge of contact with patient's skin.

Treatment Marks

Cupping	Cupping causes a more intense and thus enduring bruise by virtue of the vacuum. The bruise generally takes on the shape of the vessel, usually a circular mark, after treatment with static cupping or dark wide strips after sliding cup motion is administered.
Acupuncture	No visible markings except some occasional light bleeding after needle extraction.
Gua Sha	Usually light petechia, intensity and hue depending on the nature and duration of illness.

Stimulation Method

Cupping	Vacuum induced subcutaneous blood concentration at selected treatment areas.
Acupuncture	Hand needle manipulation, electro-impulse, electro-thermal, drug injection, moxibustion.
Gua Sha	Tonification strokes, Detoxification/Purging strokes, Moderation strokes.

Treatment Area

Cupping	Dermatome/myotome-like areas 筋经, meridians, defined acupoints.
Acupuncture	Defined acupoints, trigger points, pain reflexion points.
Gua Sha	Dermatome/myotome-like areas 筋经, meridians, defined acupoints.

General Limitations

Cupping	May be applied to body area where the anatomy offers adequate flat surface to maintain the suction that cupping requires to operate. Irregular, hairy or bony parts of the body are not candidates for cupping. Not to be administered over broken skin or on sensitive areas e.g. eye lids, genitals, breasts, throat, naval, etc.
Acupuncture	Effectiveness of treatment mainly lies with the ability of operator in selecting the appropriate combination of acupoints, in accurately locating acupoints and to elicit needling response 针感 for Qi acquisition 得气. Sensitive areas are generally avoided.

Gua Sha	Not to be administered over broken skin. Caution to be exercised when administering over sensitive areas in proximity to the eyelids, throat, naval and nipples.

Associated Risks

Cupping	The use of fire to create a vacuum in the airtight vessel, hence the name "Fire-Cupping" 火罐, runs a risk of scorching the skin if the same vessel is repeatedly applied in quick succession to the patient. The risk is apparently higher when glass vessels are used. A variant of cupping 刺絡拔罐 involves blood-letting. Usually deployed for treatment in more severe or deep seated conditions, infection risk is increased by its invasive nature.
Acupuncture	Fundamentally a treatment of invasive nature, it requires strict control in the depth of needle penetration especially for many acupoints that are located over vital organs. Mismanagement may lead to vascular perforation, organ damage and even immediate fatality.
Gua Sha	A treatment of non-invasive nature, *Gua Sha* provides wide latitude for error during execution and does not leave injuries of permanent nature especially for patients without contraindicated pre-existing conditions. A variant of Gua Sha that involves blood-letting increases infection risk.

It may be seen from the foregoing that, apart from Acupuncture, the other two external intervention techniques pose a limited risk and are deceptively simple to apply by the untrained. Make no mistake for even the apparently harmless *Gua Sha* when administered inappropriately by an over-zealous operator could end up with contusion injury to underlying soft tissues that warrant medical attention.

In a reported case of a 23-year-old man attended to by the Emergency Department for acute epiglottitis, ecchymoses were observed on the front and sides of his neck.[1] These bruises, caused by ruptured blood vessels near the surface of the skin, was clearly induced by *Gua Sha* treatment the man received earlier. Detailed examination showed an elevated hyoid bone with thickening of the retropharyngeal soft tissue. The posterior wall of the pharynx was compressed by an enlarged epiglottis, resulted in impaired speech. Although the person was traumatized, he was afebrile with normal vital signs and not in respiratory distress. The inflammation was resolved speedily with the administration of intravenous steroids.

Notwithstanding that *Gua Sha* may appear to be a gruesome and vigorous treatment, accidents like the above-mentioned case rarely occur. There are documented cases that patients suffered nausea and vertigo shortly after the administration of acupuncture. Anecdotal evidence also pointed to incidents where cupping caused elevation of vascular circulation in some patients leading to general discomfort after the session. Yet in comparison, there is a lesser incidence of such reported experiences arising from *Gua Sha* when it is administered correctly. *Gua Sha* is, therefore, a very effective and elegantly simple therapy with moderated side effects.

Glossary

Ecchymoses [plural form] — a hemorrhagic spot, larger than a petechia, in the skin or mucous membrane, forming a flat, rounded or irregular, blue or purplish patch.

Petechia — a minute, pinpoint, non-raised, perfectly round, purplish-red spot caused by intradermal or submucous hemorrhage, which later turns blue or yellow.

The epiglottis is an elastic cartilaginous structure at the root of the tongue that prevents food from entering the windpipe (trachea) when swallowing. Epiglottitis is a potentially life-threatening situation that results in swelling and inflammation of the epiglottis leading to the obstruction of the airway.

Reference

1. Tsai KK, Wang CH. Acute epiglottitis following traditional Chinese gua sha therapy. *CMAJ* **186**(8): E298 (May 13, 2014).

Topic 3

How *Gua Sha* Differs from Instrument-Assisted Soft Tissue Mobilization (IASTM)

IASTM is a western chiropractic modern-day development that involves using specialized instruments to effectively locate and treat soft-tissue dysfunctions. The Graston® Technique is one of the more popular IASTM therapy systems.

A soft-tissue injury is an impairment to the muscles, ligaments, tendons and/or fascia in the body. It is commonly caused by excessive use of a particular body part leading to chronically fatigue structure or trauma to the body that resulted in a contusion (ruptured blood vessels/bruising). It may also be caused by abrupt or uncontrolled movement. Soft tissue injuries usually result in pain, swelling, bruising and loss of function. Adhesions within the soft tissue may develop as a result of repeated strain, surgery, immobilization or other mechanisms.

Soft tissue injuries occur with varying levels of severity. Minimal over-stretching that leads to possible minor microscopic fiber tear will cause mild tenderness and swelling at the site of injury. A person with partial fiber tear will experience moderate pain, tenderness, and swelling and will not be able to apply load to the injured area without pain. In event of a complete rupture of structure, significant pain, stiffness, and swelling will cause the injured structure to be non-functional with instability of the affected joint setting in, especially weight-bearing joints like the hip, knee, and ankle.

Soft tissue injury, especially in more severe cases, will become chronic when left to heal on its own. Unfortunately, when scar tissues are formed during this self-healing process, new cells are laid down excessively and in a disorganized manner in the affected area. Myofascial adhesions so formed prevent muscles and other tissues from extending normally thereby limiting the range of motion and often time causing pain.

IASTM addresses this issue by introducing micro-trauma in a controlled manner to the affected soft tissue. This is essentially re-injuring the affected part to a lesser degree and in a controlled fashion to commence a re-healing process. In so doing it stimulates a local inflammatory response that initiates reabsorption of excessive scar tissue and facilitates remodeling of the affected soft-tissue structures in favor of normal movement.

Patients may experience soreness in the treatment area for a day or two following treatment. Bruising can but is not a common occurrence nor is desirable.

Although both techniques are derma-abrasive in nature, *Gua Sha* is in more than one way different from IASTM.

In terms of therapeutic objectives, IASTM serves to relief musculoskeletal dysfunction and pain through soft-tissue remodeling targeted at making physical changes to soft tissue or neurological stimulation designed to influence the nervous system, creating changes in neural drive to influence tissue tone and plasticity.

The guiding principle of IASTM is the identification of scar tissues or adhesions formed by the body's self-healing process after injury. The treatment is therefore localized to the site of injury. The clinician is required to perform a scanning or sweeping scrap to "feel for the adhesions" before the commencement of the actual treatment.

Gua Sha enjoys an even greater therapeutic scope that addresses ailments beyond musculoskeletal nature and its treatment has the ability to relieve pain and symptoms that are not only proximal to but also in regions far distal from the treatment zones. All told, *Gua Sha*, therefore, does what IASTM can and more!

Gua Sha's therapeutic principles are guided by the TCM Meridian Theory and Skin Theory. As *Gua Sha* can be deployed to treat a wide range of ailments, the clinician shall select the appropriate meridian(s) and acupoint(s) for treatment after evaluating the patient's condition using the Four Pillars of TCM Clinical Diagnosis 四诊.

IASTM proffers a repertoire of specialized equipment and often time employs multiple instruments within a single session.

No specific equipment is necessary for *Gua Sha* so long as the instrument offers a smooth edge of contact with the patient's skin.

In terms of execution, an IASTM clinician may perform pressure strokes in both directions and relies on feedback from the pressure strokes for interpretation of treatment effectiveness. Bruising and petechia are taken in their usual sense as capillary damage in the dermis. They are therefore not viewed as visible confirmation of effective treatment but instead indicative of excessive or over-treatment and preferably be avoided.

When applying scraping motion, *Gua Sha* is performed unidirectionally along the cutaneous area(s), the meridian-tendon 经筋 area(s), the outline of the selected meridian(s) and/or at the location of selected acupoint(s). The length, execution speed and pressure of the stroke determine if the stroke confers tonification or detoxification/dissipation effect. The appearance of petechia is a visual indication that excess heat and toxins are released through the surface. Intensities and hues of the petechia represent different manifestations of illness according to the "TCM Eight Precepts of Syndrome Differentiation 八纲辨证" — yin 阴, yang 阳, cold 寒, heat 热, superficial 表, deep-seated 里, deficiency/debility 虚, and excess 实.

Topic 4

The Etiology of Diseases from a TCM Perspective

In order to appreciate how *Gua Sha* heals, it is essential at this juncture to understand from the TCM perspective the cause of illness.

Generally, the diagnosis of diseases may be performed at three levels of complexity — cellular and molecular level, physiological level and holistic level. Modern medicine, with advanced laboratory equipment, draws its strength from cellular and molecular and physiological levels of disease evaluation. On the contrary TCM, with a history of more than 3000 years, stakes her ground on a holistic assessment of illness.

Founded on the premise that man is a microcosm as well as part of the universe, this holistic view rules that life process is interactive with and reflective of the behavior of nature. And through observation of nature, it was noted that all objects, energies, and phenomena within the universe have opposing characteristics that are relative, interdependent, mutually transformative and mutually consuming. In TCM, this interplay of two primary forces of life is represented by the Yin-Yang concept, the principles which are clearly depicted by the symbol below.

Yin and Yang are opposing imply that the characteristics of the two elements are polar in nature but relative to one another. A commonly cited example of Yin and Yang is darkness and brightness

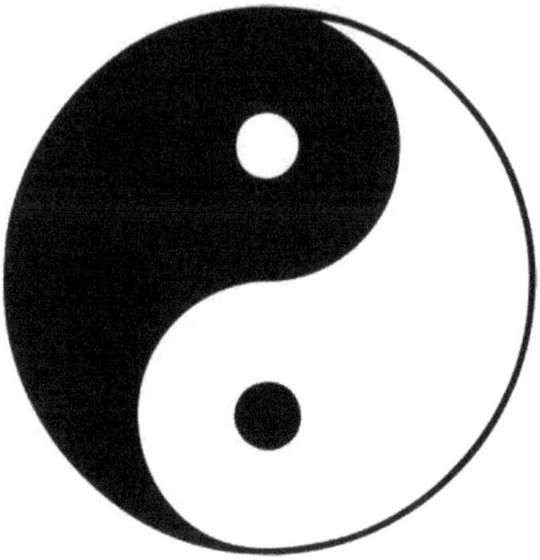

respectively. Darkness is relative to brightness and vice versa. And whilst mutually opposing 阴阳對立, they are also interdependent in that both must co-exist. One cannot perceive darkness if brightness did not exist.

Existence of the elements cannot be made absolute to the exclusion of the other. To the extent that the definition of one relies on the definition of the other, neither Yin nor Yang could subsist or thrive in exclusivity 孤阴不生, 独阳不长. This is represented in the symbol by a dark dot within the bright swirl forming part of the circle and indicative of yin existing within and engendering yang 阴阳互根. The converse is also true.

In fact, the concept of Yin-Yang is so pervasive in its application that it is adopted as the overriding principle in the "TCM Eight Precepts of Syndrome Differentiation 八纲辨证" as well as the latter-day "TCM Ten Precepts of Syndrome Differentiation 十纲辨证"

Health is an outcome of achieving a dynamic balance between these two fundamental forces of life. In a healthy state, this balance is in a constant state of flux 阴阳消長, preserving the waxing and waning of each counteracting force in a synchronized fashion without the exclusion of any one element, through a process of mutual transformation and mutual consumption 阴阳轉化.

This cyclical but harmonious balance 阴阳調和 may be skewed by both exogenous and endogenous influences. Disease occurs when the dynamic equilibrium of yin-yang within the body is displaced beyond the physiological norm and not restored within an acceptable transitional period.

Because man and nature are interconnected within the universe, any adverse change in the immediate environment would have an impact on his well-being. TCM identified Six Excesses or

Pathogenic Factors or Pernicious Elements 六淫 as the exogenous influence that will disrupt the harmonious balance in the body. The following is a brief description of the Six Pathogenic Factors.

Pathogen	Category	Disharmonizing Effects	Pathological Characteristics
Wind	Yang	Vehicle for other pathogens	Rapid/swift changing symptoms, superficial symptoms, preferentially affects superior and posterior parts of anatomy
Cold	Yin	Undermines Yang energy, obstruction of qi flow	Sudden onset of symptoms of chills, headache and body aches, pain is the signature of cold
Dampness	Yin	Undermines Yang energy, obstruction of qi flow	Sluggishness, lethargy, edema and ascites, sticky discharges, relapses, preferentially affects inferior parts of anatomy
Dehyration	Yang	Depletion of vital fluids/Yin	Closely related to Fire/Heat pathogen, general symptoms include dehydration of mucosa
Heat/Fire	Yang	Depletion of vital fluids/Yin	Heat, fire, toxins are similar in nature but of increasing intensity, general symptoms include fever, inflammation, constipation, and sores
Summer Heat	Yang	Depletion of vital fluids/Yin, depletion of qi	Combined effects of heat and dampness, general symptoms dehydration and exhaustion

Make no mistake that "wind" or "dampness" pathogen imply that wind or dampness by itself caused the disease, though climatic changes generally predispose less adaptable people to illness. It should instead be interpreted in a manner that various pathogens that thrive and propagate particularly well under that specific inclement weather condition are broadly termed or listed under that label.

Be mindful that there were no powerful microscopes or advanced laboratory equipment at the time when the classification was developed, so in hindsight, we should laud the acute observations of our forefathers made some 3000 years ago.

Exogenous influences, singularly or in concert, engender external pathogens that enter the body via the skin and the orifices. To complicate matters, external pathogens upon entering the body if left to proliferate may transform into various forms of "internal pathogens" with properties different from the original external pathogens depending on the body's constitution as well as the nature of nutrients consumed by the infected. As an illustration, external pathogens that thrive favorably in wind and heat situation will carry combined wind/heat 风热 pathological characteristics during the initial phase of the infection. However, if the person has a "damp" constitution caused by dietary habits, the subsequent symptoms developed would be inclined towards damp-heat 湿热 since wind is only a vehicle for propagation.

Beside physical adaption to the changing environment, the inability to adapt to acute or chronic psychological changes in life especially arising from exposure to traumatic events is another significant cause of illness. And this is endorsed by contemporary medical research in psychological stress.

While minor episodes of stress may be overcome by the body's natural defenses during the course of adaption to changing situations, excessive stress, acute and/or continuing over an extended period of time, can lead to health conditions of differing severity including muscle spasm, anxiety, insomnia, gastrointestinal diseases, metabolic syndrome, cardiovascular diseases, compromised immunity and even cancers.[1]

	Organ Systems					
Emotion	Viscus Cat	Viscus 脏	Bowel 腑	Element	Comment	Common Symptoms
Joy喜	Yang within Yang	Heart	Small Intestine	Fire	Heart system include brain and psychological functions.	Cardiovascular issues, Palpitation, Insomnia, Excessive dreams, Memory issues, Psychological disorders.
Anger 怒	Yang within Yin	Liver	Gall Bladder	Wood	Liver system includes haematological functions.	Breast distension, Menstrual pain, Headache, Circulation issues, Ocular conditions, Tendonitis.
Pensiveness 思	Yin within Ultimate Yin	Spleen	Stomach	Earth	Worry and Pensiveness are of similar nature but differ in intensity. Spleen is a conceptual organ in TCM, not referring to Spleen of modern medicine.	Fatigue, Appetite, Mucus discharge, Digestion, Diarrhea, Abdominal distension, Muscular weakness, Excess menstruation, Bleeding disorders.
Grief 悲 Worry 忧	Yin within Yang	Lung	Large Intestine	Metal	Lung system includes dermatological functions.	Shortness of breath, Shallow breathing, Sweating, Cough, Cold and Flu, Allergies, Dermalogical conditions.
Fear 恐 Fright 惊	Yin within Yin	Kidney	Bladder	Water	Kidney system includes genitourinary functions.	Frequent urination, Urinary incontinence, Night sweats, Lumbar pain, Tinnitus, Hearing loss, prematured aging issues, Sexual/procreation issues.

In TCM, emotions become pathological only when they are suppressed or expressed intensely beyond control or context. These excessive emotions then become endogenous influences that destabilize the Yin-Yang balance. Joy 喜, Anger 怒, Worry 忧, Pensiveness 思, Grief 悲, Fear 恐, and Fright 惊 are the Seven Emotions 七情 that when raised to unhealthy levels can cause Yin-Yang disharmony within the body.

Emotions are associated with various "organ-systems". The unresolved energy arising from a certain excessive emotion that corresponds to the organ-system and/or its meridian (energy channel) results in the manifestation of different dysfunctions when the organ-system is in a state of imbalance.

Because Fright differs from Fear in terms of anticipation to the event causing arousal of the emotion and thus a lack in reaction time for the individual, some academicians relate fright with the Gall Bladder, a "hybrid" organ in TCM characterized by jurisdiction or decision. There are, however, other schools of thought that associate fright and fear with the Kidney-system as the nature of emotions are rather similar.

As previously mentioned more than one external pathogen in combination may inflict illness. An external pathogen may also collaborate with an "innate condition" or an aggravated emotional situation to cause a disorder.

By default of a dynamically balanced organ-systems existing within us, few diseases begin as a deficient situation. Most illnesses are thus initiated by an "excess" situation. This is especially when an illness revolves around a singular organ-system.

In the larger scheme of things, organ-system imbalances may not occur in isolation. When an imbalance within an organ-system is left unchecked for an extended period of time, the position becomes chronic or *Yin-Yang mutually undermining situation* 阳损及阴. Each organ system has a pre-disposition towards either Yin or Yang as indicated in the table above. When an organ-system is in a state of disequilibrium, it will encroach upon and belabor a corresponding organ-system. The most well known of such inter-system imbalance in TCM is that of heart-kidney system disharmony, widely observed in patients with anxiety disorder, insomnia, and menopausal syndrome.

According to the Yin-Yang theory, the heart lies in the upper torso and pertains to Yang. The Five-Element theory relates the heart to fire and as fire is also of Yang nature, the heart is therefore categorized as Yang within Yang. Similarly, the kidney is located in the lower torso and pertains to Yin. As the kidney is associated with Yin-water in the Five-Element theory, the kidney is thus labeled as Yin within Yin. When in dynamic equilibrium, the spontaneous descending and ascending movement of yin and yang in the heart and kidney ensure the harmonious coordination between the two organ-systems.

Briefly, the heart-kidney system disharmony 心肾不交 has two possible pathogeneses:

a. Heart fire hyperactivity and kidney yin deficiency — generally caused by excessive consumption of kidney Yin resulting from chronic disease or sexual indulgence. Under normal circumstances, the heart Yang energy would descend to strengthen the kidney Yang energy function of keeping the kidney Yin fluid warm and propelled, thus maintaining the kidney metabolism. By the same token, the kidney Yin fluid should ascend to reinforce the heart Yin fluid in keeping the heart Yang energy in check to prevent the intense Yang energy from transforming into unrestraint heart fire when the heart becomes hyperactive.

   However, when the seamless exchange of heart fire and kidney fluid is disrupted by the suppression of Yin ascending and Yang descending, pathological conditions occur. If kidney Yin became exhausted and there is less than adequate kidney fluid for deployment to constraint the heart Yang energy, it leads to hyperactive heart fire. Meanwhile, the untamed hyperactive heart fire cannot be directed downwards to warm the kidney fluid. What remains would be the upper part of the body suffers from hyperactive heart fire, while the lower part of the body suffers from coldness and stagnation of kidney water, leading to problems like insomnia, nocturnal emissions and possibly neurosis.

b. Heart fire hyperactivity and kidney yang deficiency — unlike the previous case where the initial point of failure lies with the kidney, the heart-system is already in a hyperactive state with excessive Yang energy in this instance. This could be caused exogenously by the invasion of external pathogenic factors or triggered endogenously by emotional aggravation. In any case, the heart yang energy is entrapped and stagnated within the organ-system, turning it into uncontrollable heart fire.

   As in the previous case, the heart fire cannot be directed to help keep the kidney Yin fluid warm and mobile resulting in the Yin fluids becoming undeployable to help douse the untamed heart fire, leading to disharmony between the heart and kidney with hyperactive heart fire in the upper part of the body and deficient kidney yang in the lower part of the body.

All told, diseases are caused by disruption of the yin-yang dynamic equilibrium maintained in healthy individuals. This disruption may be caused solely by noxious external pathogens associated with the ruling exogenous influence among the Six Excesses at a given time or season. The body, however, may be made more vulnerable to invasions by external pathogens when the yin-yang dynamic equilibrium is already set to be disrupted by the endogenous influence of the Seven Emotions. Notwithstanding and given time, the Seven Emotions may also cause chronic illnesses even without the presence of external pathogens.

Disequilibrium within an organ-system may also disrupt the functionality of another organ-system resulting in more severe consequences than if the imbalance is contained within a singular organ-system.

Glossary

Six Excesses or Six Pathogenic Factors or Six Pernicious Factors refer to the same elements collectively and the terms may be used interchangeably.

TCM Ten Precepts of Syndrome Differentiation developed by Shi Jin-mo 施今墨 (28 Mar 1881–22 Aug 1969) comprises of Qi and Blood syndrome differentiation in addition to the traditional Eight Precepts of Syndrome Differentiation.

Viscus is an internal organ of the body, specifically one within the chest or the abdomen. Viscus is the singular of viscera.

Organ-system in TCM refers to an organ's functional system instead of merely the anatomical definition of the organ's somatic structure.

Five Element theory — a philosophical theory of TCM, concerning the composition and evolution of the physical universe, epitomized by the nature and the inhibition-proliferation relationships of the five elements, wood, fire, earth, metal and water, serving as the guiding ideology and methodology of physiology, pathology, clinical diagnosis, and treatment. Also known as the five-phase theory.

Pathogenesis of a disease refers to the biological mechanism (or mechanisms) that leads to the diseased state and often describes the origin and development of the disease, and whether it is acute, chronic, or recurrent.

Reference

1. Baum A, Posluszny DM. Health psychology: Mapping biobehavioral contributions to health and illness. *Annu. Rev. Psychol.* **50**: 137–163 (1999).

Topic 5

What are Meridians

TCM was born out of philosophy. Man is deemed to be a microcosm of the universe and reflective of the macrocosmic universe. When the flourishing Great Earth is drained by myriads of rivers into lakes and seas, Man was inspired to conceptualize and install irrigation systems during Agricultural China to improve harvest yield. As Earth has four seas, one in each direction, so shall the human body — the Sea of Qi 气海, the Sea of Blood 血海, the Sea of Marrow 髓海 and the Sea of Chyme 水谷之海. Meridian is an extension of this concept and akin to the unimpeded flow of life-sustaining water that feeds the bountiful land.

Meridians are energy pathways in which Qi or vital energy flow through for access to the entire body, both in human and animals. Meridians exist in symmetry and bilaterally on each side of the body, connecting acupoints beneath the skin. Meridians are named after each organ-system [viscera and bowels] they originate from. Traversing the body and with exception of the Belt Vessel 带脉, meridians run vertically and deeper while collaterals run horizontally and more superficially. Taken in totality, the meridian system forms an essential inter-connected distribution network of vital energy throughout the body.

Meridians are commonly and closely associated with acupuncture and acupoints. But the fact remains the concept of meridians was conceived independent of, developed tangentially from and even pre-existed acupoints. Qi embodies energy, intelligence and consciousness; and is beyond the single-dimensioned Western definition of energy. The notion of meridians, as suggested by Lei *et al.*, was inspired by the collective perceptions of Qi coursing through the body in a physiological state by QiGong 气功 practitioners. On the contrary, the identification of acupoints governed by the pathological principle that "acupoint is where the pain is", clearly reflects the unique feature of an acupoint as the site of pain, pathogen, and treatment.[1]

Their integration, however, happened during the Han Dynasty [206 to 220 BCE] era when the Huang Di's Internal Classics 黄帝内经 was compiled. The mapping of acupoints over established meridians resulted in the art of acupuncture gaining a firm theoretical framework that accorded its greater practical significance. In fact, even today, the age-old admonition of "miss an acupoint but never depart from its meridian 离穴不离经" is still embraced by acupuncture practitioners as a cardinal treatment guideline.

Unlike the vascular system, the meridian system is not an anatomical structure. This is not surprising as ancient Chinese philosophy with a holistic focus emphasized on functional interaction of the body in preference to Western Medicine's approach towards materialism and reductionism that borne out the precise science of Anatomy. The physical existence of meridians, though been much researched upon and somewhat validated in recent years, still remains as elusive and abstract as ever before. It is perhaps non-physical or yet to be fully observed.

In a joint project between the Heilongjiang University of Chinese Medicine and The University of Hong Kong, researchers reviewed the works of their predecessors with respect to biophysical aspects of meridians since the early 1950s till 2012 from established electronic medical databases. The desk research hopes to demonstrate the objective existence of meridians by seeking convergence in evidence identified by earlier laboratory experiments that employed different techniques in biophysics such as electric, acoustic, thermal, optical, magnetic, isotopic and myoelectric.[2]

The review showed that acoustic wave's amplitude at acupoints was significantly higher than non-acupuncture point and the waves could be transmitted along meridians with conductivity faster than that of surrounding soft tissue; though lower than bone conduction. Further, transmitted microwaves along a meridian were able to locate the next acupoint along the same meridian and the frequency ranges of the microwave transmitted in different meridians were found to be different. In addition, the frequency of microwave in cancer patients was different from that of healthy controls.[3]

The review further mentioned that tracks from infra-red radiant by an infra-red imaging system were consistent with the 14 meridians described in the ancient Chinese text and subcutaneous temperature along these tracks may be raised after acupuncture.[4] In a later study where high luminescence was employed, 14 highly distinct luminous lines on the body surface were again observed that correlated in location to the 14 regular acupuncture meridians with an overlapping rate of 92.8%.[5]

Injecting radio-isotopes into living bodies was perhaps the earliest attempt to explore and prove the physical existence of meridians. One observation was that the slow movement of the radio-isotopes along channels, besides showing similarity to the meridians mapped out in ancient Chinese literature, proved that these trace patterns are independent of the lymphatic network. Later research further demonstrated that low hydraulic resistance channels run along with the isotope-traced network where fluids may flow more efficiently in comparison to the surrounding tissues; which translates to interstitial fluid flowing along low hydraulic resistance channels.[6,7]

But not all research outcomes converged in the same direction.

Since the body is electrically charged, an obvious assumption was meridians have different electric properties. But the evidence did not conclusively support the claim that acupoints or meridians were electrically distinguishable as electrical skin resistance (ESR) at most acupoints (63%) had no significant difference when compared with that of the surrounding areas. Moreover, ESR measurement was not consistent among meridians and observations, though with high initial readings, were not sustainable over time.[8]

The studies so far suggested that meridians/acupoints have biophysical characteristics that are different from non-acupuncture points or the surrounding tissues. But these findings are outcomes from small sample-sized basic studies; some being animal studies. Notwithstanding, observations from these studies could serve as foundations to unequivocally establish the physical existence and morphology of meridians through future, large controlled experiments.

Other reviews offered yet a different but plausible perspective of meridians' structure — *"We conclude that there really are structural features along the route of the traditional meridian. But by this, we mean an orderly arrangement of normal tissues along the meridians rather than any special histological structure. In the tissue space of peripheral regions, the nerves, blood, and lymphatic vessels, and neural transmitters are concentrated along the meridians; structures in the CNS were also found to be related to meridians. Thus, it seems that the meridians are not limited to one kind of tissue or structure but are distributed around the body in different forms according to the locality."*[9]

"*Meridian system is a special channel network comprising of skin with abundant nerves and nociceptive receptors of various types, and deeper connective tissues inside the body with the flowing interstitial fluid system. These meridian channels provide efficient migratory tracks mainly due to durotaxis (also including chemotaxis) for mast cells, fibroblasts and other cells to migrate and carry out a number of physiological functions*"[10]

"*Meridians are low resistance fluid channels where various chemical and physical transports take place. The channel is called low hydraulic resistance channel and the chemical transport is named volume transmission*".[7]

Be that as it may, the establishment of meridian's anatomical structure does not in any way contribute to or diminish the value of meridians in its function and purpose. Any discovery in this direction serves no more than to satisfy the scientific curiosity of Man since the pragmatic function and utilitarian purpose of meridians are already time-honored. Empirically proven, accepted and endorsed by masses of beneficiaries not for a century in time but for more than 3000 years since its inception.

Glossary

Four Seas in the book of Miraculous Pivot《灵枢・海论》 refers to the Brain as Sea of Marrow, Stomach as the Sea of Chyme, CV17 膻中 as Sea of Qi [energy] and Chong Mai 冲脉 or Sea of 12 Channels 十二经之海 as Sea of Blood.

Chyme in Physiology is a pulpy acidic fluid which passes from the stomach to the small intestine, consisting of gastric juices and partly digested food.

QiGong is an ancient Chinese practice and healing technique involving meditation, deep controlled breathing with coordinated body posture and movement exercises. It is a martial art in its highest form when the practitioner is able to direct his Qi movement to open the channels of Conception Vessel and Governor Vessel.

Materialism is a philosophical basis that holds matter as the fundamental substance in nature, with all things including mental states and consciousness resulting from material interactions. Reductionism is an approach used in analyzing the nature of complex things by reducing them to the interactions of their parts, or to simpler or more fundamental things, akin to a 'Divide and Conquer' strategy.

Morphology is the branch of biology that deals with the form of living organisms and with relationships between their structures.

CNS refers to Central Nervous System comprising of the brain and spinal cord.

References

1. Lei L, Tung CW, Lo KC. The origin of meridians. *Chin. Med.* **5**: 71–74 (2014).
2. Li J, Wang Q, Liang H, Dong H, Li Y, Ng EH, Wu X. Biophysical characteristics of meridians and acupoints: a systematic review. *Evid. Based Complement. Alternat. Med.* **2012**: Article ID 793841, 6 pages (2012).
3. Krevsky MA, Zinina ES, Koshurinov Y, *et al.* Microwave propagation on acupuncture channels. *Acupunct. Electro-Ther. Res.* **31**(1-2): 1–12 (2006).
4. Zhang D, Wang SY, Wang CY. Determination of deep temperature under the line of high temperature along meridians. *Chin. J. Basic Med. Tradit. Chin. Med.* **7**(410): 62 pages (2001).
5. Yan ZQ, Shi YQ, Wang YZ, *et al.* Research on the biophysical features of strong luminescence phenomena in the 14 regular meridians of the human body. *Acupunct. Res.* **8**: 389–394 (1989).
6. Zhang WB, Tian YY, Li H, *et al.* A discovery of low hydraulic resistance channel along meridians. *J. Acupunct. Meridian Stud.* **1**(1): 20–28 (2008).
7. Zhang WB, Wang GJ, Fuxe K. Classic and modern meridian studies: a review of low hydraulic resistance. Channels along meridians and their relevance for therapeutic effects in traditional Chinese medicine. *Evid. Based Complement. Alternat. Med.* **2015**: 410979 (2015).

8. Kramer S, Winterhalter K, Schober G, *et al.* Characteristics of electrical skin resistance at acupuncture points in healthy Humans. *J. Altern. Complement. Med.* **15**(5): 495–500 (2009).
9. Wei H, Huang CL, Kong J. The substrate and properties of meridians: a review of modern research. *Acupunct. Med.* **17**(2): 134–139 (Dec 1999).
10. Fung CW. Probing the mystery of Chinese medicine meridian channels with special emphasis on the connective tissue interstitial fluid system mechanotransduction, cells durotaxis and mast cell degranulation. *Chin. Med.* **4**: 10 (May 29, 2009).

Topic 6

How Does *Gua Sha* Therapy Alleviate Illnesses

The human body is a microcosm of the universe. The various organ-systems within the body are closely interconnected and interact with and among themselves in a highly coordinated manner. Disorders and diseases exist because the body is thrown into a state of disharmony and imbalance, usually caused by exogenous and/or endogenous influences.

When disharmony or imbalance occurs and the organ-system resolves the disharmony expeditiously, the imbalance is deemed physiological and no disorder occurs. However, when such dynamic equilibrium is not re-established but allowed to fester, disorder will first manifest within the organ-system before affecting related organ-systems. The development of disorder normally follows a predictable pattern known as Pattern of Disharmony named according to the organ-system, meridians or pathogenic factors involved.

Meridians originate from the respective organ-systems and interconnect these 12 organ-systems in a pre-determined sequence where Qi or vital energy flows freely. In fact, the order and timing of Qi movement within this continuous meridian circuit are strictly dictated by a 24-hour energy cycle that represents the time of the day when each organ-system function optimally as the Qi arrives and remains for two hours. In the same corollary, the timing the organ-system is most vulnerable when Qi is most remote and distant. What implies here is that the repair and maintenance of an organ-system

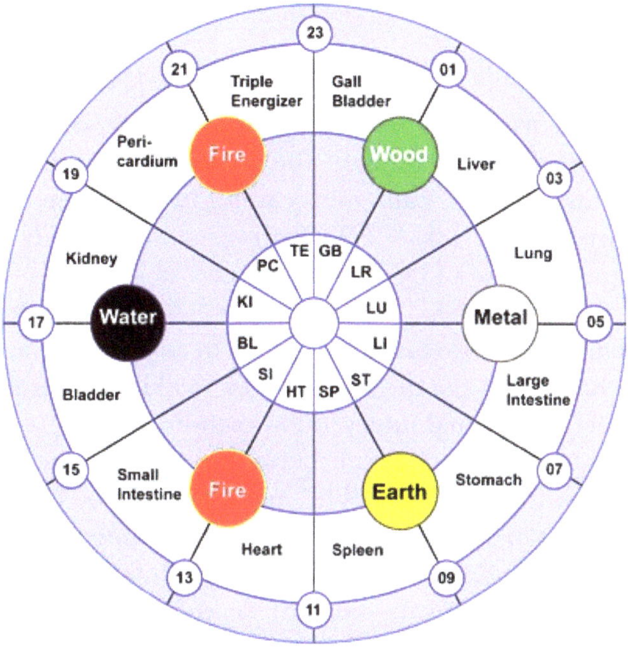

Picture credit: Pinterest.com

are time-bound and interruption means reduced ability of the organ-system to re-establish any disharmony.

The Body-Energy Cycle is a concept of the cyclical ebb and flow of energy throughout the 12 organ-systems at various defined periods. Referring to the above diagram, the liver-system is at peak functionality between 1 am and 3 am when the body is at complete rest. This augurs well with the Qi status of the small intestine-system, responsible for absorption and assimilation of nutrients, to be at its ebb. Now for someone who stayed awake beyond 11 pm and feasted on a hearty meal, it will be double-whammy as disruption will occur in both organ-systems.

Of the four different types of Qi, Nutritive Qi 营气 and Superficial Defensive Qi 卫气 course along the meridians. During the day, Superficial Defensive Qi is distributed in the skin and muscles, providing warmth and nutrition to the subcutaneous tissue, temperature control through perspiration and protection of the body against exogenous pathogens. In the evening, Superficial Defensive Qi circulates deeper within the organ-systems as the body winds down to rest.

Health is maintained when the interactions between and among the organ-systems are in harmony facilitated by open and unobstructed meridians that are the pathways connecting the organ-systems. In TCM, pathogens cannot invade when the flow of Qi is robust 正气存内，邪不可干. Pathogens in the body may only prevail when the flow of Qi is compromised 邪之所凑 其气必虚.

Qi is also the marshal of blood 气为血帅. Impediment to the flow of Qi and therefore blood and fluids in any part of the body, on the other hand, will manifest as pain or weakness 不通则痛 痛则不通. As a TCM external intervention technique, *Gua Sha* operates on the treatment principle of "addressing emergencies by first relieving its symptoms 急则治其标" and there can be no better way to put the maxim into practice than stimulating the meridians directly to clear the blockage and restore Qi flow.

Discourse on Skin in the book of Plain Questions 素问. 皮部论 theorized that the skin is an integral part of the meridian system in that meridians are connected to the skin by a web of superficial collateral vessels. The thesis went further to postulate that most diseases enter the body via the skin and accessible mucosa of orifices. When pathogens settled on the body's exposed area, the interstice structures that open rhythmically allow the entry of pathogen into the superficial collateral vessels.

When Qi flowing in the superficial collateral vessels are abound and robust, pathogens entering the body via the skin may only reside within the superficial collateral vessels. A noxious and advancing pathogen may, however, invade the meridian after overcoming the resistance of the Superficial Defensive Qi in the collateral vessels. This is the general prognosis for the invasion of pathogens through the skin for all meridians with the exception of Lesser Yin [heart and kidney] meridians where pathogens left unchecked may progress beyond the meridians and penetrate the bones. As a rule of thumb, pathogens that progress beyond the meridians will enter the organ-system accordingly.

Gua Sha seeks to alleviate illnesses expeditiously by reversing the process of disease progression mapped out in the Discourse on Skin. At least that was the thinking when the technique of *Gua Sha* was conceived. By re-opening the interstice structures and stimulating the surrounding superficial collateral vessels supplying to a selected meridian, TCM believes that an escape route is provided to harboring pathogens while improving the flow of Defensive Qi serving the meridian.

This is achieved by repeatedly "stroking" on lubricated skin with a smooth-edged instrument in a methodical and unidirectional manner to produce a moderate bruising at the selected location(s) or meridian. The repeated abrasion on the skin produces micro-trauma that activates blood circulation and dissipates blood stasis as the channel is dredged. The same repeated action also produces increased derma temperature aimed to re-open the interstice structure or pores so that pathogens and the attendant toxin produced could be expelled whilst the Qi status is enhanced. The expulsion of toxins facilitated by the invigorated Superficial Defensive Qi, manifested as petechiae and ecchymosis after treatment, help restores homeostasis or dynamic balance of yin-yang.

The therapeutic efficacy of *Gua Sha,* however, is explained by biomedical science from yet different angles. Using laser Doppler imaging and infrared thermography, Xu *et al.* were able to demonstrate *Gua Sha* significantly increases both blood flow perfusion and skin temperature immediately after scraping that persisted more than 90 minutes thereafter. Thermal conductivity along meridians and beneath tissues was found to be more efficient than other parts of the body.[1,2]

With blood flow perfusion more than doubled and skin temperature increased more than 1° centigrade above their respective baselines, *Gua Sha* effectively regulate sympathetic vasodilation and promote local blood circulation, providing relief for muscular spasm, improvement in local metabolism of tissues, reduction in tension of blood vessels and nerves, and elimination in negative impact of somatic disorders on visceral functions as well as removal of microcirculatory obstruction and blood stasis, especially for arteriole angiectasis.

In a different animal experiment, Chen *et al.* observed that *Gua Sha* could upregulate the innate and adaptive immune functions of the skin and boost response against intradermal antigens. Following the treatment, erythrocyte extravasation is induced with controlled skin tissue damage leading to wound healing process that cascaded significantly in increased ratios of immune active cells in the skin tissue especially T lymphocytes and macrophages.[3]

Although anti-inflammatory cytokine IL-4, IL-5, and IL-13 levels remained unchanged, proinflammatory cytokines TNF-α, IL-6, IL-12p70, and IL-23 were upregulated and immunosuppressive cytokines IL-10 downregulated in the cutaneous regions as well as in the systemic circulation. The same experiment further demonstrated *Gua Sha*, acted as a physical adjuvant, induced a three-fold higher IgG titer with a more Th1-biased antibody subtype profile against intradermal delivery of a model vaccine. This last observation holds special significance when *Gua Sha* is applied as an immunity booster for those with poorly functioning immune systems.

Gua Sha's therapeutic effect may well be related to its ability to ameliorate oxidative stress by upregulating Heme oxygenase-1 (HO-1) gene expression.[4]

HO-1 is a stress-induced isoform of a heat shock protein present throughout the body with highest concentrations in the spleen, liver, and kidneys. HO-1 expression is induced by oxidative stress and increasing this expression is associated with organ cytoprotection. Carbon monoxide released from heme degradation can influence vascular tone independently or influence the function of nitric oxide synthase.

Using bioluminescence imaging technology, Kwong *et al.* observed a significant upregulation of HO-1 up to 120 hours post-*Gua Sha* in transgenic mice, with peak HO-1 level at the 36th hour. The distribution pattern was represented by significant signal intensities that increased progressively over multiple organ regions encompassing the gastrointestinal tract, the genital tract, the liver, and kidneys. Upregulation of HO-1 is thought to represent an antioxidative response to circulating hemoglobin products released by *Gua Sha* in the form of petechiae and ecchymosis indicative of extravasation of blood from subcutaneous capillaries.

The upregulation of HO-1 by *Gua Sha* was again confirmed by another human case study where the treatment conferred hepatoprotection in a chronic active Hepatitis B patient presented with elevated liver enzymes ALT and AST indicative of inflammatory damage in the liver. Liver function, plasma HO-1, and T-helper (Th) cytokine balance before and after *Gua Sha* were closely monitored.[5]

Forty-eight hours after receiving *Gua Sha*, the patient registered a decline of liver enzymes (ALT and AST) indicating reduced chronic inflammation, an elevated plasma HO-1, and modulation of T-helper Th1/Th2 balance.

In a subsequent control study performed by the same scholars involving inactive Hepatitis B and non-carrier participants, *Gua Sha* did not induce any significant modulation of liver enzymes, HO-1, or cytokines.[6] The results suggest that *Gua Sha*-induced hepatoprotective effect depends on the inflammatory event or clinical stage of chronic hepatitis B. Because both active and inactive carriers were completely unaware of their liver status at the time of receiving *Gua Sha* treatment, the research protocol is effective in discounting the model that attributes *Gua Sha* therapeutic efficacy to a placebo effect due to participants' expectations. *Gua Sha* was shown to transiently reduce the inflammatory markers of liver injury in human, together with an enhancement of HO-1 which might be responsible for the hepatoprotective action.

The skin is the largest organ of the body. It is the interface most exposed to the external environment and therefore the first-line defense against external pathogens. In this regard, the therapeutic mechanism of *Gua Sha* logically is of great relevance to the immunological functions of the skin.

In the final analysis, it is apparent that the intricate web of thoughts leading to the development of *Gua Sha* was conceived by pioneering Chinese physicians with great intellectual effort and utmost wisdom. Without the benefit of modern technology, these physicians tenaciously plowed through a tortuous journey of medical discovery, connecting observation to rationality.

From activation of blood circulation to the dissipation of blood stasis, from expulsion of pathogens and toxins to the re-establishment of yin-yang homeostasis and the consequential restoration of body's Superficial Defensive Qi, they weaved a colorful yet pragmatic tapestry of profound human physiology that withstood the test of time.

With sheer mental faculty, these glorious physicians mapped out an apparently nebulous disconnected set of theories and transformed them into a rudimentary and primitive yet highly effective therapeutic protocol for benefit of the posterity.

Today, this therapy though lacking in sophistication and scientific persuasiveness in its pioneering year, have been duly validated by contemporary medicine.

Glossary

Perfusion is measured as the rate at which blood is delivered to tissue, or volume of blood per unit time (blood flow) per unit tissue mass. The SI unit for human organs perfusion is typically reported in mL/(100 g * min) or mL/(mL * min).

Angiectasis is the abnormal dilation and often lengthening of blood or lymphatic vessels.

T cells may be broadly classified as either helper T cells (Th cells, CD4+) or cytotoxic T cells (Tc cells, CD8+). Helper T cells could be further divided into two classes depending upon the specific cytokines the cells secrete in response to antigenic stimulation. Th1 cells primarily produce interferon (IFN)-γ, interleukin (IL)-2 and tumor necrosis factor (TNF)-β, whereas Th2 cells produce IL-4, IL-5, IL-6, IL-9, IL-10, and IL-13. Cytokines produced by each Th subset tend to both stimulate the production of that Th subset and inhibit the development of the other Th subset; meaning IL-2 produced by Th1 cells has the dual effect of both stimulating Th1 development and inhibiting Th2 development.

The two Th cell classes also differ by the type of immune response they produce. While Th1 cells tend to evoke cell-mediated immunity and phagocyte-dependent inflammation (against intracellular parasites such as bacteria and viruses), Th2 cells evoke strong antibody (IgG, IgM, IgA, IgE) responses, including eosinophil accumulation, but inhibit several functions of phagocytic cells (phagocyte-independent inflammation).

Because Th1 evoke cell-mediated immunity, main partner cell types are Th1, Macrophage, CD8+ and Tc cells. In contrast, Th2 evoke humoral immunity against extracellular micro-organisms, so that the main partner cell types shall, therefore, be B-cell, eosinophil and mast cells.

References

1. Xu QY, Yang JS, *et al.* The effects of scraping therapy on local temperature and blood perfusion volume in healthy subjects. *Evid. Based Complement. Alternat. Med.* **2012**: Article ID 490292, 6 pages (2012).
2. Xu QY, Yang JS, Yang L, Wang YY. Effects of different scraping techniques on body surface blood perfusion volume and local skin temperature of healthy subjects. *J. Tradit. Chin. Med.* **31**(4): 316–320 (Dec 2011).
3. Chen TT, Liu NH, Liu JX. Gua Sha, a press-stroke treatment of the skin, boosts the immune response to intradermal vaccination. *Peer J.* **4**: e2451 (Sep 14, 2016).
4. Kwong KK, Kloetzer L, Wong KK, Ren J, *et al.* Bioluminescence imaging of heme oxygenase-1 upregulation in the Gua Sha procedure. *J. Vis. Exp.* **(30)**: pii: 1385 (Aug 28, 2009).
5. Chan ST, Yuen JW, Gohel MD, *et al.* Guasha-induced hepatoprotection in chronic active hepatitis B: a case study. *Clin. Chim. Acta* **412**(17–18): 1686–1688 (Aug 17, 2011).
6. Chan ST, Yuen JW, Gohel MD, *et al.* Does Guasha offer hepatoprotective effect to chronic inactive hepatitis B carriers? A built-in design to control subject expectation. *J. Altern. Complement. Med.* **19**(9): 772–776 (Sep 2013).

Topic 7

What is *Sha*

Sha 痧 is a term with different contextual meanings.

Ancient TCM literature recorded a wide spectrum of ailments in excess of a hundred related to or caused by *sha,* many which manifested symptoms similar to our modern-day disease of tetanus 角弓反张痧, post-partum fever 产后痧, ascites 膨胀痧, intestinal adhesion 盘肠痧, migraine 头疯痧, and acute appendicitis 缩腿痈痧.

In its broad sense, *Sha* is a short-hand definition for the collective symptoms of *sha*-related illness 痧证 observed during diagnosis as well as in the post-treatment manifestations. These ailments are associated with blood stasis caused either by excess or deficiency syndrome. In excess syndrome, *Sha* is brought about by the combined effects of weather changes 八风之邪, heat convection from humid ground 湿热之气, poor nutritional status of and accumulated fatigue 饥饱劳逸 in the body that set the stage for invasion of external pathogens. The entry of pathogens from the skin suppresses the free and regular movement of Superficial Defensive Qi giving rise to blood stagnation and thus the development of *Sha*. As earlier mentioned "Where there is blockage of qi and blood, there is also pain 不通则痛 痛则不通" and pain is, therefore, one obvious presentation of *Sha*.

Sha or *sha*-related illness is, therefore, a perennial and not a seasonal disease. Its prevalence and pervasiveness during the hot summer season, however, conferred upon the disease a narrower contextual stereotype of heat stroke that the illness is often associated with.

Two observable symptoms in *Sha*-related ailments are *sha* spots on the dermis and an overall sense of general malaise with muscular discomfort in the individual. A typical presentation of the illness includes headache, fever, chest fullness, listlessness, gastro-intestinal distention, perspiration, severe thirst, joint and muscular discomfort, and pain.

According to TCM 4-Stratum Syndrome Differentiation 卫气营血辨证 for assessing severity of febrile diseases during pathogenesis, these symptoms are caused by pathogens acting on the lungs and skin during invasion of the superficial defense 卫分 layer and the build-up of internal heat resulting from intense struggle of primary Qi 正气 with the residing pathogens in the internal defense 气分 layer. This internal heat remains in the stomach and intestines with damp-heat being trapped within the spleen-system. Food consumed at this stage will be converted into phlegm (stagnated chyme), the accumulation of it at the gastro-intestinal region, unless expelled in good time, will cause distention and nausea. The disease is much easier to treat with little complications at this stage.

Sha-related illnesses may, however, develop rapidly into medical emergencies if the attacking pathogen is very virulent or if the disease is allowed to progress beyond the internal defense layer. As the pathogens penetrate into the nutrient 营分 layer, the system continues to be placed under tremendous stress. In TCM, Qi is the nutrient and the precursor of blood. Excess internal heat damages nutrient leading to high temperature, throbbing headache, tachycardia, lack of perspiration, muscle weakness or cramps, disorientation and in some cases rash outbreak and seizure; symptoms akin to severe yin-deficiency and heat stroke. The organ systems that are involved at this stage would be the heart and pericardium.

When the pathogens reached the ultimate level or the Blood 血分 layer, the continuingly generated excess heat would involve the kidneys and liver leading to wide-spread circulation disorder. Delirium, stupor, seizure or convulsion, comatose, severe rashes, shock and bleeding disorders are commonplace that correspond to the symptoms of septicemia and Disseminated Intravascular Coagulation. Progression of the disease to this stage has a poor prognosis and high mortality rate.

Sha also refers to the small reddish spots or markings 痧痕 that emerge from the deeper layers of the body to the skin surface during the course of *Gua Sha* treatment. From a biomedical perspective, *sha* is merely petechiae, a pathological abnormality arising from traumatization of the dermatological structures. When the pattern of redness is more disperse and intense, the abnormality is term ecchymosis or purpura. Ecchymosis is larger in appearance than purpura, more than 1 cm in diameter and with more diffuse borders.

It is interesting to note that contemporary medicine treats skin discolorations as lesions, as a pathological by-product, caused by extravasation of blood arising from platelet disorders, coagulation disorders or vascular disorders. When such lesions appear during treatment it implies an iatrogenic outcome.

On the contrary, the appearance of these "abnormal" discoloration during treatment is viewed positively by *Gua Sha* (and *Cupping*) practitioners. In TCM, *sha* is formed when normal Qi and blood flows are obstructed causing localized Qi stagnation, blood stasis 血瘀, and internal heat. Pathogenic factor(s) responsible for the blockage and attendant toxins are also present at these sites and when released by the action of *Gua Sha*, the normal physiological integrity of the affected area is restored.

With few adverse effects of permanent nature, *Gua Sha* is often time administered for symptomatic relief after quick assessment in an emergency situation. The attributes and characteristics of discoloration during and after treatment normally provide some confirmation of the nature of the disorder. Some attributes to look out for are:

a. General pattern of petechiae distribution together with knowledge of meridians could identify or confirm the nature of the disorder and the affected organ-system(s).

b. Locations of petechiae presented along the identified meridian(s) together with knowledge of acupoints could further pinpoint sites of Qi stagnation or blockage.
c. Elapse time taken for initial emergence of *sha* during treatment is a proxy to the degree of local Qi stagnation/blockage or the overall robustness of Qi in the patient.
d. Concentration and size of petechiae represent the severity of toxins in the body.

   Fine, dispersed petechiae reflect external pathogen and attendant toxin were residing at cutaneous level (superficial); medium-sized moderately concentrated petechiae indicate pathogen and toxin were located at the "muscles and sinews"; while large and densely concentrated petechiae demonstrate that pathogen and toxin have penetrated the "bones", i.e. extremely severe.
e. Colour of Sha may vary from light reddish-brown to almost black. Color determines the level of toxicity which is determined by virulence of external pathogens or how long-seated was the disorder.

   Liver-like red indicates a recent invasion by external pathogens, while darker red in the likeness of raw beef depicts internal heat and inflammation in the localized area. Long-seated blood stasis or internal tissue scarring are represented by very dark red to purplish spots.

Liver Red

Dark Red

Purplish/Very Dark Red

f. Elapse time taken for post-treatment fading of skin discoloration is indicative of the vigor of blood circulation, the flow of Qi and therefore recuperative power of the patient. Normally, skin discoloration begins to fade from the second day after treatment and shall disappear completely after five days.

That the appearance of *sha* after treatment correlates with the amount of toxins the body is unable to normally evacuate, does it imply the amount of *sha* surfaced during treatment be as much as possible? Or is less *sha* better than more? This matter shall be addressed under the topic of *Gua Sha* technique.

Glossary

Phlegm 痰饮 in TCM has a very broad meaning that encompasses matters beyond the thick viscous substance secreted by the mucous membranes of the respiratory passages. It refers to any humoral, fluid or semi-fluid substance generated by the body arising from a pathological incident caused by the coalesce of poorly distributed body fluids associated with compromised Qi flow.

Iatrogenic means relating to errors and omissions during medical treatment.

"Muscle, sinews and bones" in this order are various connotations used as proxies by ancient Chinese to indicate increasing severity of an ailment.

Topic 8

How Meridians Named and Distributed in the Human Body

The overriding precept in TCM is the concept of dynamic equilibrium within Yin and Yang. These universal polarities are reflected in all aspects of the discipline including human surface anatomy.

When it comes to assigning Yin-Yang to a whole upright human body, the rule of thumb is that the upper body is Yang in relation to the lower body, which is Yin. Similarly, anything posterior of the mid-axillary line is Yang and anything anterior of the mid-axillary line is Yin.[1] "Yang is the part of the body exposed to the sun when toiling the earth during mid-day and anything otherwise shall be Yin". At least this was believed to have been disseminated to the laypeople for eons since China became an agricultural economy.

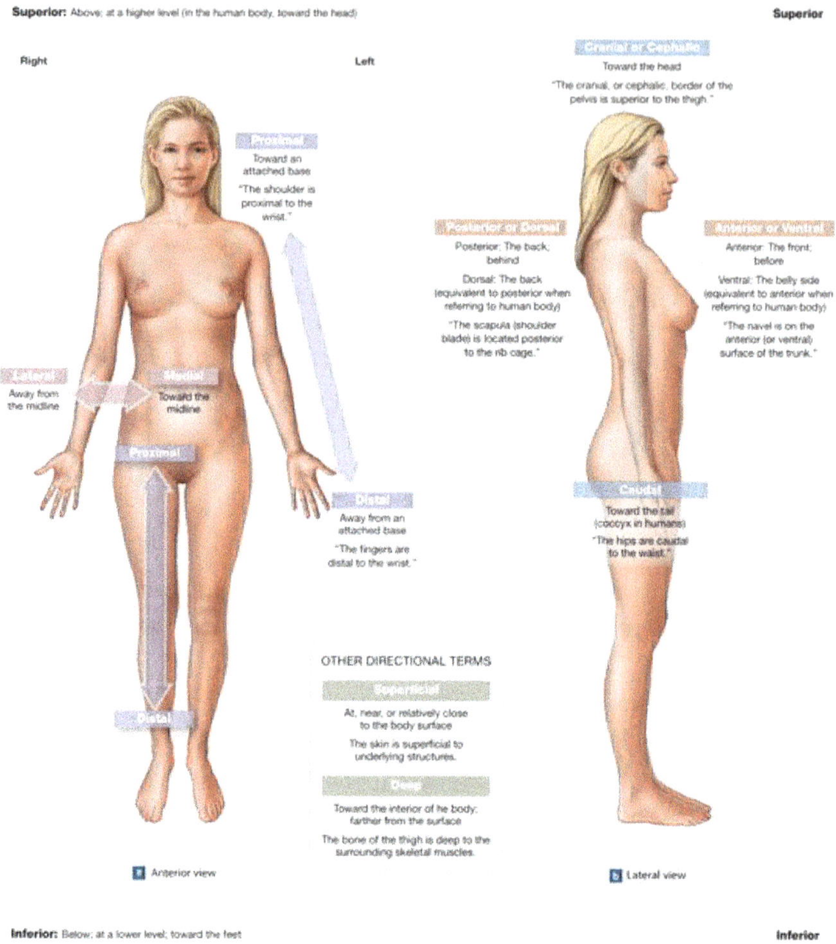

Picture credit: https://www.earthslab.com/wp-content/uploads/2017/01/Directional-Terms-1.jpg

For an upright body with hanging arms and forward-facing palms, this roughly translates to the softer, paler, less hairy regions of the body, found on the front of the trunk and the medial surface of the limbs, abdomen, chest, and throat to be Yin surfaces. The rougher, darker, more hairy surfaces that are found on the postero-lateral aspect of the limbs, the back of the trunk and the head shall then be Yang.

This segmentation in the surface anatomy provides the primary basis of naming the meridians that navigate the body. The Yin and Yang meridian names are further qualified by the relative intensity of mid-day solar exposure on the six surfaces of each limb as illustrated in the transverse section of a limb below:

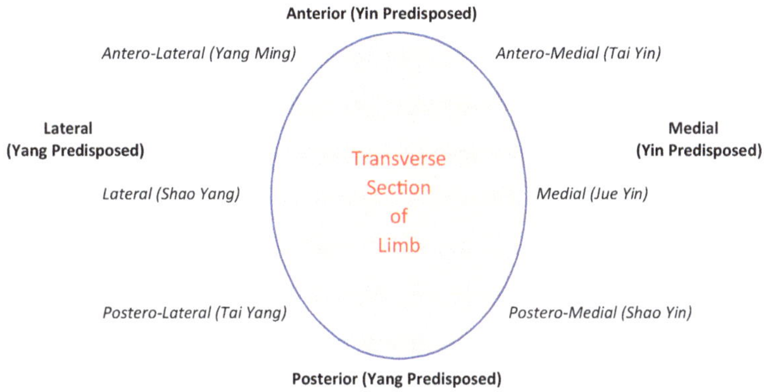

	Limb	Qualifier	Meaning	Organ System	Solar Exposure	Location on Limb	Flow Order
Yin	Hand	Tai Yin	Greater Yin	Lung	Least Exposed	Antero-Medial Surface	1
	Hand	Jeu Yin	Transiting Yin	Pericardium	Moderately Exposed	Medial Surface	9
	Hand	Shao Yin	Lesser Yin	Heart	Most Exposed	Postero-Medial Surface	5
Yang	Hand	Tai Yang	Greater Yang	Small Intestine	Most Exposed	Postero-Lateral Surface	6
	Hand	Shao Yang	Lesser Yang	Triple Energizer	Moderately Exposed	Lateral Surface	10
	Hand	Yang Ming	Rising Yang	Large Intestine	Least Exposed	Antero-Lateral Surface	2
Yin	Foot	Tai Yin	Greater Yin	Spleen	Least Exposed	Antero-Medial Surface	4
	Foot	Jeu Yin	Transiting Yin	Liver	Moderately Exposed	Medial Surface	12
	Foot	Shao Yin	Lesser Yin	Kidney	Most Exposed	Postero-Medial Surface	8
Yang	Foot	Tai Yang	Greater Yang	Bladder	Most Exposed	Postero-Lateral Surface	7
	Foot	Shao Yang	Lesser Yang	Gall Bladder	Moderately Exposed	Lateral Surface	11
	Foot	Yang Ming	Rising Yang	Stomach	Least Exposed	Antero-Lateral Surface	3

In the table above are 12 regular meridians named by Yin-Yang characteristics, the limbs they course through as well as the organ-systems they originate from. An example arising from this naming convention would be the Hand Tai Yin/Greater Yin Meridian of the Lung. Details of these 12 regular meridians will be covered as separate topics in this book.

There are yet another 8 extraordinary meridians that have no direct connections to the organ systems and, with the exception of the Governor Vessel 督脉 and Conception Vessel 任脉, share acupoints with the regular meridians. The other six extraordinary meridians are Thoroughfare/Penetrating Vessel 冲脉, Belt Vessel 带脉, Yin Heel Vessel 阴跷脉, Yang Heel Vessel 阳跷脉, Yin Link Vessel 阴维脉, and Yang Link Vessel 阳维脉.

By definition, the Yin and Yang regions should be the surface anatomical zones served by the yin and yang meridians respectively. Matters, however, get complicated and inconsistent when one traces the pathways of these meridians as they course through the human body. Most of these inconsistencies occur with the Leg Yang meridians though.

A trained acupuncturist would attest that the Rising <u>Yang</u> Stomach meridian courses through the abdomen and chest that is clearly a Yin zone of the trunk. The Lesser <u>Yang</u> Gallbladder meridian also intrudes slightly into the Yin surface of the trunk. The Transiting <u>Yin</u> Liver meridian feeds the dorsum of the foot, a <u>Yang</u> surface. All six Yang meridians serve various parts of the face, a *presumed* Yin region by virtue of its anterior orientation.

Some of these departures may, however, be explained by evolution theories and embryological development.

When life was found on Earth some 3.6 billion years ago, the earliest life form was marine dwelling. Fast forward 3.0 billion years, some creatures developed bilateral symmetry for the first time, that is they have a distinct top and bottom as well as a front and back. During the Cambrian explosion, fish became the first known vertebrates and the genesis of all land-walking vertebrates (tetrapods). Fish then developed jaws during the Devonian period as part of morphology driven by survival. Jawed fish further evolved with time into two surviving groups — the cartilaginous fish and the bony fish. The cartilaginous fish remain in the seas to be the sharks of today and the bony fish further evolved into ray-fin fish and lobed-fin fish. Ray-fin fish are the myriads of fish species inhabiting both fresh and salt waters today. The lobed-fin fish, however, compelled by ecological and competitive pressures, sought existence on land. Powered by fleshy fins and internal bone structure, they adapted to the demands of land habitation without losing their aquatic abilities to become amphibians. Of course, evolution did not stop here for the amphibians progressively developed into land dedicated reptiles, reptiles into mammals and mammals into man. This is the evolution of man over a period of 530 million years in a single paragraph.

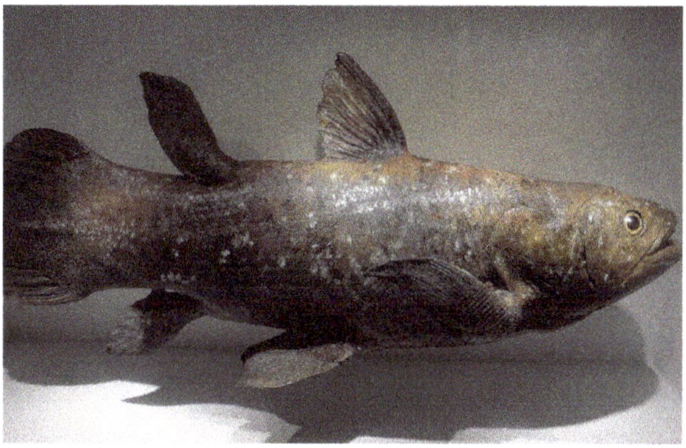

The coelacanth, a prehistoric lobed-fin fish and living fossil from the Devonian Period

Evolution is the necessity of survival and existence. Morphology is thus justified purely by functionality. In this respect, it is observed that the basic body plan of the modern fish is no different from that of her pre-historic cousin with the ventral aspect characterized by softer tissues covering internal organs while the dorsal aspects comprise mainly of firmer musculature of the back and including the face above the jaw. The modern fish, however, has a subtle color difference on the exterior between the dorsal and ventral aspects.

Yin-Yang division in surface anatomy is very much akin to the dorsal-ventral distinction in the body plan of the fish. Except that over the course of evolution, the dorsal features have migrated forward such that the eyes now face the anterior instead of being located on the sides. The jaw, however, remains the demarcation for the dorsal-ventral boundary which implies that the human face above the jaw shall be Yang territory, justifying convergence of all six Yang meridian at the face. The consistency of Yin-Yang division to the dorsal-ventral distinction also supports the notion that Yin meridians that serve the ventral aspects have a stronger effect on organ-systems when stimulated while Yang meridians that course the dorsal aspects have a stronger effect on locomotion or mobility when stimulated.

Without going into the intricacies of embryology, perhaps an easier approach to explaining embryological development would be to imagine a person lying prostrate on the floor attempting to imitate the position of a crouching frog. Referring to the above diagram depicting the Transverse Section of a Limb, the medial part of the limbs in contact with the floor corresponds to the Yin areas. However, to provide the more powerful locomotion and improved support required for purely land habitation later in life, our limbs are gradually orientated to the current positions as the embryo develops.

In terms of distribution, the three Yin meridians of the hand originate in the chest and course towards the extremity of the arms while the three Yang meridians of the hand ascend from the extremity of the arms to converge at the head. The three Yang meridians of the Leg, however, originate in the head and course towards the extremity of the leg while the three Yin meridians of the Leg ascend from the extremity of the leg to terminate at the anterior torso. The layout of these meridians would be more lucid to all when each meridian is discussed individually in detail in subsequent topics.

The Conception Vessel originates in the lower abdomen and descends to exit at the center of perineum before ascending along the midline of the anterior torso to terminate at the chin. An internal part of this Conception Vessel continues upwards to terminate below the eyes.

The Governor Vessel originates in the lower abdomen and exits at the rear of the anus, sending one branch forward to meet the Conception Vessel. The main portion of the meridian ascends along the midline of the back to the top of the head and then descends along the midline of the face to a point that approximates the upper lip.

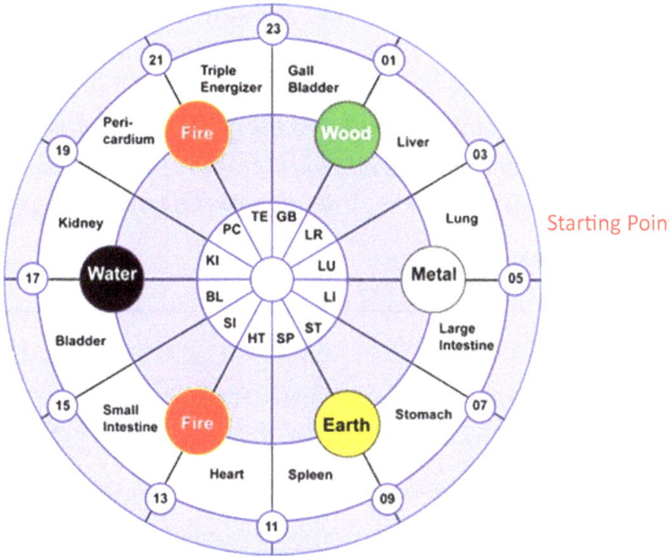

Picture Credit: Pinterest.com

In terms of direction, sequence and timing of Qi flowing around the body via the 12 meridians, it "traditionally" commences from the Lung (LU) meridian and courses to the Large Intestine (LI) meridian, Stomach (ST) meridian, Spleen (SP) meridian, Heart (HT) meridian, Small Intestine (SI) meridian, Bladder (BL) meridian, Kidney (KI) meridian, Pericardium (PC) meridian, Triple Energizer (TE) meridian, Gall Bladder (GB) meridian and the Liver (LI) meridian in this order.

It is instructional to note that each meridian may have one or more branches aside from its main trunk. When the trunk or branch making up the meridian is subcutaneous, it may be located from surface anatomy 外行部分. The others may be lying deep within the body 内行部分, the purpose of which is to connect a meridian to its related organ-system as well as another meridian.

Although the WHO has simplified the meridian names by merely referring to the organ-systems associated with the meridians, it would be extremely helpful for readers in practice to be able to recall meridian names in accordance with the full naming nomenclature. This is because the full naming convention embodies locational reference of the meridian relative to other parallel meridians running along the same part of the body. An example is the Hand Tai Yin Meridian of the Lung should be interpreted as a meridian traversing along the *medial* part of the *arm above its centreline*. Similarly, the Hand Shao Yin Meridian of the Heart traverses along the *medial* part of the *arm below its centreline.*

Glossary

Anterior refers to the front while posterior refers to the back.

Medial refers to a position nearer to the mid-line of the body while lateral refers to a position further from the mid-line of the body.

The mid-axillary line is an imaginary line dropped from the mid-point of the armpit or axilla.

Reference

1. Discourse in the True Words of the Golden Chest, Plain Questions, Chapter 4, *Huang Di's Internal Classics.*

Topic 9

The Greater Yin Lung Meridian of the Hand

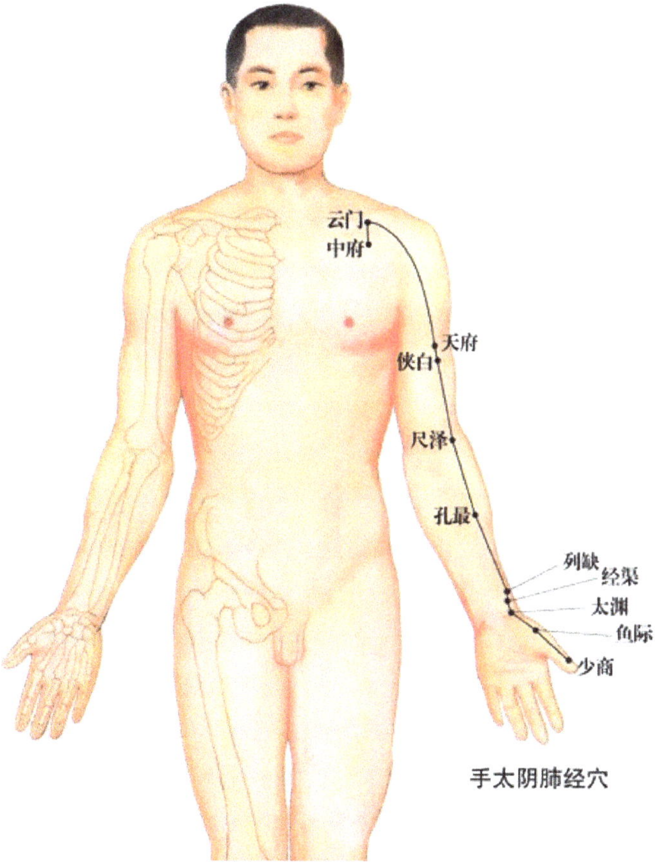

The Lung Meridian (LU) has 11 acupoints.

Internally, this Meridian originates from the mid-energizer 中焦 in the torso and descends towards the Large Intestine before ascending to circumvent the stomach, rising through the diaphragm and anchoring itself onto the Lung-system including the throat.

The superficial part of the pathway, as illustrated, surfaces near the deltopectoral groove and descends towards the medial aspect of the upper arm where it crosses the cubital crease. It then continues to course above the radial artery towards the wrist and emerges at the medial side of the tip of the thumb (LU11 少商). A branch of the Meridian sprouting from about an inch above the wrist flexion crease makes a connection with the Large Intestine Meridian on the index finger.

This Meridian is employed in the treatment of respiratory-related issues and localized upper limb musculoskeletal conditions where the Meridian courses.

Acupoints to note — LU1 中府, LU5 尺泽, LU6 孔最, LU7 列缺, LU9 太渊, LU10 鱼际 and LU11 少商.

Topic 10

The Rising Yang Large Intestine Meridian of the Hand

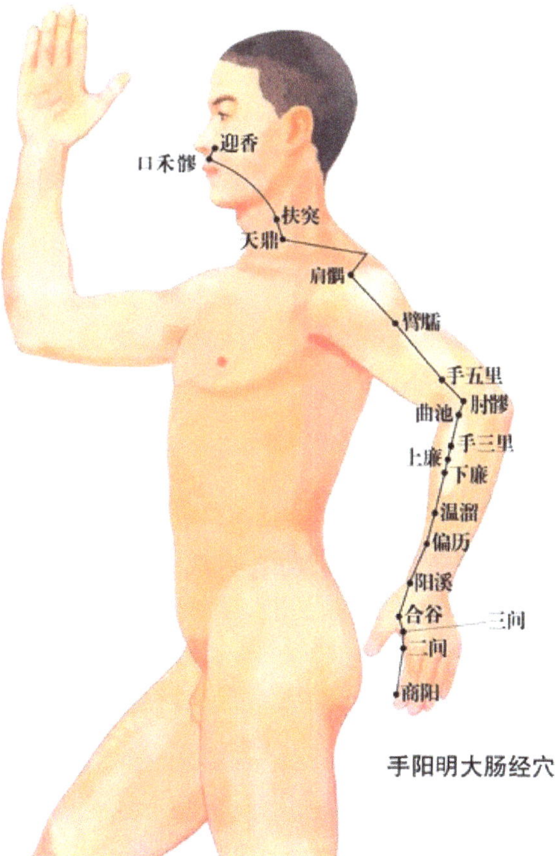

The Large Intestine Meridian (LI) has 20 acupoints.

Commencing from the tip of the index finger (LI1 商阳), this Meridian courses between the thumb and index finger along the radial aspect of the forearm before proceeding along the lateral side of the forearm adjacent to the lateral epicondyle and along the anterolateral side of the upper arm, until it reaches the highest point of the shoulder. It then travels to C7 region of the spine, the conference of Yang meridians, before descending through the supraclavicular fossa, connecting the Lung, passing through the diaphragm and anchoring itself at the Large Intestine. An upward branch of the Meridian tracks anteriorly and medially across the shoulder, the neck and across the face and cheek where it then curves around the upper lip and crosses the midline to the opposite side of the face. It ends at the side of the nose (LI20 迎香), where it connects with the Stomach Meridian.

This Meridian is employed in the treatment of intestinal related issues, Ear Nose and Throat issues, febrile-like ailments and localized upper limb musculoskeletal conditions where the meridian courses.

Acupoints to Note — LI4 合谷, LI10 手三里, LI11 曲池, LI12 肘髎, LI13 手五里, LI14 臂臑, and LI15 肩髃.

Topic 11

The Rising Yang Stomach Meridian of the Foot

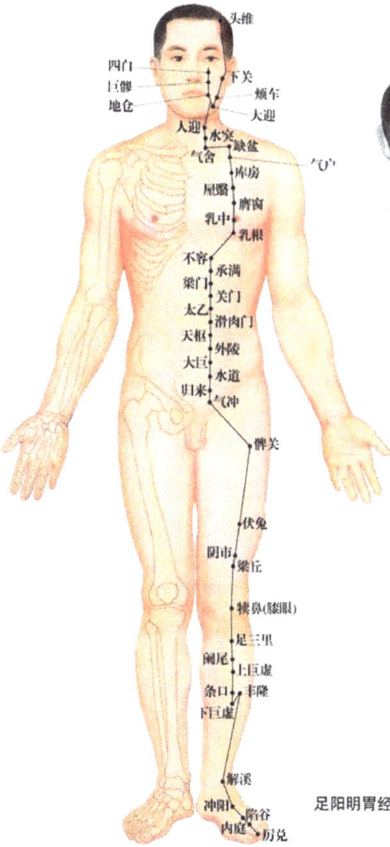

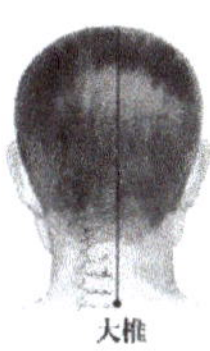

足阳明胃经穴

The Stomach Meridian (ST) has 45 acupoints.

Ascending from the end of the Large Intestine Meridian at the side of the nose, the Stomach Meridian crosses the Bladder Meridian at the medial canthus (inner corner) of the eye and runs down to the mid-lower jaw. From there, it travels toward the posterior of the mandible, then ascends in front of the ear and follows the anterior hairline until it reaches the corner of the forehead before terminating at the middle of the forehead above the hairline.

A branch of the Meridian from the lower jaw travels down the anterior aspect of the neck towards the clavicle and enters the supraclavicular fossa. At the supraclavicular fossa junction, this branch bifurcates into a deep-lying branch and a more superficial "straight-line" branch. The deep-lying branch passes through the diaphragm and connects the Meridian to the stomach and spleen. The "straight-line" branch descends the chest in line with the nipple before deflecting medially towards the midline where it runs 3 finger-width and in parallel with the Conception Vessel to the inguinal groove. It then courses laterally to descend along the anterior aspect of the thigh to the knee before traveling further down along the anterolateral border of the tibia to the dorsum of the foot before terminating at the lateral side of the tip of the second toe (ST45 厉兑). At the dorsum of the foot, the Meridian branches out to the medial side of the great toe to connect with the Spleen Meridian.

This Meridian is employed in the treatment of gastrointestinal ailments, ocular, nasal issues and medical conditions associated with locations along where the Meridian courses.

Acupoints to Note — ST2 四白, ST3 巨髎, ST4 地仓, ST5 大迎, ST6 颊车, ST7 下关, ST16 膺窗, ST18 乳根, ST29 归来, ST31 髀关, ST32 伏兔, ST34 梁丘, ST36 足三里, ST37 上巨虚, ST38 条口, ST39 下巨虚, ST40 丰隆, ST41 解溪, and ST44 内庭.

Topic 12

The Greater Yin Spleen Meridian of the Foot

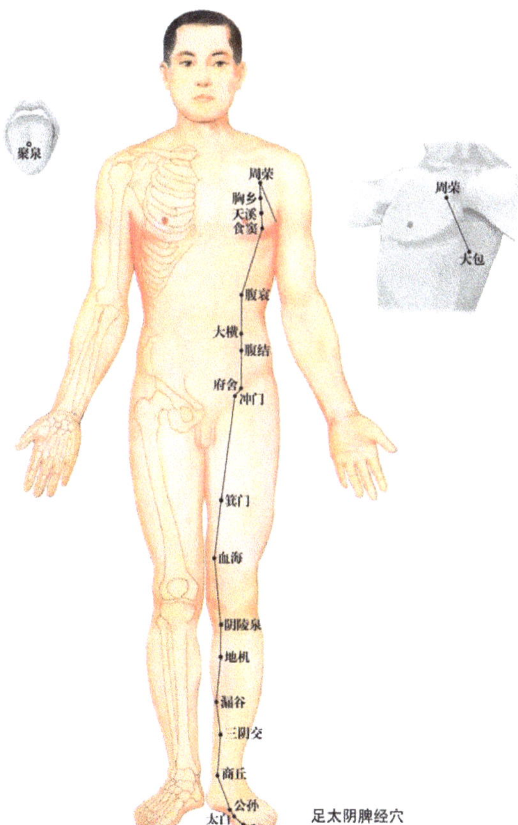

足太阴脾经穴

The Spleen Meridian (SP) has 21 acupoints.

Commencing from the medial aspect of the tip of the great toe (SP1 隐白), the Spleen Meridian travels along the medial aspect of the foot at the junction between the red and white skin, then ascends anteriorly to the medial malleolus up to the medial aspect of the leg while crossing the paths of the Liver Meridian and Kidney Meridian (SP6 三阴交). Coursing upwards along the anterior medial aspect of the thigh, it enters the inguinal region ascending the anterior of the abdomen. Upon entering the abdomen, it continues upward crossing briefly into the path of Conception Vessel. It then makes a lateral detour to connect up with the Stomach, then anchors itself with the Spleen before making another lateral detour to ascend along the esophagus and terminates at the tongue. As the Meridian rises toward the tongue, a branch, however, turns inferiorly to terminate at a point in the 6th intercostal space along the mid-axillary line (SP21 大包).

From the Stomach, a deep-lying branch of the Meridian travels toward the chest, passes through the diaphragm to connect with the Heart Meridian.

This Meridian is employed in the treatment of gastrointestinal, gynecological and genital ailments as well as medical conditions associated with locations along where the Meridian courses.

Acupoints to Note — SP1 隐白, SP2 大都, SP3 太白, SP4 公孙, SP5 商丘, SP6 三阴交, SP8 地机, SP9 阴陵泉, SP10 血海, SP12 冲门, SP14 腹结, SP17 食窦 and SP18天溪.

Topic 13

The Lesser Yin Heart Meridian of the Hand

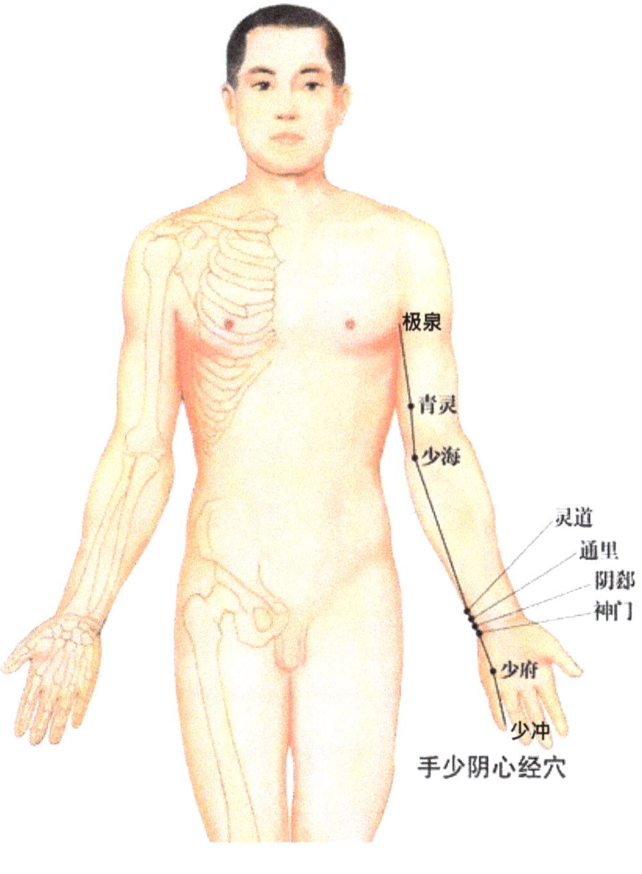

The Heart Meridian (HT) has 9 acupoints.

Internally, this Meridian originates from the heart in the torso and after passing through the diaphragm, descends toward and connects with the Small Intestine. An ascending branch from the heart passes alongside the esophagus to terminate at the eye.

Another branch of this Meridian travels laterally and crosses the Lungs to reach the center of axilla under the arm. From the axilla, it continues to course along posterior border of the medial aspect of the upper arm, passes through the cubital region (elbow) and down the forearm where it then crosses the inner side of the wrist and palm and terminates at the medial aspect of the tip of the little finger (HT9 少冲) to connect with the Small Intestine Meridian.

This Meridian is employed in the treatment of cardiothoracic and neurological ailments as well as medical conditions associated with locations along where the Meridian courses.

Acupoints to Note — HT3 少海, HT6 阴郄 and HT7 神门.

Topic 14

The Greater Yang Small Intestine Meridian of the Hand

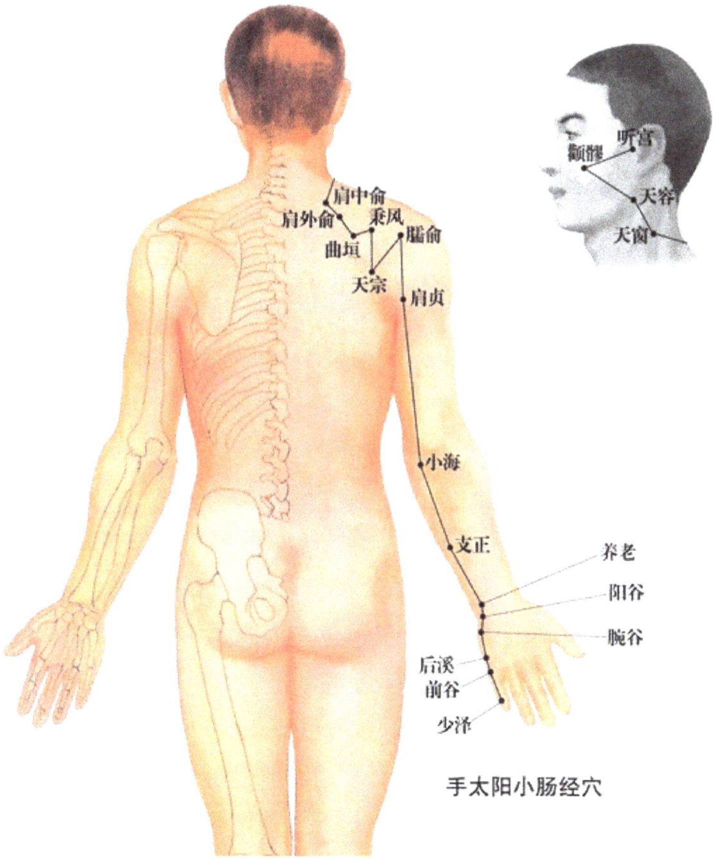

手太阳小肠经穴

The Small Intestine Meridian (SI) has 19 acupoints.

Commencing from the tip of the little finger (SI1少泽), the Small Intestine Meridian travels proximally along the ulnar border of the hand dorsum upward to the posterior border of the lateral aspect of the upper arm, passing adjacent to the medial epicondyle and upward until it reaches the back of the shoulder. It continues to zig-zag across the scapula to C7 of the spine before turning down to the supraclavicular fossa where the Meridian splits into 2 branches aside from the trunk. The trunk descends to connect the Heart, continues along the esophagus, passing through the diaphragm and circumventing the stomach before terminating at the Small Intestine.

From the supraclavicular fossa where the Meridian splits into 2 branches, one branch ascends the neck to the zygomatic bone (cheek), passes the outer canthus of the eye before turning around to terminate at the anterior of the tragus of the ear (SI19 听宫). Another branch traverses the zygomatic bone to the medial canthus of the eye to connect with the Bladder Meridian.

This Meridian is employed in the treatment of ocular, ear, throat, neurological and febrile-like ailments as well as musculoskeletal conditions associated with locations along where the Meridian courses.

Acupoints to Note — SI3 后溪, SI8 小海, SI9 肩贞, and SI11 天宗.

Topic 15

The Greater Yang Bladder Meridian of the Foot

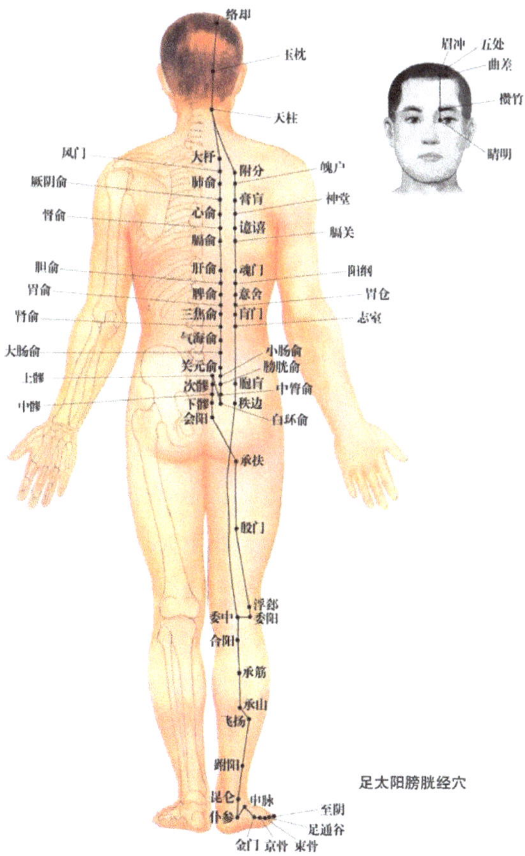

足太阳膀胱经穴

The Bladder Meridian (BL) has 67 acupoints.

Commencing from the medial canthus of the eye (BL1 睛明), the Bladder Meridian passes over the forehead to the cranial vertex before descending the back of the head and neck where it bifurcates above the posterior hairline into two branches. At C7 of the spine, one branch extends parallel downward and about 2 finger-width to the midline of the spine to the lumbar region and zig-zag to reach the 4th sacral foramen (BL34 下髎). As this branch descends, it makes a connection to the Kidney and the Bladder. The other branch travels from the posterior aspect of the neck downward along the medial border of the scapula and about 4 finger width in parallel to the midline of the spine to reach the gluteal region.

From the gluteal region, the two branches descend along the posterior aspect of the thigh, briefly crossing each other, before converging at the popliteal fossa (BL40 委中). The joint meridian continues to the posterior aspect of the gastrocnemius muscle (calf) and further to the posterior inferior aspect of the lateral malleolus (BL60 昆仑), traveling along the lateral side of the foot and terminating at the lateral side of the tip of the little toe (BL67 至阴)where it connects with the Kidney Meridian.

This Meridian, that runs the entire length of the body, is extensively employed in the treatment of febrile-like illnesses, wide-ranging ailments, and organ dysfunctions as well as musculoskeletal conditions associated with locations along where the Meridian courses.

Acupoints to Note — BL2 攒竹, BL7 通天, BL13 肺俞, BL14 厥阴俞, BL15 心俞, BL17 膈俞, BL18 肝俞, BL23 肾俞, BL37 殷门, BL39 委阳, BL40 委中, BL54 秩边, BL57 承山 and BL60 昆仑.

Topic 16

The Lesser Yin Kidney Meridian of the Foot

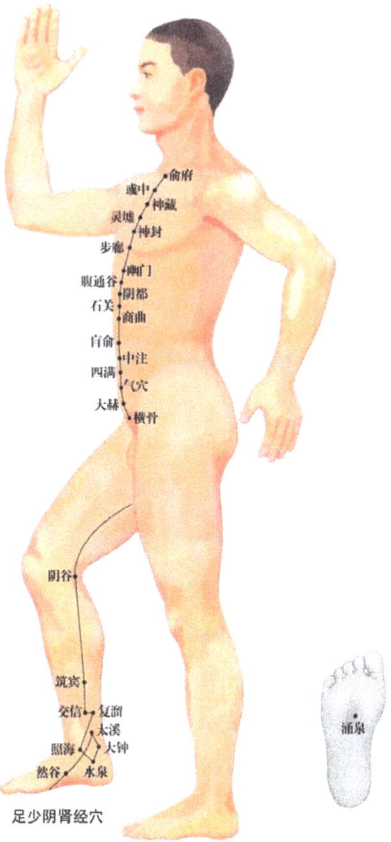

The Kidney Meridian (KI) has 27 acupoints.

Commencing from the inferior aspect of the little toe, the Kidney Meridian runs medially through a depression in the lower aspect of the tuberosity of the navicular bone (middle of the sole) toward the arch of the foot (KI1 涌泉). Ascending from the arch, it navigates behind the medial malleolus and encircles the malleolus then rises along the medial side of the leg (KI7 复溜), passes the medial side of the popliteal fossa and ascends further along the posterior-medial aspect of the thigh until it enters the body near the sacrum. Rising internally in line with the lumbar spine it connects with the kidney before descending to the connect with the bladder. From the superior border of the symphysis pubis (pubic area), the Meridian tracks upward, a finger width in parallel to the abdominal midline (KI11 横骨)but diverging at the diaphragm, to terminate at the inferior border of the clavicle (KI27 俞府).

Internally, a second branch emerges from the kidney, moves upwards and passes through the liver, diaphragm, lungs, and throat, finally terminating at the root of the tongue. Another minor branch divides from the lung to connect with the heart and the Pericardium Meridian.

This Meridian is employed in the treatment of gynecological and genital ailments and kidney, lung and throat dysfunctions as well as musculoskeletal conditions associated with locations along where the Meridian courses.

Acupoints to Note — KI1 涌泉, KI3 太溪, KI6 照海, KI7 复溜, KI10 阴谷 and 12 大赫.

Topic 17

The Transiting Yin Pericardium Meridian of the Hand

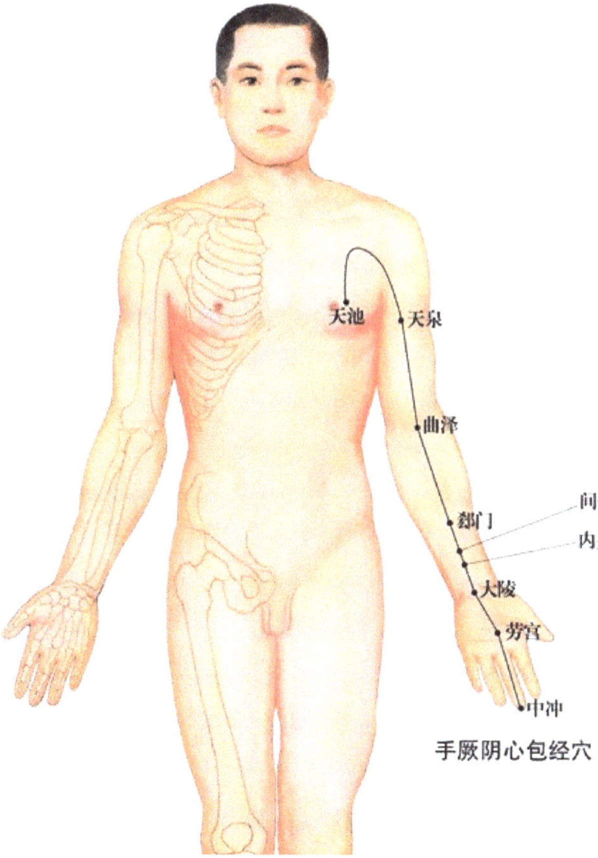

The Pericardium Meridian (PC) has 9 acupoints.

Originating in the chest, the Pericardium Meridian connects the Pericardium internally before descending through the diaphragm to the lower abdomen, connecting with the Upper Energizer, Mid-Energizer and the Lower Energizer along the pathway (not illustrated).

A branch from the Meridian then ascends to the axillary fossa and travels along the medial aspect of the upper arm, passing through the cubital fossa (PC3 曲泽) and descending further down the middle of forearm (PC6 内关) to enter the palm before terminating at the tip of the middle finger (PC9 中冲). From the palm, a connecting branch also extends to join with the Triple Burner Meridian at the end of the ring finger.

This Meridian is employed in the treatment of cardiothoracic, gastric and neurological ailments as well as musculoskeletal conditions associated with locations along where the Meridian courses.

Acupoints to Note — PC3 曲泽 and PC6 内关.

TOPIC 18

The Lesser Yang Triple Energizer Meridian of the Hand

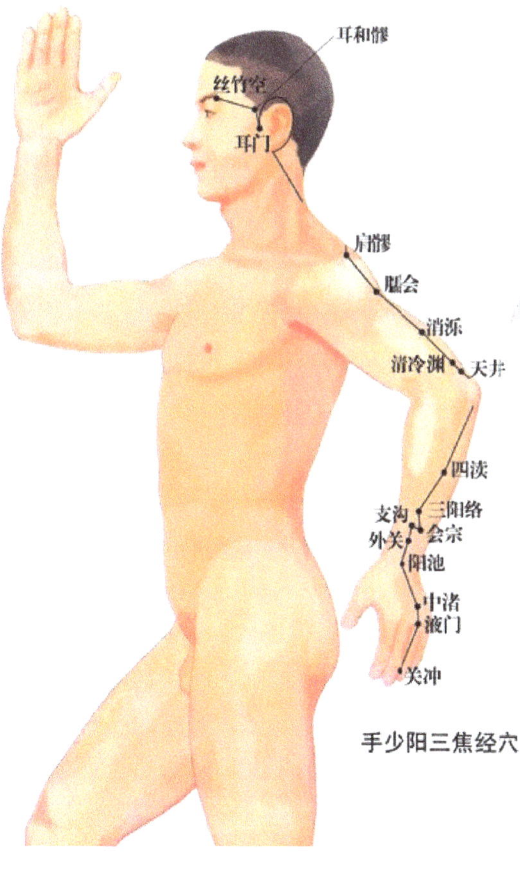

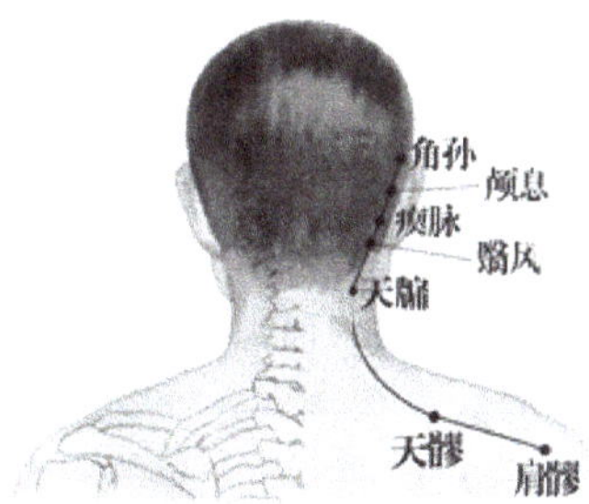

手少阳三焦经穴

The Triple Energizer Meridian (TE) has 23 acupoints.

Commencing from the outer tip of the ring finger (TE1 关冲), the Triple Energizer Meridian travels upward between the fourth and fifth metacarpal bones and along the dorsal side of the wrist and the lateral side of the forearm between the radius and ulna (TE5 外关), passing through the olecranon (elbow). It then navigates along the lateral aspect of the upper arm to reach the shoulder region before crossing over and enters the supraclavicular fossa. It then descends to the region mid-point between the nipples to connect with the Pericardium and reaching further down to pass the diaphragm and connect the three Energizers.

From the chest, the Meridian retraces its pathway through the supraclavicular fossa and navigates up the side of the neck, encircling the posterior border of the ear (TE17 翳风) to reach the superior aspect of the ear. Ascending from the tip of the ear (TE20 角孙) to the corner of the forehead, it then descends to the cheek before terminating at the lower eye region. A branch emerging from the inner ear crosses path with the Meridian at the cheek and terminates at the lateral end of the eyebrow (TE23 丝竹空) where it connects with the Gall Bladder Meridian.

This Meridian is employed in the treatment of thoracic, ear, eye, throat and febrile-like ailments as well as musculoskeletal conditions associated with locations along where the Meridian courses.

Acupoints to Note — TE2 液门, TE3 中渚, TE4 阳池, TE5 外关, TE6 支沟, TE10 天井, TE14 肩髎, TE17 翳风, and TE23 丝竹空.

TOPIC 19

The Lesser Yang Gall Bladder Meridian of the Foot

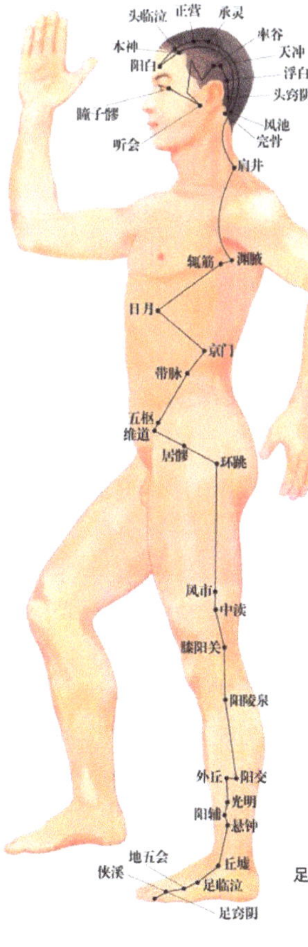

足少阳胆经穴

The Gall Bladder Meridian (GB) has 44 acupoints.

Commencing from the lateral canthus of the eye (GB1 瞳子髎), the Gall Bladder Meridian descends to the anterior aspect of the ear where it ascends to the corner of the forehead and then navigates downward posterior to the ear before arcing forward to the forehead at the midpoint of the eyebrow. It then returns above the hairline (and above the previous arcing) to the lateral side of the neck. On reaching the top of the shoulder (trapezoid) it travels laterally to C7 of the spine before crossing over to enter the supraclavicular fossa. From there it further descends to the axilla and crosses the lateral side of the rib cage and abdomen near the femoral artery in the inguinal region (pubic area), moving posteriorly to the gluteal region.

A branch of the Meridian enters the ear from its rear and emerges at the anterior of the ear (GB2 听会) to reach the lateral canthus of the eye. It then descends to encircle the cheek before traveling downward to the supraclavicular fossa before entering the chest to connect with the liver and gall bladder. It continues further down to the pubic area to merge with the earlier branch at the side of the hip.

The merged branches then descend along the lateral side of the thigh to the lateral side of the knee, along the anterior aspect of the fibula (GB34 阳陵泉) to reach the anterior of the lateral malleolus (GB40 丘墟). Following the dorsum of the foot, it terminates at the lateral side of the tip of the fourth toe (GB44 足窍阴).

A minor branch sprouts from the Meridian at the dorsum of the foot to connect with the Liver Meridians between the large and second toe.

This Meridian is employed in the treatment of febrile-like, ear and eye ailments as well as musculoskeletal conditions associated with locations along where the Meridian courses. The Gall Bladder Meridian is much favored for the management of headaches and neuropathic pains because of the extensive distribution of points on the lateral aspects of the head as well as its reach to major nerve pathways.

Acupoints to Note — GB14 阳白, GB20 风池, GB30 环跳, GB31 风市, GB34 阳陵泉, GB39 悬钟, GB41 足临泣 and GB43 侠溪.

Topic 20

The Merging Yin Liver Meridian of the Foot

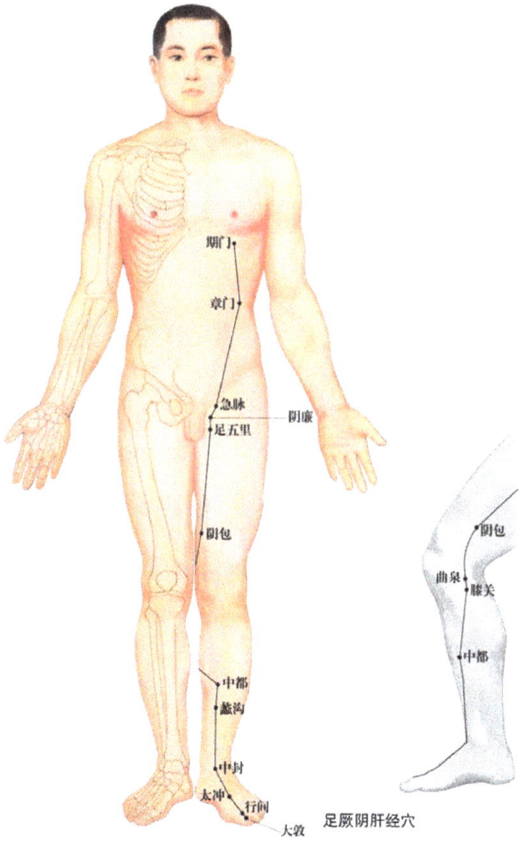

足厥阴肝经穴

The Liver Meridian (LR) has 14 points.

Commencing from the lateral side of the great toe (LR1 大敦) and goes across the dorsum of the foot, the Liver Meridian crosses the anterior aspect of the medial malleolus (ankle) and continues to ascend along the lower leg and the thigh medially into the pubic region. Continuing the path of ascent, the Meridian encircles the external genitalia and crosses the midline up to the lower abdomen. It then extends upward across the abdomen to reach the lower chest laterally where it connects the Liver and Gall Bladder before passing through the diaphragm and ascends to the throat posteriorly. From here it enters the nasal region and rises through the optic region of the brain, then the forehead to connect with the Governor Vessel at the cranial vertex. A minor branch of the Meridian extends from the optic region of the brain to encircle the inner lips.

From the Liver, a branch of the Meridian ascends to cross the diaphragm to the Lungs to connect with the Lung Meridian.

This Meridian is employed in the treatment of hepatic, gynecological and genital ailments as well as musculoskeletal conditions associated with locations along where the Meridian courses.

Acupoints to Note — LR1 大敦, LR2 行间, LR3 太冲, LR4 中封, LR5 蠡沟, LR6 中都, and LR8 曲泉.

TOPIC 21

The Conception Vessel

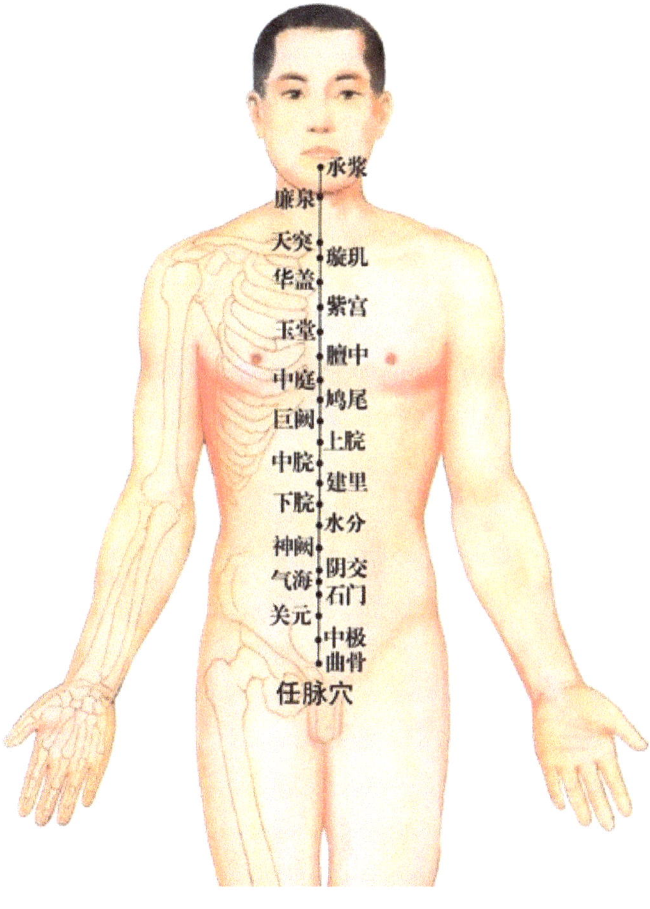

The Conception Vessel (CV), one of the eight extraordinary meridians, has 24 acupoints.

Originating from the lower abdomen, the Conception Vessel descends to center of the perineum (CV1 会阴) before rising anteriorly to the pubic region and then extends along the anterior midline of the torso until it reaches the mandible (lower jaw) where at the center of the mentolabial groove directly below the lip (CV24 承浆), it bifurcates into two branches. These branches terminate after entering the infra-orbital margin (lower eyelid region).

The Conception Vessel is a long meridian that runs the entire length of the torso that contains many vital-organ systems. The Meridian also represents the convergence of all Yin meridians. In this regard, this Meridian is employed extensively in the treatment of many ailments as well as for tonification purposes.

Acupoints to Note — CV17 膻中, CV22 天突, and CV24 承浆.

Topic 22

The Governor Vessel

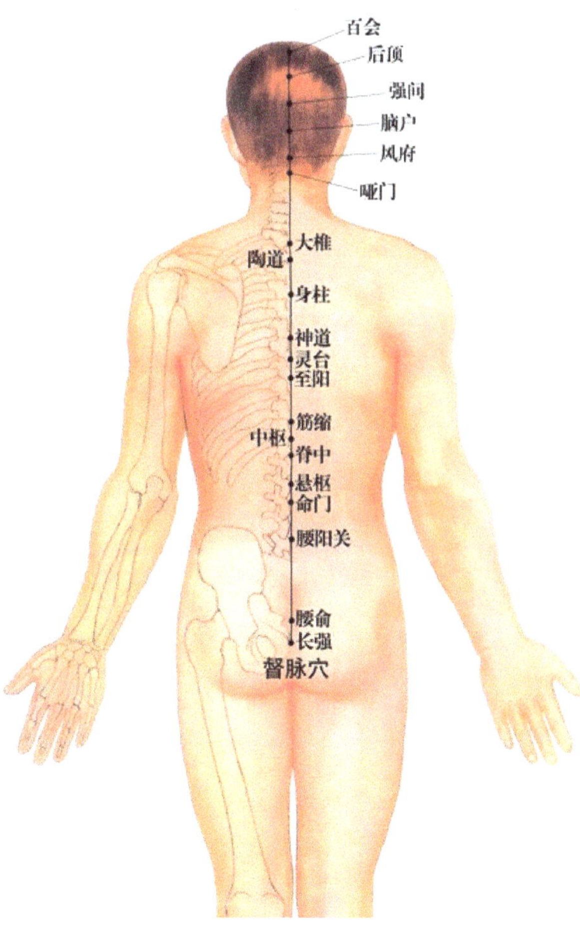

The Governor Vessel (GV), one of the eight extraordinary meridians, has 28 acupoints.

Originating from the lower abdomen, the Governor Vessel descends to the midpoint between the tip of the coccyx bone and the anus (GV1 长强) before ascending posteriorly along the spinal column until it reaches the nape of the neck (GV15 哑门). After crossing the cranial vertex, it continues its downward path over the face and along the nose bridge (GV25 素髎) to terminate at the junction of the gum and the labial frenulum of the upper lip (GV28 龈交).

The Governor Vessel is a long meridian that runs the entire length of the spinal column and the head. It also represents the convergence of all Yang meridians. In this regard, the Governor Vessel is generally employed in the treatment of musculoskeletal conditions of the spine, vertigo and the management of febrile-like ailments.

Acupoint to Note — GV14 大椎 and GV16 风府.

Part 2
Treatment Protocols

Topic 23

Techniques for *Sha* Extraction

Sha extraction may be performed with or without the assistance of instruments. *Gua Sha* is one therapy that can be performed with the aid of easily available apparatus or even improvisations.

Bare Hand Techniques

Without engaging the use of apparatus, there are generally four different bare hand techniques — pinching 挟痧法, pulling 扯痧法, slapping 拍痧法 and squeezing 挤痧法. Bare hand techniques are non-invasive and particularly useful when applied to treatment spots that are small or difficult to access.

a. Pinching — with this method, the operator first curls his hand into a loosely held fist with a hollow in the palm. Applying a pinching force from the middle and index fingers that are reinforced by the thumb, the skin and muscles at the lightly lubricated treatment surface of the patient are picked up and then slid outwards before being released in quick succession. A light sound created by the snapping of the index and middle finger as the skin slips away would be emitted with every successful pinch at the point of release.

   The above procedure should be repeated six to seven times at the same spot until a skin discoloration appears and remains consistent.

This method may be applied to both meridian or acupoint *Gua Sha* treatment.

b. Pulling — with this method, the thumb and the index finger are used to lift the skin and its subcutaneous tissue at the treatment surface of the patient before releasing the grip spontaneously. After wetting the thumb and forefinger, this procedure is repeatedly executed in quick succession until the epidermis subjected to this procedure shows a consistent skin discoloration.

   The technique may also be executed using three fingers with the index and middle fingers and the thumb opposing for improved grip and force. Unlike the Pinching method, this method being "more gentle and friendly" to the skin at the point of contact is often used in treatment where the selected area is sensitive. This method may be applied in both meridian or acupoint *Gua Sha* treatment.

   The Pulling method may also be used for the early detection of heat-stroke by gently applying the technique to the area above the nasal bridge or dorsum of the hand between the 1st and 2nd metacarpal bones.

c. Slapping — with this method, the treatment surface of the patient is repeatedly slapped with the relaxed hand of the operator in quick succession until the treatment site yields a slight bruising. The patient should feel a sensation of pain, itch, numbness or distention at the treatment site. The intensity of the slap impact may be adjusted by the degree of relaxation of the wrist of the slapping hand as well as the coordination of the operator's shoulder.

   The Slapping method should be applied judiciously on the merit of the situation and delivered only by trained hands. Serious injuries including fatalities have been reported of the very young and the very ill patients who were subjected to this technique.

d. Squeezing — with this method, the operator uses the thumb and index finger of one hand to squeeze the treatment site in an orderly and repetitive manner until skin discoloration appears as rows of circular dots. For greater pressure and speed, both hands may be applied at the same time.

Instrument-Assisted Techniques

Instrument-assisted techniques require the use of different apparatus to draw out *sha* in the form of skin discoloration or waste-laden blood from the patient. These techniques may be further classified as invasive and non-invasive methods.

In invasive methods, the treatment site is often perforated to release waste-laden blood. In this regard, the standard required for disinfection of the treatment site is held more stringently when invasive methods are applied. Patients' immediate response to treatment may also be exaggerated and intense as invasive methods are perceived to be more painful. Because of the inherent risks, patients with pre-existing conditions of compromised immunity or bleeding disorders shall not be subject to these treatment methods. Invasive methods should, therefore, be executed strictly by trained operators who understand the scope of therapeutic application. There are generally two different invasive methods — picking method 挑痧法 and releasing method 放痧法.

Invasive methods

a. Picking method — with this method, the treatment site must be thoroughly disinfected to prevent infection. Similarly, the procedure must be executed under sterile conditions using a disposable diabetic lancet or disposable hypodermic needle. Other improvisations, like sewing needles and use of primitive sterilization protocols, are not recommended under normal situation. The operator shall don disposable surgical gloves or thoroughly disinfect his hands before the treatment.

   The perforation protocol involves the operator pinching the flesh at a spot of the treatment site with one hand before superficially puncturing the pinched flesh with a sterile instrument and rapidly withdrawing the instrument with an upward picking motion. This process is repeated three times in succession at each spot. The broken skin is then squeezed to release a small amount of blood before being cleaned with a sterile cotton ball.

This method should be reserved only for the treatment of deep-seated or latent *sha*, of which other less invasive methods are incapable of drawing out.

b. Releasing method — unlike the picking method where perforation is confined to intradermal level, this method may only be appropriate for treatment sites where there are superficial blood vessels like the cubital fossa (inner elbow), axilla (armpit), popliteal (back of knee) and temporal regions as well as extremities of the limbs. Another point of differentiation is the releasing method is generally targeted at selected acupoints.

   In a nutshell, the method involves identifying a treatment site, disinfecting it, perforating some minor blood vessel and extracting a limited amount of blood from the puncture.

   This protocol should be strictly performed by trained professionals in a clinical setting as it is a form of therapeutic phlebotomy or blood-letting.

Non-invasive methods

The treatment site is not perforated when instrument-assisted non-invasive methods are employed. These methods are always considered safer options and may, therefore, be delivered by informed operators.

Gua Sha or derma abrasive scraping is by far the most commonly adopted technique in and is considered the safest of *sha* extraction and disposal methods. One reason for its popularity is that the resources required for *Gua Sha* in terms of equipment and operator skill are not demanding as the treatment may be delivered at various levels of sophistication, from basic cutaneous scrapping, meridian dredging to selective acupoint scraping. In this regard, *Gua Sha* is also the most versatile of the methods.

As earlier mentioned, the method can be applied at different levels of competency. In its most primitive and basic form that was imparted to laypeople, *Gua Sha* involves only cutaneous scrapping and meridian dredging. The operator needs only to identify the major meridian pathways distributed in the body as treatment sites and master the basic scraping techniques and he is good to go.

In the more refined and latter-day method, *Gua Sha* is extended to the scraping of acupoints which is much akin to acupuncture except that this is done with *Gua Sha* apparatus in substitution to needles. In this regard, the operator's level of knowledge in respect of meridians and acupoints is raised by many notches since the location of acupoints is a much more precise exercise when compared to merely identifying the approximate pathways of meridians.

In terms of hand techniques for acupoint *Gua Sha*, three popular methods are acupoint scrapping, acupoint 'press-and-hold' and acupoint jabbing.

Acupoint scrapping is deployed when two or more acupoints, to be treated concurrently, are located along the same meridian or on different but parallel meridians. The first scenario is similar to meridian scrapping but executed for only a designated portion of the meridian. An example would be to perform acupoint scrapping from ST36 to ST39 for ST36 足三里, ST37 上巨虚 and ST39 下巨虚 instead of attempting 'press-and-hold' protocol for the three acupoints separately.

The second instance is when the acupoints having a similar function are treated concurrently to reinforce therapeutic effect, e.g. scrapping the antecubital fossa region activates two acupoints L5 尺泽 and PC3 曲泽 for rapid heat dissipation. The same applies to the popliteal region where three acupoints BL39 委阳, BL40 委中 and KI10 阴谷 reside.

For effectiveness, the acupoint scrapping line should run about one cm above and below the prescribed acupoints on parallel meridians. For acupoints residing on the same meridian, the scrapping line should course continuously through the all prescribed acupoints and about one cm above the first indicated acupoint and one cm below the last indicated acupoint.

The other two acupoint methods, 'press-and-hold' and jabbing are designed to stimulate an isolated acupoint by applying the sharp corner of a handheld instrument with focussed energy over the selected spot to clear an obstructed pathway.

In the acupoint 'press-and-hold' method, steady pressure is applied incrementally with the instrument's edge being held in place over the contact point momentarily for up to two seconds before making a gradual withdrawal. This action is then repeated rhythmically for about 10 times for each acupoint. The instrument may be held at an angle though.

The acupoint jabbing method is much similar to the 'press-and-hold' method except for two differences — timing and pressure. The contact area of the instrument to the skin is much reduced by holding the instrument vertically which exerts a higher pressure on to the selected acupoint and that the instrument is withdrawn immediately when the desired pressure is achieved by the operator.

For both methods, the pressure exerted should be steadily incremental during application as well as gradually decreasing when withdrawing.

Notwithstanding, cutaneous scrapping, meridian dredging, and acupoint scraping methods are not mutually exclusive in an application and may be performed on different parts of the body or even over selected parts of the same treatment area within the same therapy session. These methods merely characterize plane (cutaneous), line (meridian) and point (acupoint) geometry of *Gua Sha* methods respectively.

<u>Press-Stroke Fundamentals</u>

a. Deliberate superficial bruising or skin discoloration of any intensity may be expected but on no account shall the skin surface be broken resulting from *Gua Sha* treatment.
b. The treatment area shall be sufficiently lubricated before the commencement of treatment to facilitate rhythmic stroking and prevent breaking of the skin.
c. Cutaneous scraping should be performed in the motion of a unidirectional, constant-pressure, straight and rhythmic press-stroke. A press-stroke is performed by firmly landing the smooth contact surface of the instrument at an angle to the skin of the treatment site before running off the instrument a short distance of about 12 cm along the skin under constant force.
d. There are occasions when press-strokes are performed with speed but do not *rush* the strokes. There is a major difference between performing the stroke with speed and *rushing the stroke*

that may yield outcomes ranging from favorable therapeutic relief to increased discomfort and even aggravated symptoms for the patient.

e. Press-strokes are repeatedly applied to the same spot at the treatment area until a consistent bruising or skin discoloration is obtained before moving on to the adjacent spot at the treatment area.
f. The force applied behind each stroke is to be held constant but for repeated delivery of strokes to the same spot, the intensity of force should be increased gradually so as not to elicit muscular spasm at the treatment spot.
g. The rule of thumb for *Gua Sha* is from top to bottom (head towards foot), from medial to lateral (mid-line outwards), from dorsal(back) to ventral(front) and upper to lower limbs. An example of complete body treatment would flow from head to neck, to back, to lumbar, to sacrum before turning to the chest, to medial upper limbs, to lateral upper limbs, to medial lower limbs, and to lateral lower limbs. Exception for the top to bottom rule is when the patient suffers from edema or varicose veins and in this instance, the direction of strokes shall be reversed. Facial *Gua Sha* for beauty is also performed upwards.
h. When applying *Gua Sha* to limbs, joint areas should be met with reduced pressure.
i. In meridian dredging, the established convention is to perform the routine on the left side of the patient's body before repeating the same, in mirror-image, for the right side.

Topic 24

Advanced Press-Stroke Variants In *Gua Sha*

Like in any manual technique, the basic press-stroke in *Gua Sha* is a fundamental skill that any *Gua Sha* practitioner should familiarize and internalize. The basic press-stroke is the bedrock upon which other advanced variants are developed.

To reiterate, the basic press-stroke comprises a scraping motion performed in the following manner:

a. Unidirectional — strokes for a specific spot may be repetitive but no stroke for a treatment area shall be retraced, reversed in direction or back-tracked in terms of the motion. This is an immutable rule in *Gua Sha* therapy.
b. Straight — a press-stroke shall generally be performed in a short straight line. Curve press-strokes are permitted as an advanced variant.
c. Rhythmic — press-strokes may be performed fast or slow but when executed in quick succession, should do so without a sense of haste.
d. Constant-pressure — from the point in time of contact between the instrument and the skin, the force applied for each press-stroke shall be constant. Notwithstanding, the force applied may be progressively increased to avoid muscular spasm at the treatment site.

Advanced press-stroke variants are developed from the interplay of rhythm and stroke pressure.

a. Light Stroke — a light stroke is achieved by maximizing the contact area between the skin and instrument at the treatment area, maintaining a slow stroke rhythm and moderating the force applied such that no pain or discomfort is felt by the patient. Although this is deemed to be a novice's stroke, it is always appropriate for application to *Yin* surfaces of the body, for children, the elderly and the infirmed.
b. Heavy Stroke — in a heavy stroke, the contact area between the skin and instrument at the treatment site is reduced, the stroke rhythm is condensed and the force applied is progressively increased to patient's tolerance breakpoint. Needless to say, treatment sites for application of heavy strokes shall be fleshy and on the *Yang* surfaces of the body. Regularly deployed to relieve painful conditions of soft tissues, it is appropriately used for the young and the physically strong.
c. Fast Stroke — refers to repetitive strokes executed with a rhythm in excess of 30 times per minute with varying but constant stroke pressure. When executed with higher stroke pressure, fast strokes can be used for quick relief to body aches at fleshy areas and for the physically strong. In combination with light stroke pressure, fast strokes are applied to *Yin* surfaces of the body and for those with a weak constitution.
d. Slow Stroke — refers to repetitive strokes executed with a rhythm not exceeding 30 times per minute with varying constant stroke pressure. When executed with higher stroke pressure, slow strokes can be used for quick relief to body aches at fleshy sites and for the physically strong. In combination with light stroke pressure, slow strokes are applied to *Yin* surfaces of the body and for those with a weak constitution.
e. Arc Stroke — refers to a stroke of which the scraping direction is in the shape of an arc thereby leaving an arc-shaped bruising. Arc strokes are applied to follow the contour of the body as in the sides of the shoulder following the neck and the intercostal

spaces (between the ribs). Modified arc (circular) strokes are also used for the umbilical or abdominal area. Short arc strokes are also employed in breaking up internal scarring, muscle knot or myofascial trigger point; similar to Instrument Assisted Soft Tissue Mobilization technique.

f. Reversed-directional Stroke — refers to a stroke or a series of strokes executed contrary to the direction dictated by the conventional rule of *Gua Sha*. As a rule of thumb, *Gua Sha* shall be performed in the direction of top toward the bottom and medial toward lateral. For the avoidance of doubt, reversed-directional stroke means that scraping is performed from the bottom towards the top and from lateral to medial. This exception shall only be applied in situations where there are varicose veins in the lower extremities, edema in the lower extremities, engorgement of mammary glands or when treatment is done in a conventional manner would yield unsatisfactory outcomes. The reverse scraping operation should employ light and slow strokes, starting from the proximal end of the heart and gradually extending to the distal end. The direction of each stroke should, however, be from the distal to the proximal end for the purpose of promoting venous return and reducing edema or pain.

The diagram below epitomizes the interplay between stroke rhythm and stroke pressure in producing press-strokes with varying purposes.

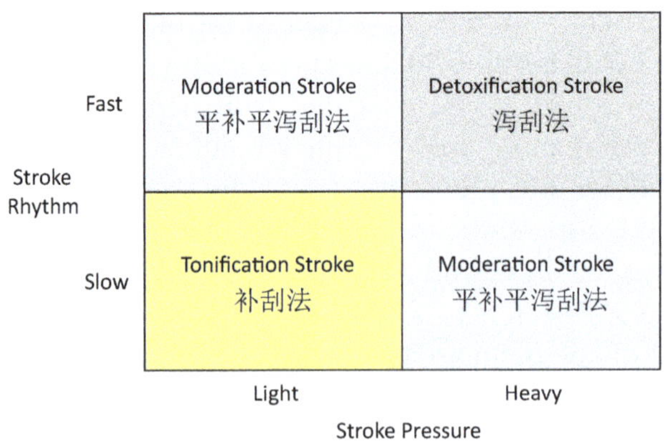

There are yet other ways, when applicable, that the practitioner may choose to reinforce tonification and detoxification strokes by varying the treatment duration, the direction of the press-stroke with reference to the flow of the selected meridian(s) as well as the number of acupoints selected during treatment. In the end, the treatment will be evidenced by the differing hue, texture, and intensity of Sha manifestation

	Stroke Pressure	Stroke Rhythm	Treatment Duration	Meridian Direction	Acupoint Selection	*Sha* Manifestation
Tonification	Light	Slow	Short	Compliant	Few	Light & Shallow
Detoxification	Heavy	Fast	Long	Opposing	Many	Heavy & Patchy

From the foregoing, it may be obvious that these advanced variants are designed to meet two primary objectives — to provide relief to disorders by either tonifying the body via raising Qi level or detoxifying the body through extracting and evacuating pathogenic substances. While weak stimulation boosts tonification, strong stimulation promotes detoxification. Detoxification has anti-inflammatory 消炎, analgesic 镇痛 and anti-pyretic 解热 effects. The body's Yin-Yang balance is therefore re-established when such objectives are achieved.

Disease in humans is caused mainly by the disorder of the blood and/or vital energy. While blood is tangible and less susceptible to speedy repair, Qi which is intangible has a much shorter recovery window. Qi is the driving force underlying blood circulation. Blood and Qi are congenial twins and maintain a symbiotic relationship. Blood without an appropriate level of Qi results in blood stasis. The ensuing delay in supply of nutrients to as well as the removal of toxins from organ-systems cannot, therefore, keep the body in a healthy state. Similarly, Qi relies on blood for sustenance, without which Qi shall perish and so shall the body.

If for any reason *Gua Sha* may provide rapid relief, it is attributed to the ability to re-invigorate the Qi mechanism 气机 that has been exhausted or spent due to severe or chronic illness. Or perhaps for a situation that requires the speedy evacuation of pathogenic substances obstructing the normal flow of Qi and impeding the operation of the Qi mechanism. In any case, when the Qi mechanism is being prevented from performing its role in controlling the spontaneous emergence and withdrawal 升降沉浮 of vital energy, disease occurs.

The human body has a self-healing mechanism. Through a process of compensation and re-balancing, the body achieves harmony within itself as well as with the external environment. There are however times when such imbalances tipped the scale and a little external help is required to restore equilibrium. *Gua Sha* is the little boosting force that helps reinstate the dynamic equilibrium.

Topic 25

Apparatus for *Gua Sha* Therapy

Because *Gua Sha* was a natural healing folk remedy, the specifications for Gua Sha instrument are less than demanding. In fact, any apparatus having a smooth rounded edge that is large enough to offer a comfortable grip by the operator would fit the bill.

In this regard, there exists a wide scope of improvisation if proper instruments are not available. Many authors suggest using a metal spoon or a worn-out coin as a *Gua Sha* tool but such improvisation hardly meets the criteria of "smooth rounded" edge. A high-quality minted spoon, regardless of finish, is still a smooth thin edge that when repetitively ran over a treatment spot will invariably cause micro-tears in the epidermis. In this sense, a ceramic or porcelain Chinese soup spoon would serve as a better option. Another feasible alternative is to use the top facing edge of a metal twisting lid from a jam jar as a smooth rounded contact to the skin. The author has also once used the smooth bottom of a tall but thick, drinking glass as an effective *Gua Sha* instrument. The options are indeed only limited by one's imagination, sense of pragmatism and creativity.

The most commonly available professional instrument used for *Gua Sha* is the "*gua sha* ban" 刮痧板 (means *gua sha* board literally). These may be fashioned out of Bian stone 砭石, jade, water buffalo horns, rose quartz or even animal bones. Medical grade stainless steel IASTM instruments which can be expensive may also be used for *Gua Sha*.

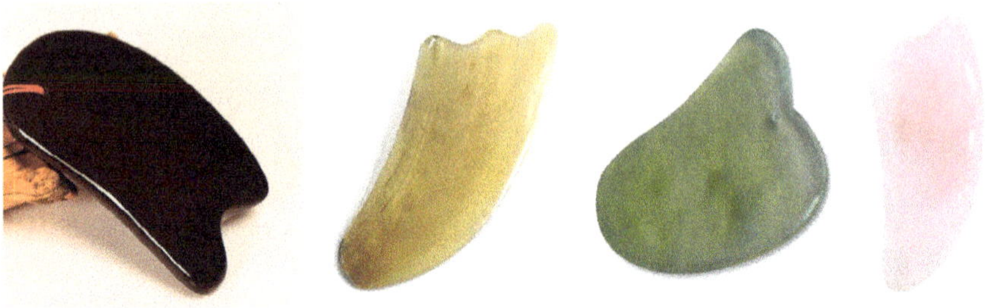

Bian Stone Water Buffalo Horn Jade Rose Quartz

The material which the *Gua Sha* instrument is fashioned is less critical in determining the outcome of the treatment as compared to the skills level of the operator. Notwithstanding, some natural healing practitioners believe that the choice of material does contribute to the efficacy of the therapy.

Sibin Bian stone from Sishui-Shandong 泗水-山东 is considered the material of choice for *Gua Sha* tools. As a polished rock, Bian stone has low hardness, is colored gray-black at its surface but deep gray at the section. Petrological and mineralogical studies showed that its compactness, graphite (carbon), anatase (titanium dioxide) and pyrite (iron sulfide) content enhance thermal conductivity, thermoelectric performance, infrared absorption and reflection properties. With a vertical far-infrared emittance up to 0.923 in the 8–14 μm spectral zone, it is capable of stimulating blood activity, dissipating blood stasis and regulating blood circulation in the human body owing mainly to its excellent thermal emission capability.[1]

Gua Sha tools are often weighted to facilitate the application of consistent pressure during press-strokes by practitioners performing the procedure. Grip is another consideration in the choice of build material. Bian stone is the heaviest in weight among the commonly selected materials for fashioning *Gua Sha* tools. Its compactness and low hardness provide a smooth contact surface for the patient yet offering a firm grip on the instrument for the operator especially when the hands become greasy during the *Gua Sha* process. All these considerations make Bian stone *Gua Sha* tools the choice of professionals.

Water Buffalo Horn is the next best material for generic *Gua Sha* tools when genuine Bian stone from Sishui-Shandong is not available. *Cornu Bubali* (water buffalo horn) is an animal-derived product which is widely used in TCM for dispelling heat, relieving convulsions and cooling blood; detoxification properties that many *Gua Sha* practitioners believe that may be leveraged upon to reinforce the therapeutic effect of treatment if the *Gua Sha* instrument made of Water Buffalo Horn.

Of course, it is hardly conceivable that these same effects be conferred upon a patient in any considerable way via *Gua Sha* even though it has been scientifically proven that *Cornu Bubali*, when imbibed, exhibits antipyretic activity in both infectious and non-infectious hyperthermia situations through enhancing antioxidation enzyme activities, decreasing prostaglandin E_2 production and protecting microvascular cells against hydrogen peroxide-induced toxicity.[2]

A disadvantage in using water buffalo horn as a material is that it is the lightest in weight among generally selected materials.

Gua-Sha tools fashioned out of Jade and Rose Quartz are generally reserved for aesthetic treatment. Apart from having a delicate built quality appearance, the materials indeed provide the most refined contact surface that confers confidence upon even the most discerning patient that the equipment will not cause micro-lacerations. Aside from cost consideration, the disadvantage in the use of these materials is that tools built out of them are difficult to grip once in contact with lubricants, but such a disadvantage is moderated when light quick press-strokes are usually used in aesthetics Gua *Sha*.

Apart from an instrument, Gua Sha therapists require a lubricant to be applied to the treatment site so that the instrument may glide across the skin smoothly during each stroke and thus reduce the incidence of micro laceration after repeated press-strokes.

Pragmatically, the choice of lubricant may have a telling effect on the outcome of the therapy especially if the objective of the treatment is therapeutic. Again, there is a wide ambit for improvisation aside from seeking out specialized *Gua Sha* preparations so long as the selection bases are predicated on purpose and function.

Two objectives for lubricating the treatment surface before performing press-strokes are primarily for dermal protection and administration of topical medication as an added benefit.

The largest and perhaps one of the toughest organs of the body, the skin barrier, can still breakdown when subject to repeated "abuse". The treatment area in *Gua Sha* may at times be very extensive that covers a significant part of the entire body. As such it is necessary to protect the skin's lipid barrier and in so doing, retain moisture content and prevent extensive infection during and after the treatment process.

When deciding on dermal protection effect of a lubricant against physical trauma, a major consideration is the viscosity of the product. By and large, the greater the viscosity, the greater the protective effect against derma abrasion.

Different types of press-stroke require differing amounts of glide or surface tension and thus viscosity of lubricant makes an appreciable difference in the effectiveness of the press-stroke. Generally, higher viscosity lubricants that offer greater drag and less glide are more appropriate for heavy and slow press-strokes while thinner lubricants that allow for more glide with less surface tension are suitable for light and quick press-strokes. Higher viscosity lubricants, because of the drag effect, further provide greater stroke control during acupoint *Gua Sha* when the operator needs to focus on more precise treatment sites.

Transdermal Drug Delivery (TDD) is a painless method of delivering topical medication by applying the formulation directly onto intact and healthy skin to produce a slow, controlled, systemic effect. The drug initially penetrates through the stratum corneum and then passes through the deeper epidermis and dermis without drug accumulation in the dermal layer. When the drug reaches the dermal layer, it becomes available for systemic absorption via the dermal microcirculation. Transdermal absorption has many advantages including the elimination of hepatic first-pass and avoidance of degradation in the gastrointestinal tract.

The efficacy of TDD is a function of the surface area available to the application as well as the relative surface temperature of the treatment site. In this regard, *Gua Sha* treatment that engages large dermal surface area provides an excellent platform for transdermal absorption. With suitable topical medications being easily integrated into skin lubricants, TDD can favorably augment the therapeutic outcomes of the treatment. And in acupoint *Gua Sha* where the treatment sites are small, it appears that placement of topical medication at close proximity to an acupoint enhances drug absorption.[3] Research in heat-enhanced transdermal drug delivery whose dominant mechanism is heat-induced local vasodilation and acceleration of skin blood flow also support Gua Sha's efficacy of absorption.[4–6] Transdermal absorption may, however, be altered if lesions, burns or skin breakdowns are present at the application site.

Gua Sha lubricants could, therefore, be merely pure lubricants or carrier lubricants for medicinal additives. Pure lubricants with various degree of viscosity may either be organic or inorganic. Petroleum-based products are inorganic whereas coconut oil, olive oil, sweet almond oil, and other plant-based oils are organic. Most natural oils are non-comedogenic which means they do not cause pore-clogging.

Medicinal additives used in therapeutic *Gua Sha* are herbal extracts that may be broadly classified as antipyretic (fever-reducing), analgesic (pain-relieving), detoxicant, Qi enhancing and blood stasis dispelling. There are however other herbal additives employed in aesthetics *Gua Sha* and *Gua Sha* for wellness. The table in the next topic, which by no means exhaustive, provides some popular herbs used under the various categories.

One caveat prudent to note for any informed *Gua Sha* operator is the possibility of patient allergy to the skin lubricant, be it pure lubricant or carrier lubricant with medicinal additives. If time permits, it is advisable to perform a simple allergy skin test with the intended lubricant/medicinal additive on the inner arm of the patient before applying the same on the patient extensively.

Peanut oil was one of the early improvised skin lubricants adopted in *Gua Sha* treatment. It is however strongly not recommended as it is possible for a peanut-derived product, especially expeller pressed or extruded or cold-pressed type, to trigger a life-threatening systemic anaphylactic response in a patient. People with a peanut allergy may also have cross-reactivity with soy. Soy oil is also not recommended due to its propensity to turn rancid due to rapid oxidative deterioration.

Glossary

Hyperthermia is elevated body temperature, i.e. fever due to failed thermoregulation when a body produces or absorbs more heat than it dissipates. Extreme temperature elevation is a medical emergency requiring immediate attention to avert disability or death.

Stratum corneum is the outermost epidermal layer of the skin, consisting of dead or keratinized cells (corneocytes) and is the major barrier to chemical transfer through the skin.

Vasodilation is the widening of blood vessels, more precisely the diameter of the interior vessel called the lumen, caused by relaxation of the muscular walls of the vessels resulting in a decrease of blood pressure.

References

1. Xie X, Wang F, Sun Z, Lo PL, Kong KC, Xie N. Petrological and mineralogical studies of the Sibin Bian-Stone, a material for making acupuncture tools in ancient China. In: Broekmans M (ed.) *Proceedings of the 10th International Congress for Applied Mineralogy (ICAM)*. Berlin, Heidelberg: Springer (2012).
2. Liu R, Wang M, Duan JA. Antipyretic and antioxidant activities of the aqueous extract of Cornu bubali (water buffalo horn). *Am. J. Chin. Med.* **38**(2): 293–306 (2010).
3. Wang YM, Gao JH, Lu B, Peng J, Bin F, Cui JJ, *et al.* Comparison of the effects of carbamyl-beta-methylcholine chloride administered by intravenous, intramuscular and intra-acupuncture point injections. *J. Tradit. Chin. Med.* **32**: 93–98 (2012).
4. Xu QY, Yang JS, Zhu B, Yang L, Wang YY, Gao XY. The effects of scraping therapy on local temperature and blood perfusion volume in healthy subjects. *Evid. Based Complement. Alternat. Med.* **2012**: Article ID 490292, 6 pages (2012).
5. Xu QY, Yang JS, Yang L, Wang YY. Effects of different scraping techniques on body surface blood perfusion volume and local skin temperature of healthy subjects. *J. Tradit. Chin. Med.* **31**(4): 316–320 (Dec 2011).
6. Hull W. Heat-enhanced transdermal drug delivery: a survey paper. *J. Appl. Res. Clin. Exp. Ther.* **2**(1): (Winter 2002).

TOPIC 26

Popular Herbs Used with Skin Lubricant to Enhance *Gua Sha*

It is not the intention of this book to share the process of extraction and concentration of herbal effective components for *Gua Sha* as there are many convenient options that one may avail oneself. One such option is the use of essential oils. Essential oils are mainly used in Aromatherapy and of late TCM has also developed its own line of herbal essential oils. Wheresoever the sources of such essential oils, it is important to note that the essential oils must be obtained from organic sources and not through chemical combination.

Gua Sha treatment provides an effective platform for transdermal drug delivery. Fundamentally, the choice of an herb(s) for treatment shall be based on matching therapeutic properties of the herb(s) to the diagnosis of the disorder. In addition, treatment efficacy could be further enhanced if the herbs(s) selected be affiliated with the meridian 归经 that courses through the treatment area.

Such precision treatment though preferable is often time made difficult in practice due to economic reasons. Most essential oils have to be diluted many folds before use and many being aromatic have expiry dates. Even for a professional outfit, unless it offers other treatment modalities that use essential oils heavily, it is not plausible to stock a wide repertoire of oils that closely target specific diagnosis.

A suggested alternative is to select an herbal essential oil that has a wide spectrum of usage, both in terms of meridian affiliation 归经 as well as therapeutic properties. Examples would be Red sage 丹参 for improving circulation, Gardenia 栀子 for febrile illnesses, Astragalus 黄芪 for wellness and White Angelica 白芷 for aesthetics. For carrier lubricant, one could opt for coconut oil or even Vicks Vaporub, the latter contains menthol, camphor and eucalyptus oil that come in handy for relief of influenza and body aches.

As mentioned earlier, it is not advisable to apply essential oils without dilution. Using essential oils neat or undiluted greatly increases the risk of sensitization that may appear as anything from a slight rash to contact dermatitis or even life-threatening anaphylaxis. The face, neck, and chest are the common places that manifest adverse reactions. Those with pre-existing conditions of auto-immunity (a disorder of adaptive immune system), auto-inflammation (genetic mutation of the innate immune system), allergies or chronic skin disorders shall only use essential oils of higher dilution ratio than the norm. A safer approach perhaps is to adopt dose escalation when the concentration of essential oil is gradually increased to avoid the occurrence of severe allergies.

As a rule of thumb, essential oils should be diluted to form a working blend as follows:

For every 1% increase in concentration, 1 drop of essential oil should be added to every 5ml or 1/6 oz of carrier lubricant.

An interpretation of this dilution guideline would be for a 3% dilution, 3 drops of essential oil are added to every 5ml or 1/6 oz of carrier lubricant. Similarly, for 10ml or 1/3 oz of carrier lubricant, 2 drops of essential oil shall be added to achieve a dilution of 1%.

Dilution factors shall also be used with caution. The appropriate concentration to be applied is indeed situational. Dilution factor normally used for the body has to be moderated for facial applications simply because the facial skin is much more sensitive. Similarly, if the application is intended for an extensive surface of the body, one may wish to increase the dilution to avoid transdermal drug overdose.

Botanical Name	Common Name		Meridian	AT	CM	Therapeutic Properties
Ocimum basilicum	Basil	罗勒	L, S, ST	*	*	Anti-inflammatory, promote circulation, dispel dampness, detoxicant
Commiphora myrrha	Myrrh	没药	H, LV, S	*	*	Anti-inflammatory, promote circulation, anti-embolism, analgesic
Boswellia sacra	Frankincense	乳香	H, LV, S	*	*	Anti-inflammatory, promote circulation, anti-embolism, analgesic, invigorate Qi
Gardenia jasminoides Ellis	Gardenia	栀子	H, LV, L, ST, TE	*	*	Anti-inflammatory, promote circulation, analgesic, anti-pyretic, dispel dampness
Hyssopus officinalis	Hyssop	藿香	L, S, ST	*	*	Dispel dampness, gastro-intestinal issues
Jasminum sambac F	Jasmine	茉莉花	LV, S, ST	*	*	Regulate qi, dispel dampness
Juniperus rigida S	Juniper	杜松	LI, K	*	*	Arteriosclerosis, dispel dampness, analgesic
Cymbopogon citratus	Lemon grass	香茅	L, ST	*	*	Anti-inflammatory, promote circulation, dispel dampness, analgesic
Matricaria chamomilla	Chamomile	黄春菊	L, H, ST	*	*	Anti-inflammatory, analgesic, anti-pyretic, sedative

(*Continued*)

(*Continued*)

Botanical Name	Common Name		Meridian	AT	CM	Therapeutic Properties
Rosae rugosae F	Rose	玫瑰花	LV, S	*	*	Regulate qi, promote circulation, analgesic
Cinnamomum cassia	Cinnamon	肉桂	H, LV, S, K	*	*	Promote circulation, invigorate Qi, analgesic, tonify Yang
Eugenia caryophyllata T	Clove	丁香	S, ST, K	*	*	Anti-inflammatory, tonify Yang
Angelica sinensis	Dong quai	当归	H, LV, S	*	*	Promote circulation, analgesic, tonify blood, laxative
Vitex agnus-castus	Vitex	蔓荆子	—	*		Estrogen progesterone equilibrant
Artemisia argyi	Mugwort	艾叶	LV, S, K	*	*	Anti-inflammatory, promote circulation, regulate qi
Lavandula angustifolia	Lavender	熏衣草	—	*		Anti-inflammatory
Helichrysum italicum	Immortelle	蜡菊	—	*		Anti-haematoma
Atractylodes lancea	Cang zhu	苍术	S, ST	*	*	Dispel dampness, anti-rheumatic, anti-aging, anti-oxidant

Ligusticum wallichii	Lovage root	川芎	LV, GB, PC		*	Promote circulation, analgesic, invigorate qi, vasodilator
Bergamot	Bergamot	佛手	L, LV, S, ST	*	*	Qi stagnation esp Liver, mucolytic, dispel dampness, regulate liver
Zingiber officinale R	Ginger	生姜	L, S, ST, H	*	*	Anti-inflammatory, anti-oxidant, promote circulation, invigorate qi
Rhodiola rosea L	Golden root	红景天	L, H	*	*	Promote circulation, anti-pyretic, regulate qi, detoxicant, adaptogen
Paeonia lacti flora	Chinese peony	白芍	L, S	*	*	Analgesic, tonify Yin
Angelica dahurica	White angelica	白芷	L, ST		*	Aesthetics use against melasma or acne, skin astringent, improve complexion
Astragalus membranaceus	Milkvetch	黄芪	S, L		*	Diuretic, elevate Yang, immuno-modulator, promote qi, anti-oxidant
Ganoderma lucidum	Reishi/ Lingzhi	灵芝	L, H, S		*	Immuno-modulator, anti-tumor, anti-platelet
Mentha haplocalyx B	Peppermint	薄荷	L, LV	*	*	Anti-pyretic, regulate liver, dispel liver stagnation
Eucommiae ulmoides C	Eucommia bark	杜仲	LV, K		*	Anti-hypertensive, regulate Qi, tonify LV, K, improve metabolism

(*Continued*)

(*Continued*)

Botanical Name	Common Name		Meridian	AT	CM	Therapeutic Properties
Bupleurum chinensis R	Thorowax	柴胡	LV, GB		*	Anti-pyretic, regulate liver, dispel liver stagnation, elevate Yang
Dryobalanops aromatica G	Borneo camphor	冰片	H, S, L		*	Anti-pyretic, analgesic
Corydalis remota Fisch	Yanhusuo	延胡索	H, LV, S		*	Promote circulation, invigorate Qi, analgesic
Paeonia suf fruticosa Andr	Peony root bark	牡丹皮	H, LV, K		*	Anti-pyretic, invigorate circulation, dispel blood stasis
Carthamus tinctorius	Safflower	红花	H, LV	*	*	Promote circulation, anti-embolism anti-pyretic, detoxicant
Salvia miltiorrhiza	Red Sage	丹参	H, LV	*	*	Anti-inflammatory, promote circulation, anti-embolism, anti-pyretic, sedative
Curcuma longa	Tumeric	姜黄	LV, S	*	*	Anti-inflammatory, promote circulation, invigorate qi, analgesic
Curcuma phaeocaulis Val	Curcuma	莪术	LV, S	*	*	Same as curcuma longa but more potent, anti-oxidant, anti-tumor

Notes: Meridian Key — L: Lung, LI: Large Intestine, ST: Stomach, S: Spleen, H: Heart, K: Kidney, PC: Pericardium, TE: Triple Energizer, LV: Liver, AT: available as Aromatherapy essential oils, CM: available as Chinese Medicine essential oils from internet traders.

TOPIC 27

Gua Sha Protocol in Practice

Gua Sha may be performed at various levels of sophistication and effectiveness which is limited only by the skill and competency of the operator. At the most basic level, cutaneous and meridian-tendon 经筋 scrapping are performed to give rapid relief to a patient. At a higher level of sophistication, selected acupoints may be scrapped and meridian dredged to provide a targeted remedy to specific disorders.

But *Gua Sha,* even in its most primitive form, is very effective as having unobstructed meridians is the hallmark of health. An acupoint is a specific juncture along a meridian and is analogous to a kink along a river where silt tends to accumulate when water flow slackened. In the same corollary, *sha* has a propensity to gather at acupoints along a meridian; with certain acupoints being more predisposed. In this regard, dredging a meridian has almost the same effect as scrapping selected acupoints located on the meridian; very similar to a 'shotgun versus rifle' approach. In fact, one would often observe *sha* concentration at various acupoints along a meridian after dredging it. For this reason, *Gua Sha* practitioners share the same cardinal treatment guideline as acupuncturists in that "miss an acupoint but never depart from its meridian 离穴不离经".

Acupoint scrapping has merit in the economy of operation. Instead of dredging a number of meridians to relief a specific ailment, a skilled operator could select and scrap the precise acupoint(s) across these meridians to address the disorder. Acupoint scrapping, however, requires accurate diagnosis of an ailment as pre-requisite. Acupoint scrapping and meridian dredging are not mutually exclusive treatment protocols.

The following are the recommended steps for the proper performance of *Gua Sha*:

Diagnosis — is the basis for appropriate *Gua Sha* treatment; in fact for any form of therapeutic treatment. Diagnosis may be to detect *sha* presence *per se* or identify the cause of a disorder. The presence of *sha* at the site of pain may be detected via test *Gua Sha* performed with a few press-strokes locally. Under normal conditions, no skin discoloration may appear but when *sha* is present, a few well-executed strokes over the site of pain will cause *sha* to surface and be vividly displayed.

Detection of *sha* alone may be an adequate diagnosis for simple complaints of common body aches but the determination of the cause of the disorder is mandatory for more complex symptoms. More importantly, the operator must ensure that the patient's condition is not contraindicated for *Gua Sha*.

From *Gua Sha* perspective, illnesses should at least be identified by attributes of cold 寒, heat 热, superficial 表, deep-seated 里, deficiency/debility 虚, and excess 实. In TCM, the general principles of treatment are warm the cold 寒者热之, cool the heat 热者寒之, expel the superficial 客者除之 and eliminate the deep-seated 留者攻之.[1] These principles are augmented by learnings from acupuncture advocating purge the excess 泻其有余, tonify to rectify deficiency 补其不足, moderate the deficiencies and excesses 调其虚实 to unblock the meridians 以通其道.[2]

Putting principles into practice, *Gua Sha* effectively provides detoxification strokes for purging excesses, tonification strokes for rectifying deficiencies and moderation strokes for rebalancing a hybrid situation of excess and deficiency (Refer Advanced Press-Stroke Variants In *Gua Sha*). Moderation press-stroke has an added advantage that it may be safely executed in the event of doubt in or lack of clarity during diagnosis.

An ailment being superficial or deep-seated is related to the pathogenesis of the disease and directly translates into the duration of a treatment session and length of the treatment course. By and large, a longer treatment session, and perhaps repeated treatment is necessary to address an ailment with the deep-seated issues. The texture and color of *sha* released during a treatment session provide a hint as to how deep-seated is the illness. The speed of the patient's recovery is another indication if a course of treatment is recommended.

Strictly speaking, Gua Sha as a technique does not address the hot or cold attribute of a disease. However, acupoint scrapping at judiciously selected acupoints and dredging meridians that course through these acupoints will. These acupoints normally rest on Yang meridians and some frequently used acupoints are GV16 风府, GV14 大椎, BL11 大杼, BL12 风门, GB20 风池 and EX-HN5 太阳. Moreover, herbal additives to the skin lubricant may also contribute to the alleviation of symptoms associated with hot or cold attributes of an ailment. Gardenia, Chamomile, Golden root, Peppermint, Thorowax, Peony root bark, and Red sage are herbs with antipyretic properties that will ease excess heat accumulated in the body. More of these herbs are listed in a table under an earlier topic.

Information Exchange — *Gua Sha* treatment, regardless of how light-handed it was executed, would doubtlessly leave a series of markings on a patient's body. In some advanced countries that are less informed about this treatment protocol, *Gua Sha* markings are associated with physical abuse. Do not assume that the patient has agreed to the therapy even when the service is offered *pro bono* to an acquaintance. One cannot expect how the sequence of post-therapy events may act out that could prejudice the operator.

It is always prudent to provide an informative and brief explanation of the *Gua Sha* process to the patient prior to obtaining informed consent. The explanation should include possible reactions during and after the therapy, emphasizing on the appearance of transient skin discoloration that may be socially objectionable to the patient. The consent may not necessarily be in writing. The operator is protected so long as there is a positive intimation from the patient to proceed with the therapy.

The practitioner when seeking informed consent from the patient should attempt to probe for pre-existing medical conditions, drug history, and allergies and reactions. Such disclosures would allow the practitioner to assess if the patient is a suitable candidate for *Gua Sha* and the use of herbal additive(s) contemplated. Perhaps the practitioner should use this opportunity to observe other characteristics of the patient like physique, age, state of mind in order to moderate his treatment protocol.

Setting — patient privacy is foremost in the list of considerations when it comes to making a choice for a location where the therapy is to be delivered. To some extent, the intended treatment site(s) of the patient will be exposed and nothing short of an enclosed area is therefore appropriate. The enclosed space shall preferably be tranquil, well ventilated and adequately lighted to give the patient a sense of calmness and relaxation. Lighting is also important for the operator to ascertain if a consistent *sha* texture and density have been achieved for a treatment spot before moving on to the next. If mechanical ventilation supplied with the enclosed space cannot be adjusted to a comfortable level, the patient shall be position away from the direct draft of ventilation to avoid rapid loss of body heat.

Depending on the location of the treatment site(s), *Gua Sha* may be performed on a patient either seated or lying down. Furniture available at the setting may not be a 'show-stopper' but is important enough to affect the quality of service delivery. Be mindful that *Gua Sha* protocol is a continuous, steady and rhythmic *sha* extraction process and any interruption resulting from a major postural change of the patient or operator may yield less than desirable results. Sitting or lying down a patient on a cold hard floor is not recommended unless for no better alternative. And even under such a situation, one should at least attempt to insulate the loss of body heat through patient contact with the bare flooring.

Equipment — *Gua Sha* may be performed with or without the use of an instrument. Bare hand *Gua Sha* though when executed correctly is as effective as when performed with an instrument, it is, however, less elegant and more painful. It should, therefore, be deployed only when there is absolutely no scope for equipment improvisation.

Always disinfect Gua Sha instruments and clean the intended treatment site before treatment to prevent infection or cross-contamination. The hands of the operator shall also be duly disinfected before making contact with the patient for the same reason.

Whilst the specifications for *Gua Sha* equipment is not demanding and any hand-held implement with a smooth rounded contact edge and a comfortable grip suffice, the instrument must be capable of being disinfected. Having said that, the same standard of disinfection should also apply without exemption to specialized *Gua Sha* implements before being used on a patient.

By disinfection, this section refers to the decontamination of equipment for non-invasive *Gua Sha*. Because the equipment is to be applied onto intact skin, and by virtue of the treatment process would not cause any visible lacerations, the standard for equipment disinfection is less stringent than sterilization. The simplest way is to wash the instrument with soap and running water for a minute, drying the instrument with a clean disposable towel before applying it immediately on a patient. Another option is to wash the equipment in the normal way, dry it with a clean disposable towel and wipe the instrument with a cotton ball soaked with 75% ethyl alcohol prior to using it.

Skin Lubricant — the choice of skin lubricant has been extensively discussed in an earlier topic. Save for the head (hair) portion, never perform *Gua Sha* on bare dry skin. The treatment area, however, should not be damp and any perspiration should be duly removed before applying a skin lubricant.

Skin lubricant serves two major functions — dermal protection and as a carrier of transdermal medication. The level of dermal protection against physical abuse offered by a skin lubricant is correlated to the lubricant's viscosity. Higher viscosity, however, means higher cohesive force between lubricant's molecules, making the lubricant less desirable as a carrier for transdermal medication. Higher viscosity lubricants facilitate heavy and slow press-strokes as well as acupoint *Gua Sha* where greater stroke control is desired.

Whilst there are relative pros and cons in the use of high viscosity lubricants, be mindful that high viscosity means these lubricants cannot be pumped out of a container in the way lighter lubricants may. High viscosity lubricants can, therefore, be kept in wide throat containers only. In a clinical setting where patient hygiene is paramount, the practitioner should cultivate the habit of not double-dipping into the jar to minimize contamination.

The practitioner should not discount the possibility of a patient being allergic to the skin lubricant or the combined carrier lubricant and medicinal additives and take necessary precaution to prevent it. The use of peanut or soy-derived products as skin lubricant should always be avoided.

Treatment — it is always prudent to carefully note and confirm presenting symptoms with the patient prior to treatment. Where pain and movement restriction exist, the practitioner should test the range of movement for the patient to note for comparison with the increase in movement range and comfort level post-treatment. The intended treatment site(s) should also be examined for lacerations, lumps, inflammation, varicose veins and any anomaly so that appropriate measures may be taken.

Even without contraindications, the patient must nevertheless arrive in a qualified state before treatment. No therapy should be rendered to anyone immediately after a heavy meal or in a state of severe hunger. There should be a lapse of at least 30 minutes between mealtime and commencement of treatment. No therapy should also be rendered to anyone in a state of extreme exhaustion (applies to heat stroke as well).

Unless the patient is very ill, the practitioner should maintain an open dialogue or some form of communication with the patient throughout the treatment session and noting any cue of discomfort arising from the posture of the patient during treatment or the application of excessive force during press-stroke. Having a dialogue during treatment also put the patient at ease to facilitate therapy as well as provides early warning to the operator before an adverse reaction occurs.

From the diagnosis of the patient's disorder, the practitioner should map out the meridian(s) to be dredged and the acupoints to be scrapped prior to commencement of the treatment. The operator should also be completely familiar with the technicalities regarding the therapy which are described in

"Press-Stroke Fundamentals" under the topic "Techniques for *Sha* Extraction".

As far as feasible, the treatment area should be well lubricated before delivering press-stroke. Not more than 20 uninterrupted press-strokes should be applied to a specific spot within the lubricated treatment site before a consistent *sha* texture and skin coloration surfaced. Once achieved, move on to the adjacent spot within the treatment area and repeat the protocol.

Always begin press-stroke for each spot gently before gradually increasing the intensity of force for subsequent strokes to a point of slight discomfort but within pain threshold of the patient. Stroke lengths should be extended as far as the anatomy permits and what pragmatism allows. This pressure should then be held constant until *sha* appears. Be mindful that on no account shall the skin surface be broken during or after *Gua Sha* treatment.

As a general caveat, apply less forceful press-strokes during treatment at Yin regions of the body.

The practitioner should be mindful to maintain between the treatment surface and the *Gua Sha* tool an angle of fewer than 90 degrees when manipulating with the instrument. Applying drag force before the point of contact would prevent the undesirable "bobbing" when the instrument moved over an uneven surface. For a seasoned practitioner, strength should be derived from the coordinated action of sinking the shoulder 沉肩, relaxing the elbow 垂肘, rotating the wrist 运腕 and conducting the focussed energy to the fingers 透指 grasping the instrument. By focussing motion at the wrist and beyond, the force so transmitted would be continuous yet supple 持续而柔, light yet firm 轻而不浮, weighty yet not stagnated 重而不滞 and penetrating as well as telling 渗透有知. "Telling" means that the patient would respond with a feeling of distention 胀 and soreness 酸 with slight pain 痛 at the treatment area.

Do not force the situation when no skin discoloration or *sha* appears after about 20 strokes. There will be occasions where *sha* appeared after a treated spot is abandoned. The operator should proceed to the adjacent spot at the treatment area and continue with the protocol.

Gua Sha therapy, when appropriately delivered, provides major relief to the presenting symptoms of the patient. The entire therapy session should not exceed 20 minutes. Any session longer than 30 minutes hour may be more harmful than beneficial.

Post-Treatment — A logical and obvious post-treatment procedure is reinstatement, which means lightly cleaning off the remaining lubricant from the treatment area(s) with a clean disposable paper towel to avoid staining the apparel of the patient.

The last thing a practitioner wants is to invite negative impressions of the therapy that require immense corrective effort or damage control. It is therefore imperative to visually show the patient the extent and magnitude of skin discoloration to reinforce the pre-treatment message that these are not traumatic bruises but normal *sha* markings that fade within days. In so doing, the patient will be not surprised by the appearance of skin discoloration when he subsequently discovers the same in privacy.

The patient should also be rested for about 10 minutes after treatment. During this stabilization period, the patient should be offered a room-temperature drink, preferably plain water, to replenish lost fluids and facilitate the flushing of toxin in the body when an obstruction in the flow of Qi is removed. The patient should also be advised to cover up the treatment area(s) from exposure to draft and to avoid shower at least an hour after treatment.

The patient should be advised that, for the same treatment area(s), the therapy should not be repeated until the skin coloration or *sha* markings have completely faded. For situations where no *sha* markings are manifested, a lapse of three days should still be imposed before *Gua Sha* be attempted again. In the event the situation merits another round of treatment before earlier markings have faded, the practitioner shall select a fresh area adjacent to the unfaded markings or previously unexplored acupoints along the same meridian.

References

1. *Huang Di's Internal Classic*, Suwen (Plain Questions), Chapter 74.
2. *Huang Di's Internal Classic*, Lingshu (Miraculous Pivot), Chapter 71.

TOPIC 28

Contra Indications for *Gua Sha* Therapy

Gua Sha, from a TCM perspective, has therapeutic effects of invigorating circulation and dissipating blood stasis, regulating organ functions, relaxing musculature and evacuating toxins.

Modern science has validated similarly that *Gua Sha* therapy significantly increases both blood flow perfusion and skin temperature that effectively regulate sympathetic vasodilation and promote local blood circulation. It could also up-regulate the innate and adaptive immune functions especially T lymphocytes and macrophages. Its ability to induce more Th1-biased antibody subtype also facilitate the modulation of T-helper in promoting a healthy Th1/Th2 balance. Finally, the therapy ameliorates oxidative stress by up-regulating heat shock protein Heme oxygenase-1 (HO-1) gene expression.

Gua Sha, with its profound and wide-ranging effects, however, may not be an appropriate therapeutic application under some circumstances. The following situations are deemed to be contraindicated:

a. During pregnancy — avoid abdominal, pelvic and nipple areas
b. Menstruation — no heavy strokes for abdominal and pelvic areas
c. Bleeding tendencies — Haemophiliac diseases (lacking in clotting factors), thrombocytopenia (lacking in platelets), aplastic anemia, etc
d. Installed implants — pacemaker or internal defibrillator

e. Critical hepatic disorders — cirrhosis, ascites, and severe peripheral edema
f. Diabetes with healing issues
g. Reduced renal function — severe renal insufficiency, fluid retention, and patients undergoing hemodialysis or continuous ambulatory peritoneal dialysis
h. Acute injury of connective tissue and tendons, fractures and surgical suture sites — may only be administered after full recovery
i. Under alcoholic or drug intoxication
j. Malnutrition state, extremely weak or advanced age
k. Contagious diseases
l. Abdominal pain of unknown origin
m. Ailments relating to sensitive or mucosal areas — avoid eyes, lips, tongue, naval, moles, genitals and nipples

For the following ailments, caution to be exercised during treatment even after the acute phase:

a. Cardiac arrhythmias (chronotropic incompetence, bradycardia, tachycardia, abnormal electrocardiogram), obstructive cardiac diseases (aortic stenosis, mitral stenosis, pulmonary embolus, hypertrophic cardiomyopathy, ventricular dysfunction), angina
b. Cerebrovascular accident (CVA), seizures and/or epilepsy, severe anxiety attack
c. Auto-immune diseases

Simply put, *Gua Sha* therapy is not for everyone.

Glossary

Chronotropic incompetence is broadly defined as the inability of the heart to increase its rate commensurate with increased activity or demand. Common among patients with cardiovascular disease, it causes exercise intolerance that impairs quality-of-life and thus an independent predictor of major adverse cardiovascular events and overall mortality.

Topic 29

Recovery Actions for Exceptional Situations During Treatment

Although *Gua Sha* treatment is generally very safe, some patients may react adversely during or after treatment. These exceptional situations are seldom life-threatening and can be effortlessly overcome if timely and appropriate recovery measures were administered to the patient.

In clinical settings, exceptional situations manifest themselves as giddiness, vertigo, palpitation, sudden excessive perspiration, pallor, weakness, paresthesia (tingling/numbness sensation at extremities), nausea and possibly fainting.

Fainting or syncope, a fairly common event, is the transient loss of consciousness caused by a temporary reduction in blood flow to the brain. The brain's blood supply can be interrupted for a number of reasons and may either be cardiac-related or non-cardiac related; with virtually all potentially life-threatening kinds of syncope in the cardiac-related category.

Cardiac-related syncope may be easily avoided if a general evaluation was carefully made prior to treatment to eliminate candidates with contra-indication of cardiac arrhythmias and obstructive cardiac diseases. Once such screening is performed, the operator can reasonably be assured that whatever happened subsequently, it is unlikely to be an imminent life-threatening situation.

Neurological, metabolic and vasomotor conditions are among the non-cardiac related causes of syncope.

Neurological conditions, though have serious consequences, are infrequent and account for less than 1% of syncopal episodes. Transient Ischemic Attack, Subclavian Steal Syndrome, Normal Pressure Hydrocephalus and Epileptic Seizures are some neurological conditions. These conditions are also contra-indicated and caution be exercised if *Gua Sha* is to be performed.

Transient Ischemic Attack (TIAs) is caused by blood flow blockage in the vertebrobasilar arteries responsible for supply to the brainstem, the part of the brain responsible for maintaining consciousness.

Subclavian Steal Syndrome (SSS), a more severe disorder than typical vertebrobasilar insufficiency, arises from retrograde (reversed) blood flow in the vertebral artery or the internal thoracic artery resulting in deprivation of blood supply to the brain. This is caused by proximal stenosis (narrowing) and/or occlusion of the subclavian artery.

Normal Pressure Hydrocephalus (NPH), more common among the elderly, is an abnormal build-up of cerebrospinal fluid (CSF) in the brain's ventricles or cavities when the normal flow of CSF throughout the brain and spinal cord is obstructed, causing the ventricles to expand and put pressure on the brain.

Epileptic seizures are often confused with neurological conditions due to the common manifestation of temporary loss of consciousness. However, an obvious differential diagnosis would be the typical involuntary movements usually accompanying a seizure.

Metabolic causes of syncope include hypoxia (reduced oxygen level in the blood usually relating to lung or heart disease), hyperventilation accompanying severe anxiety reactions or panic attacks and severe hypoglycemia (low blood sugar) associated with diabetes.

Vasomotor syncope, though comprising the majority of fainting incidents and yet be managed safely, occurs in two forms, vasovagal syncope, and orthostatic hypotension.

Vasovagal syncope, caused by a temporary glitch in the autonomic nervous system that regulates heart rate and blood pressure, accounts for more than 80% of all syncopal episodes. The onset of an external trigger could temporarily disrupt the autonomic nervous system resulting in a fall in blood pressure and diminished blood supply to the brain. The trigger may be an unpleasant sight, sudden pain, objectionable smell, etc; all could be defused by pre-conditioning the first-time patient via succinct briefing and visual introduction of equipment before treatment.

In people with orthostatic hypotension, normal blood pressure cannot be maintained when there is an abrupt postural change; usually immediately after standing up from a prone or supine position. If blood pressure fell beyond acceptable tolerance (>20mm Hg systole >10mmHg diastole), one may lose consciousness while attempting to maintain an upright posture. Orthostatic hypotension is often seen in older people and is commonly caused by prescription drugs. Other possible triggers include dehydration, diabetes and neurological conditions such as Parkinson's disease.

A related condition, prone to people below the age of 45, is postural orthostatic tachycardia syndrome (POTS). While POTS also produce low blood pressure, this is caused by an extremely rapid heart rate upon standing.

Appropriate clinical settings and choice of patient's posture during treatment are countermeasures against vasomotor syncope.

The following is a recommended recovery protocol in the event of syncope:

a. Stop *Gua Sha* treatment immediately.
b. Assist or ease the patient into a supine position.
c. Do not adopt a modified Trendelenburg position or Passive Leg Elevation (PLE) where the body is left supine but with feet raised above head level.[1,2]
d. If the patient is unconscious or non-responsive, tap face briskly to revive the person.
e. If the patient is vomiting, turn face to the side to avoid choking on the vomitus.
f. If the patient is not breathing, apply CPR and immediately switch to prescribed CPR protocol until breathing and consciousness are restored.

g. When dizziness has abated, offer a room-temperature isotonic drink to the patient.
h. If dizziness persists, massage acupoint GV20 百会, GV26 水沟, PC6 内关, ST36 足三里, KI1 涌泉 and CV6 气海 selectively or in any combination.
i. Instruct the patient to rest quietly for 20 mins after he comes around. Stay with the patient until the condition is stabilized to prevent possible falls.

Syncope, in most cases, is a transient condition with little long-term repercussions. Notwithstanding, it may also be indicative of a serious or even life-threatening underlying medical condition that has yet to present itself. It is therefore mandatory to advise the patient to consult his regular physician at the earliest opportune time.

Glossary

Trendelenburg position became common practice in various healthcare settings such as emergency rooms, operating theatres, post-anesthesia care units, and critical care units. The controversy surrounding its use in hypotensive situations lies in whether blood moving from the extremities to the central part of the body contributes to hemodynamic stability and whether there are adverse effects that outweigh benefits. Potential harmful effects include increased intracranial pressure, decreased lung expansion/lung volumes caused by upward diaphragmatic push, baroreceptor effects promoting a false sense of blood flow improvement leading to vasodilation and a decreased response to the hypotensive state.

The American Heart Association (AHA) and the American Red Cross in a 2010 revised consensus document for first aid treatment reported the use of Trendelenburg position in patients with shock lacks sufficient evidence and is unable to make a recommendation.[3]

The National Association of Emergency Medical Technicians (NAEMT) and the American College of Surgeons in their Prehospital Trauma Life Support Manual recommend using the supine position for the management of patients with shock, explicitly discouraging Trendelenburg position or its variants.[4]

References

1. Bridges N, Jarquin-Valdivia AA. Use of the Trendelenburg position as the resuscitation position: to T or not to T? *Am. J. Crit. Care* **14**(5): 364–368 (2005).

2. Ballesteros Peña S, Larrad AR. Does the Trendelenburg position affect hemodynamics? A systematic review. *Emergencias* **24**: 143–150 (2012).
3. Markenson D, Ferguson JD, *et al.* First Aid: 2010 American Heart Association and American Red Cross Guidelines for First Aid. *Circulation* **122**: S934–S946 (2010).
4. Prehospital Trauma Life Support Committee of the National Association of Emergency Medical Technicians in collaboration with the Committee on Trauma of the American College of Surgeons. *PHTLS: Prehospital Trauma Life Support, 6th ed.* Mosby (2008).

Topic 30

Meridian Principles Underlying the *Gua Sha* Therapy

Gua Sha is a TCM external intervention technique that, because of its simplicity in application, became a popular ancient folk remedy. It can, however, be practiced at various levels of sophistication, all which delivers effective and rapid therapeutic relief to a wide range of contemporary ailments.

At its most fundamental level, *Gua Sha* is performed at the cutaneous and meridian-tendon 经筋 regions. By adhering to some simple yet intuitive rules, the layperson with some mastery of instrument manipulation can safely provide treatment with predictable and favorable outcomes.

At the intermediate level, meridian dredging becomes an essential module of *Gua Sha* therapy. Things get a little more complex as the operator is required to understand the distribution of meridians, their flow direction and the time of the day when the meridians ebb and flow.

Delivering *Gua Sha* at an advanced level requires the practitioner to master the knowledge of both meridians and acupoints.

Before exploring the topic of frequently used areas for *Gua Sha* therapy, it is beneficial to present some important aspects of meridians.

a. Meridian-Tendon Assembly 经筋 — These are muscle-tendon-fascia organized around the 12 principal meridians forming a structure of its own. They exist along the surface of muscles and tendons, running from joint to joints. Though they are specifically associated with and generally mirror the pathway of principal meridians, they are however not physically connected to any internal organ due to their superficial nature. Like their principal meridians, the Yang meridian-tendons are distributed on the dorsal aspect of the surface anatomy whilst the Yin meridian-tendons are concentrated on the ventral surface of the body. Being part of the body's musculature and thus a site of energy expenditure, the meridian-tendon assembly is nourished by their principal meridians and also provides biofeedback to the internal organs via the principal meridians.
b. Flow and General Connection — The Yin meridians of the Hand originate from the chest and terminate at the hand where they connect with the Yang meridians of the Hand. From the hand, the Yang meridians of the Hand ascend to the Head where they connect with the Yang meridians of the Foot. From the head, the Yang meridians of the Foot descend towards and terminate at the foot where they connect with the Yin meridians of the Foot. At the foot, the Yin meridians of the Foot, ascend and terminate at the chest. In this regard, all Yang meridians converge at the head and all Yin meridians meet at the chest.

Similarly, the Conception Vessel forms a circular entity with the Governor Vessel.

The table below summarises the general direction of flow of the 12 meridians. It would be helpful for the operator to commit to memory the general flow direction of meridian types as these have profound implications for tonification/detoxification press-strokes in *Gua Sha* therapy.

Meridian Type	Direction of Flow
Yin meridians of Hand	Chest to Hand
Yang Meridians of Hand	Hand to Head
Yang Meridians of Foot	Head to Foot
Yin meridians of Foot	Foot to Chest

c. Pairing and Specific Connection — Meridians connect internal organs and are pathways that Qi travels along to nourish the organs and allow communication among these organs. Meridians are paired on the premise of organ-systems as well as their Yin-Yang relationship. Recalling that the Yin-Yang relationship was based on the relative intensity of solar exposure discussed in "How are Meridians Named and Distributed in the Human Body", one can observe the following relationships from the table below:

   i. The flow order depicts the sequence of connection of individual meridians commencing from the Lung Meridian and ending at the Liver Meridian.
   ii. In terms of surface anatomy, the continuous flow serves three distinct sectors in the order of anterior, posterior and the intermediate area. Within each area, four meridians course longitudinally from top to bottom, starting and ending with Yin meridian with the same qualifier. The connecting Yang meridians within each sector also bear the same qualifiers.

Limb	Qualifier	Organ System	Solar Exposure	Location on Limb	Flow Order	Timing
Hand	Tai Yin	Lung	Least Exposed	Antero-Medial Surface	1	3 - 5am
Hand	Yang Ming	Large Intestine	Least Exposed	Antero-Lateral Surface	2	5 - 7am
Foot	Yang Ming	Stomach	Least Exposed	Antero-Lateral Surface	3	7 - 9am
Foot	Tai Yin	Spleen	Least Exposed	Antero-Medial Surface	4	9 - 11am
Hand	Shao Yin	Heart	Most Exposed	Postero-Medial Surface	5	11 - 1pm
Hand	Tai Yang	Small Intestine	Most Exposed	Postero-Lateral Surface	6	1 - 3pm
Foot	Tai Yang	Bladder	Most Exposed	Postero-Lateral Surface	7	3 - 5pm
Foot	Shao Yin	Kidney	Most Exposed	Postero-Medial Surface	8	5 - 7pm
Hand	Jeu Yin	Pericardium	Moderately Exposed	Medial Surface	9	7 - 9pm
Hand	Shao Yang	Triple Energizer	Moderately Exposed	Lateral Surface	10	9 - 11pm
Foot	Shao Yang	Gall Bladder	Moderately Exposed	Lateral Surface	11	11 - 1am
Foot	Jeu Yin	Liver	Moderately Exposed	Medial Surface	12	1 - 3am

d. Timing of Qi Flow — Qi, within the unbroken meridian circuit, flows uninterrupted in a 24-hour cycle commencing at the Lung Meridian for a two-hour duration before reaching the Large Intestine Meridian. This Qi movement shall then transit to the subsequent meridians until it completes its journey at the Liver

Meridian before restarting the entire cycle again. All said, the flow of Qi across the 12 meridians over 24 hours divided the circadian clock into 12 meridian time zones.

It is cogent to note that pain arises when the flow of Qi is impeded 不通则痛 痛则不通 and thus pain occurring at a consistent and predictable timing of the day is indicative of some obstruction along the part of the meridian during which the Qi is either due to arrive, in-transit or about to depart. As a rule of thumb, if the pain occurred predictably at the earlier hour of the meridian time zone, it is appropriate to treat the meridian associated with that time zone as well as the meridian of the preceding time zone. As an example, if the pain occurred consistently between 3 pm and 4 pm daily, it would be prudent to treat both the Small Intestine Meridian and the Bladder Meridian as the pain could be caused by either a tapering flow of Qi along the Small Intestine Meridian or an obstruction in the Bladder Meridian that impeded Qi arriving from the Small Intestine Meridian. Similarly, a pain between 4 pm and 5 pm should receive treatment for both the Bladder Meridian and the Kidney Meridian.

TOPIC 31

Frequently Used Areas/ Patterns for *Gua Sha* Therapy

Frequently used regions for *Gua Sha* therapy generally refer to the Cutaneous regions and Meridian-Tendon Assembly. These are targeted regions for fundamental level treatment that require adherence to fewer operating rules. By and large, so long as the operator performs the protocol from top to bottom, left to right and medial to lateral, all will be good.

The operator should be mindful that Cutaneous *Gua Sha* and Meridian-Tendon Assembly *Gua Sha* are not mutually exclusive to Acupoint Gua Sha but often time used in conjunction with one another to reinforce the therapeutic effect.

In the following text, the word "Dredge" is reserved exclusively for meridian referenced locations.

<u>Head Region</u>

TCM regards the head as "the confluence of the Yang 诸阳之会" which implies it is a site for regulating all six Yang Meridians as well as the Governor Vessel. The brain is also termed "the sea of marrow 髓海" which is derived from kidney essence and nourished by food nutrients. The brain is also held to be "the dwelling of the *Shen* or Lucid Soul 元神之府" which means the head is closely connected with other parts of the body, and all the organs are responsible for nourishing it.

The head connects with the internal organs through the meridians and collaterals. GV20 百会 located at the head's vertex, is the crossroad for Governor Vessel, Bladder Meridian, Gall Bladder Meridian, Triple Energizer Meridian, and the Liver Meridian. The head also has orifices that communicate with the external environment directly. When external and/or internal factors impede the flow of Qi in meridians, disturb nutrient supply to the head and obstruct orifices in the head, disorder occurs.

Patient posture — Seated upright and relaxed

Execution — Moderation press-stroke, avoid skin lubrication, head immobilization at the occipital region, observation of *sha* appearance not mandatory.

1. Four Spirit Extension

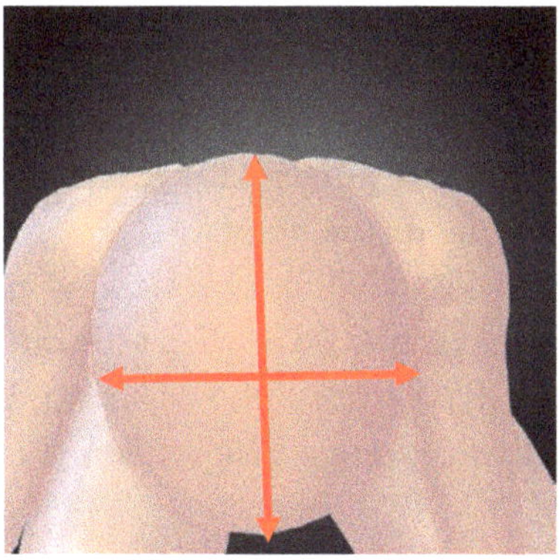

Press-stroke outwards from GV20 百会 in the direction of every point in EX-HN1 四神聪. GV20 rests on the midsagittal or medial line, at the intersection of the line connecting the right and left ear apices. Forward stroke towards the anterior hairline, backward stroke to the occipital protuberance, left and right outward strokes to reach the tip of the ears.

Indicated for insomnia, tension headache, hypertension, post cerebrovascular accident conditions, seizure, neurological developmental delay, dizziness, memory improvement.

2. Trident Comb

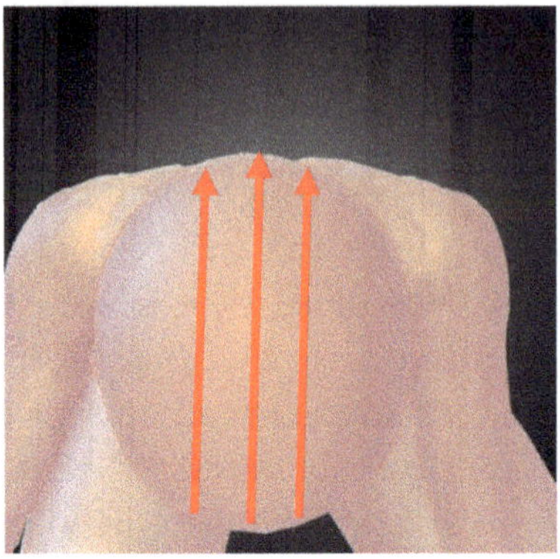

Press-stroke from anterior hairline to the occipital bone, the medial line passes through GV20 百会. The two lateral stroke paths should be two finger width from the medial line in alignment with the Bladder Meridian.

Indicated for neurosis, tension headache, dizziness, memory improvement.

3. Lesser Yang Plough

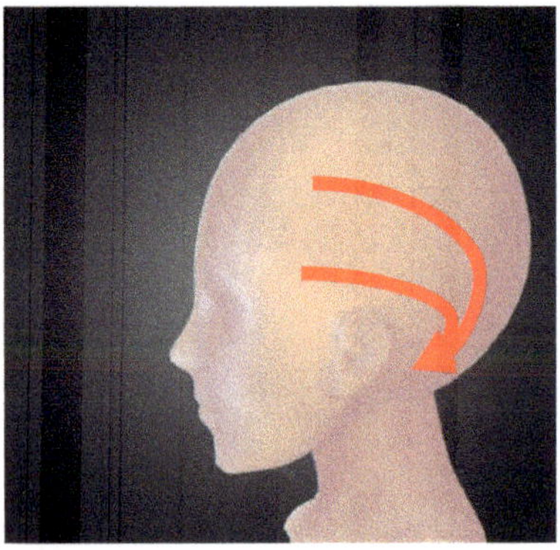

The top stroke pathway commences from ST8 頭維, passes the midpoint between GV20 百会 and the apex of the ear and arch downwards to GB20 风池. ST8 is located at the corner of the forehead and a finger width posterior to the anterior hairline. GB20 is located at the depression created between the origins of the Sternocleidomastoid and Trapezius muscles, at the junction of the occipital and nuchal regions, posterior head.

The bottom stroke commences from EX-HN5 太阳 following a curved pathway over the ear, passing through GB8 率谷 and arch downwards to meet the top stroke at GB20 风池. GB8 is located superior to the apex of the auricle and two-finger width within the hairline.

Indicated for migraine headache, nervous tension, dizziness, trigeminal neuralgia, palsy, hearing loss, motion sickness.

4. Occipital-Cervical Sweep Lines

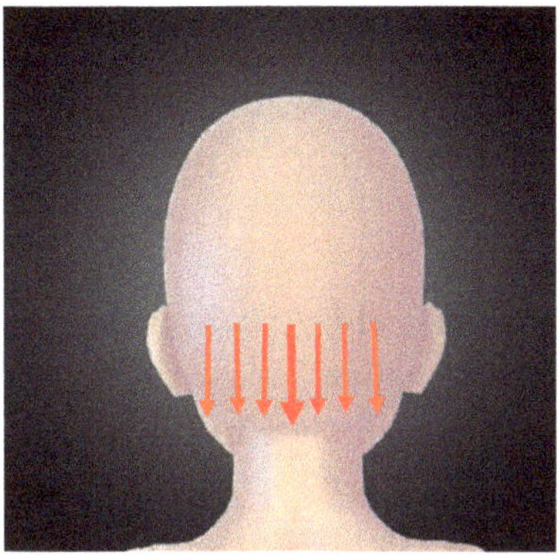

The principal line of Occipital-Cervical Sweep Lines extends medially from occipital protuberance GV17 脑户 to GV15 哑门. Secondary lines run bilaterally to cover the entire sub-occipital musculature region, particularly to include GB20 风池.

GV15 is located below the spinous process of the first cervical vertebra (C1). GV17 is located at the posterior head and two-finger width directly above the external occipital protuberance.

Indicated for hypertension, post cerebrovascular accident conditions, post-concussion issues, sensorineural hearing loss, post-nasal drip, neurosis, incontinence.

<u>Dorsal Region</u>

This is the most commonly used region in *Gua Sha.*

The Dorsal Region is traversed by two Yang meridians, namely the Governor Vessel (GV) and the Bladder (BL) Meridian. The GV "regulates" the Yang meridians such that active Defensive Qi can be raised and mobilized via the Yang meridians in the body. The GV may also be manipulated to address conditions involving the spine and/or brain or relieve tension and pain along this pathway. As the longest and most complex meridian, the BL meridian serves extensively the dorsal region of the body.

Comprehensive *Gua Sha* for the Dorsal Region is often done in the order of Shoulder Sweep, Governor Vessel Dredge, Para-Vertebral Dredge, Upper Bladder Meridian Dredge, Trapezius Sweep and, when necessary, the Sacral V Dredge and Iliac Contour Sweep Lines. As these regions are Yang aspects of the body, the effectiveness of treatment is evidenced by the appearance of *sha* discoloration.

Patient posture — Seated upright and relaxed or preferably prone position

Execution — Press-stroke type selection based on diagnosis, skin lubrication mandatory, observation of *sha* discoloration preferable.

1. Governor Vessel Dredge Line

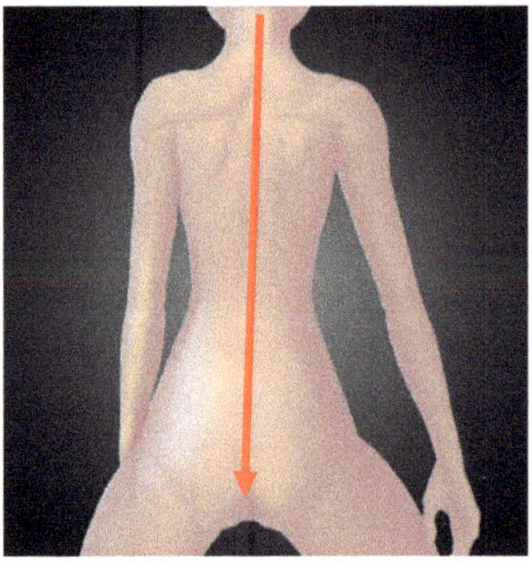

Single press-stroke pathway medially on the spine from C1 to S5 passing through all acupoints lying along the Governor Vessel from base of the skull to sacral hiatus. Less forceful press-strokes when traversing over the spine.

Indicated for muscular spasm of the back, fever, influenza, heat stroke, fatigue and a wide range of illnesses as follows:

C1-C4 — head and face
C1-C7 — neck
C3-T7 — upper limbs
T1-T7 — heart, lungs
T8-L2 — stomach, liver, gall bladder, "spleen"
T10-L5 — lumbar
L2-S2 — lower limbs
L3-S4 — intestinal, kidney, urological, reproductive

Notes on the Spinal Column Surface Anatomy

The human spinal column consists of 33 vertebrae divided into 3 segments: presacral, sacrum and coccyx.

Presacral — 7 cervical (C1-C7), 12 thoracic (T1-T12) and 5 lumbar (L1-L5) totaling 24 vertebrae

Sacrum — 5 fused sacral (S1-S5)
Coccyx — 4 fused vertebrae (unreferenced)

The presacral vertebrae allow both rotational and torsional movements rendering the vertebral column flexible.

The 7 cervical vertebrae form the neck with C1 supporting the skull.

The 12 thoracic vertebrae each support a pair of ribs, with the first 10 (T1-T10) being part of the rib cage. T11 and T12 support floating or free ribs.

The spinous processes of the spinal column are palpable in the median furrow of the back. The spinous process is a long slender and sloping bony projection from the vertebra to the opposite of the vertebra below. The spinous process of C6, C7, and T1 are very prominent and may be made more conspicuous by the forward flexion of the neck. In the thoracic region, the spinous process of each vertebra extends to the level of at least the body of the vertebra below. The inferior angle of the scapula is frequently at the level of the spinous process of T7. A horizontal plane between the highest points of the iliac crests is usually at the level of the spinous process of L4.

2. Para-Vertebral Dredge Lines

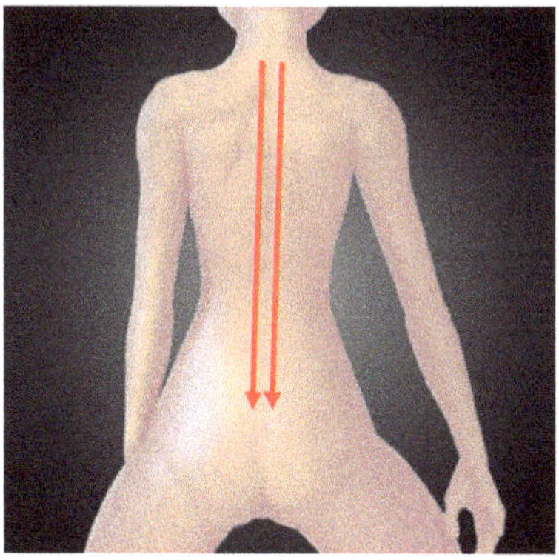

Para-Vertebral Dredge lines overlay the EX-B2 夹脊 acupoints. There are 34 acupoints in total with 17 on each side situated laterally to the lower border of the spinous processes of T1 to L5 and one-finger width from the medial line. These dredge lines may also be extended superiorly to include both splenius capitis muscles of the neck from C1 to C7.

Indicated for quick relief for spine-related ailments.

3. Superior Bladder Meridian Dredge Lines

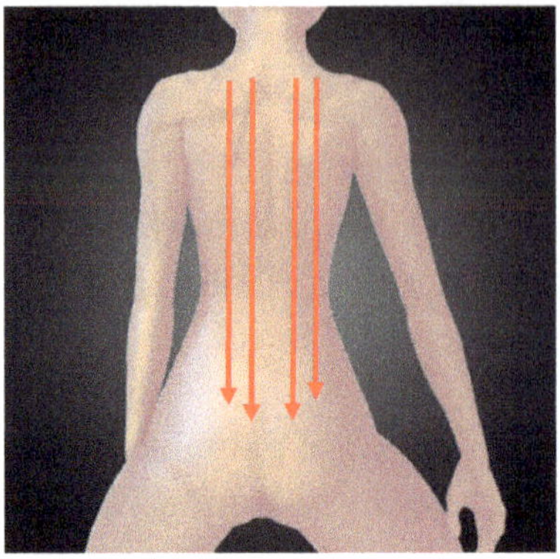

As the longest meridian, the Bladder Meridian courses from head to heels. This book identifies the Superior Bladder Meridian Dredge Lines with pathways two-finger and four-finger widths laterally parallel to each side of the spine from T1 to L5.

Indicated for the treatment of a wide array of illnesses similar to those treated by the Governor Vessel Dredge. For this reason, the Governor Vessel Dredge is often time performed prior to the Superior Bladder Meridian Dredge and Para-Vertebral Dredge.

Generally, the treatment is performed from top to bottom, medial to lateral, left to right.

4. Shoulder Sweep Lines

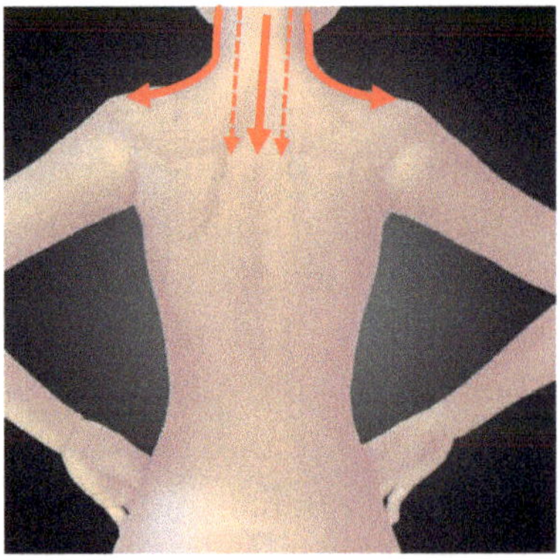

The central sweep line runs medially from the occipital bone to T3. The adjacent sweep lines, originating from GB20 风池, run along the shoulders to pass GB21 肩井 and terminate at LI15 肩髃.

GB21 is located midway between the spinous process of C7 and the acromion process, at the highest point of the trapezius muscle. LI15 is located anterior and inferior to the acromion, on the upper portion of the deltoid muscle, in a depression formed when the arm is in full abduction.

The splenius capitis muscles of the neck may also be scrapped if necessary (broken line arrows).

Indicated for neck muscle spasm, influenza, fever, headache, and respiratory issues.

5. Trapezius Sweep Lines

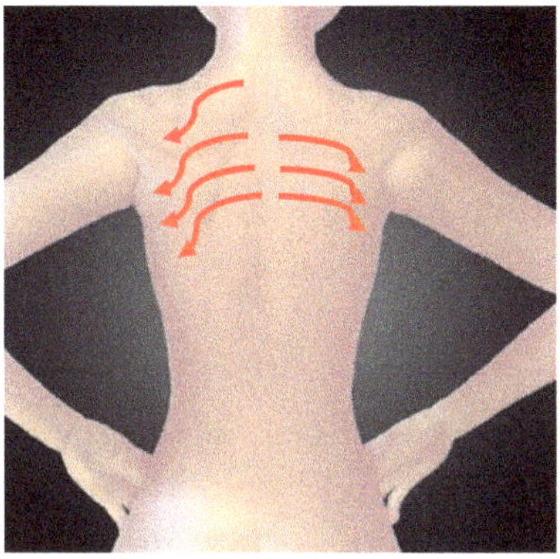

The Trapezius Sweep Lines run bilaterally from T1 to T11 and follow the natural contour of the dorsal intercostal spaces. As usual, the run direction should be top to bottom and medial to lateral. The entire upper back may be scrapped if necessary.

For more effective treatment, the operator should attempt to determine the trigger point(s) where *sha* discoloration is more intense.

Indicated for intercostal neuralgia, respiratory problems, cardiovascular discomfort, gastro-related issues, gall-stone induced discomfort, and uplifting natural immunity.

6. Back Rejuvenation Dredge Lines

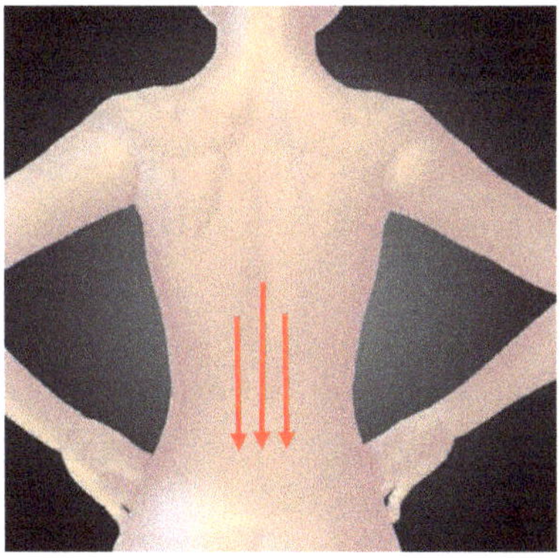

The Back Rejuvenation Dredge Lines lie between T11 and L4 with the central line running along the Governor Vessel and the two lateral lines two-finger width from the Governor Vessel along the Bladder Meridian.

Indicated for lumbar spasm, hearing loss, intestinal, kidney, urological, reproductive and intestinal issues.

<u>Ilio-Sacral Region</u>

The Ilio-Sacral Region includes the ilium and the sacrum and, for the purpose of *Gua Sha*, extends from the Iliac crest to the sacral hiatus. The sacrum is the home of Bladder Meridian's Eight Crevice acupoints 八髎 generally used to address intestinal, urological and reproductive disorders.

Gua Sha for the Sacral Region is often done in the order of Sacral V Dredge Lines and Iliac Contour Sweep Line. As these regions are Yang aspects of the body, the effectiveness of treatment is evidenced by the appearance of *sha* discoloration.

Patient Posture — Prone position

Execution — Press-stroke type selection based on diagnosis, skin lubrication mandatory, preferable to witness surfacing of *sha* discoloration.

1. Sacral V Dredge Lines

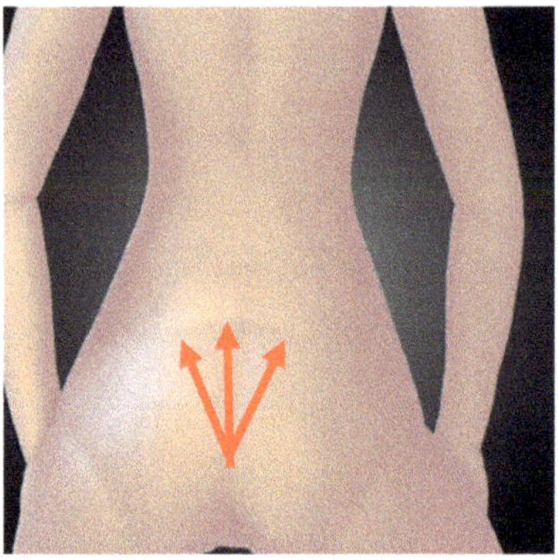

The Sacral V Dredge Lines originate from GV2 腰俞 and branch upward in three directions, the central one along the Governor Vessel to terminate at GV3 腰阳关 or L4 with two flanking lines fanning outwards bilaterally to cover the entire sacrum and the Bladder Meridian's Eight Crevice acupoints 八髎 from BL34 下髎 (4th sacral foramina) to BL31 上髎 (1st sacral foramina).

Indicated for urological disorders, reproductive issues, intestinal issues, uterine prolapse, and benign prostate hyperplasia. Promotes labor. Facilitates fecal and urinary evacuation in the elderly.

2. Iliac Contour Sweep Lines

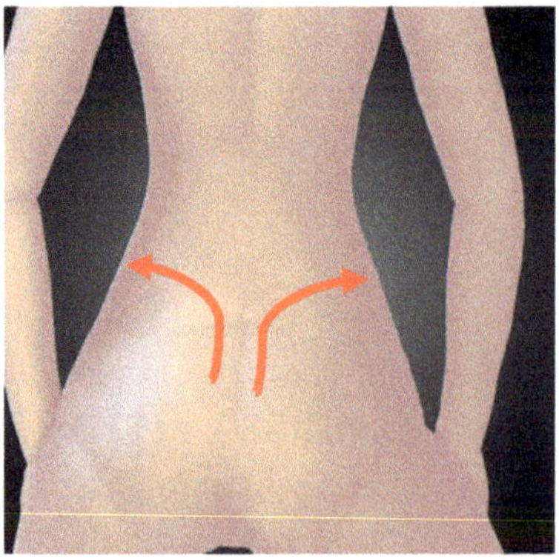

The Iliac Contour Sweep Lines, as described by the name, originate bilaterally from BL32 次髎 and ascend along the upper border of the iliac crest.

BL32 is located at the second posterior sacral foramen within the sacrum, a triangular bone in the lower back formed from fused vertebrae and situated between the two hip bones of the pelvis.

Indicated for iliolumbar pains, and sciatica.

Ventral Region

The Ventral Region, for purpose of *Gua Sha*, consists of both the chest and abdomen and is traversed by three Yin meridians, the Conception Vessel (CV), the Kidney Meridian (KI) and the Spleen Meridian (SP) and a Yang meridian, the Stomach Meridian (ST). The CV, in conjunction with the Governor Vessel, provides a closed conduit that facilitates the continuous movement of Qi within the body. As the "Sea of Yin", the CV regulates all other Yin meridians.

Since the Yin aspects of the body primarily constitute the Ventral Region, the practitioner should be mindful not to exert excessive force during press-stroke. What is deemed to be appropriate force has been duly discussed in an earlier section. The effectiveness of treatment is not necessarily evidenced by the appearance of *sha* discoloration.

Patient Posture — Seated upright and relaxed or preferably supine position

Execution — Press-stroke type selection based on diagnosis, skin lubrication mandatory, registration of *sha* discoloration not mandatory.

1. Sternal Sweep Line

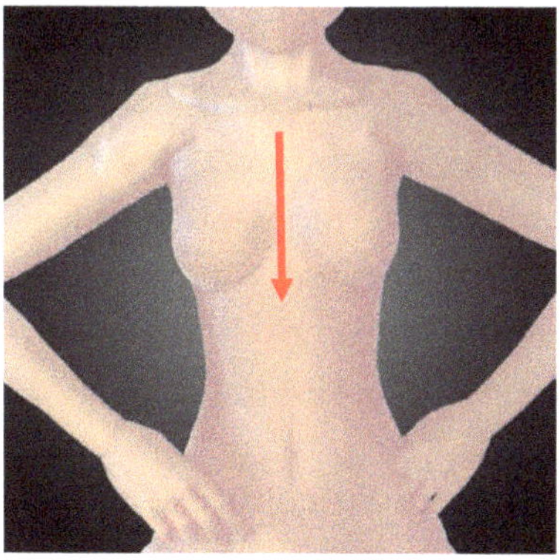

The Sternal Sweep Line, extending from the manubrium to Xiphoid Process, lies medially over the Conception Vessel and passes through CV17 膻中 the crossroad of Spleen, Kidney, Small Intestine, and Triple Energizer meridians. Indicated for cardiovascular disorders, respiratory issues, immunity improvement, diaphragm issues like hiccups, lactation insufficiency, breast engorgement, and menopausal syndrome.

2. Ventral Intercostal Space Sweep Lines

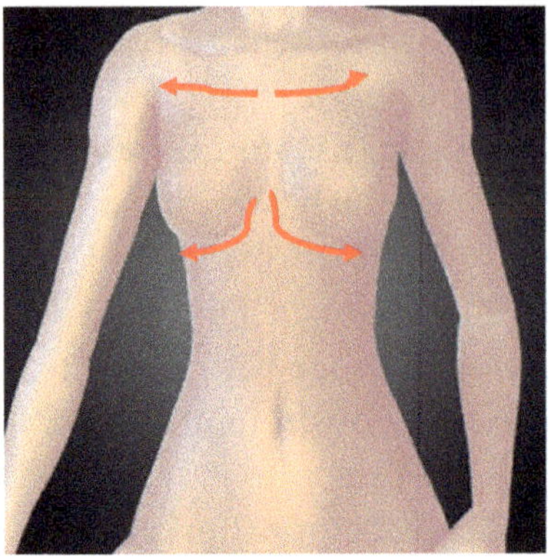

The Ventral Intercostal Space Sweep Lines run bilaterally from T1 to T11 and follow the natural contour of the intercostal spaces whilst avoiding the nipples. As usual, the run direction should be top to bottom and medial to lateral.

Indicated for intercostal neuralgia, respiratory problems, cardiovascular discomfort, gastro-related issues, gall-stone induced discomfort, and uplifting of natural immunity.

3. Epigastric-Umbilical Sweep Lines

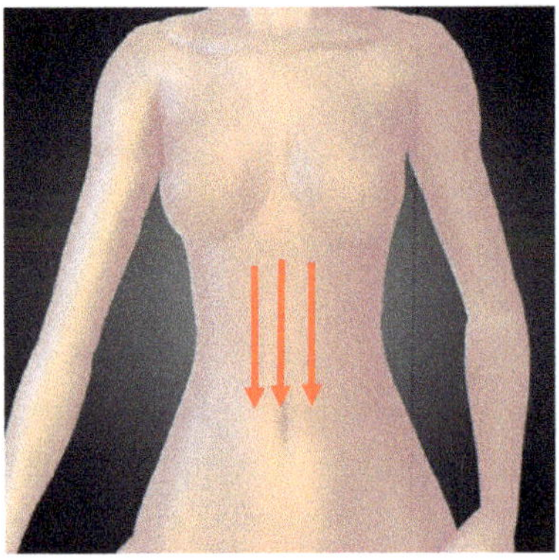

The Epigastric-Umbilical Sweep Lines, extending from the Xiphoid Process to the umbilicus, has three lines. The central line lies medially over the Conception Vessel from CV15 鸠尾 to CV8 神阙 and embodies three vital acupoints for gastric-related ailments — CV10 下脘, CV12 中脘, and CV13 上脘. Secondary lines run three-finger widths bilaterally from ST19 不容 to ST25 天枢 of the Stomach Meridian.

ST19 is located on the abdomen three finger widths lateral to the midline and eight finger-widths above the umbilicus. ST25 is located on the abdomen and three finger widths lateral to the umbilicus.

Indicated for cholecystitis, wide-ranging gastro-intestinal disorders, menopausal syndrome, and chronic liver inflammation.

4. Umbilical-Pubic Sweep Lines

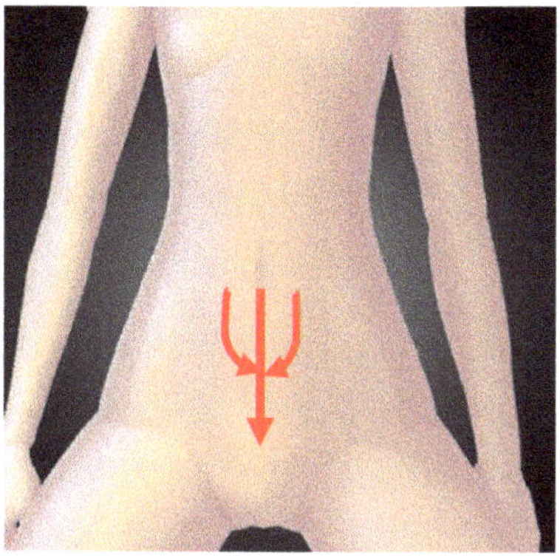

The Umbilical-Pubic Sweep Lines, extending from the umbilicus to the pubic symphysis, has three lines. The central line lies medially over the Conception Vessel from CV8 神阙 to CV2 曲骨 to include three vital resuscitation acupoints CV3 中极, CV4 关元 and CV6 气海. CV2 lies on top of the notch in the center of the superior border of the pubic symphysis, above the external genitalia and in front of the bladder.

Secondary lines run three-finger width bilaterally from ST25 天枢 through ST28 水道 of the Stomach Meridian to meet at CV4. ST25 is located on the abdomen and three finger widths lateral to the umbilicus. ST28 is located on the lower abdomen, four finger widths inferior to the umbilicus and three finger widths lateral to the anterior midline.

Indicated for weight loss, gastrointestinal ailments, and reproductive disorders.

5. Abdominal Spiral Sweep

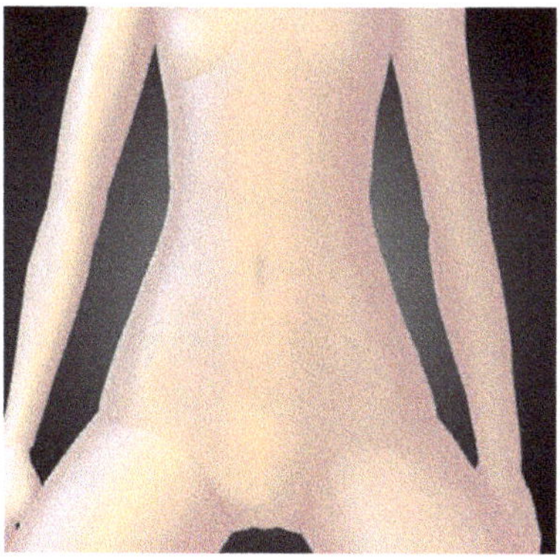

The Abdominal Spiral Sweep originates from the umbilicus and spiral progressively outwards in a clockwise manner to reach superiorly the Xiphoid Process and the pubic symphysis inferiorly.

The treatment is normally administered with both bare hands using a continuous sweeping motion.

Indicated for general immunity improvement, nutritional malabsorption, and constipation.

6. Clavicular Sweep Lines

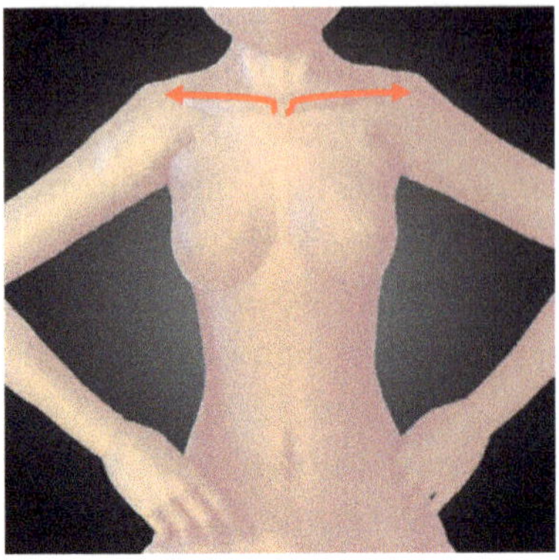

The Clavicular Sweep Lines originate bilaterally from the Jugular Notch of the Sternum and traverse along the two clavicles to terminate at the acromioclavicular joint near the tip of the shoulders.

Caution should be exercised when performing press-stroke as the sweep line is close to the trachea (windpipe). Stroke pressure shall also be moderated considering the sweep is performed above the collar bone which can be very painful. Moderation press-stroke recommended.

Indicated for respiratory problems, diaphragmatic spasm, and loss of voice.

Topic 32

Meridian Dredging

There are 12 Principal meridians and eight Extra meridians in the human body.

The 12 Principal meridians comprise of three Yin meridians of Hand, three Yang meridians of Hand, three Yang meridians of Foot and three Yin meridians of Foot; all having a distinct direction of flow. Of the eight Extra meridians, the more frequently used ones are the Conception and Governor Vessels.

In terms of delivery, meridian dredging is very similar to cutaneous and meridian-tendon assembly scrapping. Except for two differences.

a. Greater precision required in the identification of the location of the meridian pathway coursing through the body; and
b. The direction of flow of the meridian — scrapping consistent with the direction of the meridian flow tonifies whilst doing so in the opposing direction detoxifies.

An operator intending to execute meridian dredging must be versed with the mapping of the meridians and its direction of flow with reference to the surface anatomy of the human body. A summary of the meridian flow direction is tabulated below:

Meridian Type	Direction of Flow	Relative Stroke Force
Yin meridians of Hand	Chest to Hand	Light
Yang Meridians of Hand	Hand to Head	Heavy
Yang Meridians of Foot	Head to Foot	Heavy
Yin meridians of Foot	Foot to Chest	Light
Conception Vessel	Pubic symphysis to Chin	Light
Governing Vessel	Sacral hiatus to Head	Light

As the head and torso have been exhaustively covered by different press-stroke combinations discussed earlier, meridian dredging appears to have greater application at the limb regions. The graphic below illustrates the direction and pathway of dredging for the Lung Meridian.

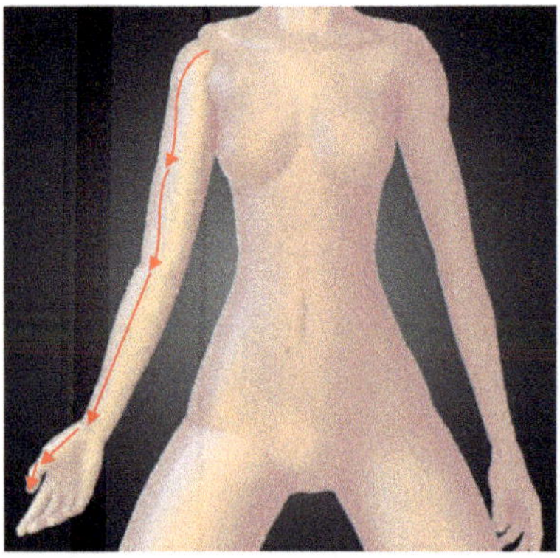

The following table summarises the general treatment areas served by the respective meridians.

Limb	Qualifier	Meaning	Organ System	Meridian Specific Treatment Areas	Other Treatment Areas
Hand	Tai Yin	Greater Yin	Lung	Thoracic, Respiratory	
Hand	Jeu Yin	Transiting Yin	Pericardium	Thoracic, Cardiovascular, Gastric	Neurological
Hand	Shao Yin	Lesser Yin	Heart	Thoracic, Cardiovascular	Neurological
Hand	Tai Yang	Greater Yang	Small Intestine	Occipital, Ocular, Ear, Throat, Neck, Shoulder	Fever, Neurological
Hand	Shao Yang	Lesser Yang	Triple Energizer	Lateral, Ocular, Ear, Throat	Fever, Neurological
Hand	Yang Ming	Rising Yang	Large Intestine	Forehead, Facial, Ear, Nasal, Throat, Oral	Fever
Foot	Tai Yin	Greater Yin	Spleen	Gastro-Intestinal, Reproductive, Urological	Abdominal
Foot	Jeu Yin	Transiting Yin	Liver	Hepatic, Anterior Genital, Gynae, Urological	Abdominal
Foot	Shao Yin	Lesser Yin	Kidney	Kidney, Intestinal, Reproductive, Urological	Respiratory, Throat
Foot	Tai Yang	Greater Yang	Bladder	Occipital, Ocular, Neck, Spinal	Fever, Neurological
Foot	Shao Yang	Lesser Yang	Gall Bladder	Lateral, Ocular, Ear, Intercoastal	Fever
Foot	Yang Ming	Rising Yang	Stomach	Forehead, Facial, Gastro-Intestinal, Throat, Oral	Fever, Neurological
Conception Vessel				Thoracic, Respiratory, GI, Reproductive,	Resuscitation, Neurological, Tonification
Governor Vessel				Head, Thoracic, Respiratory, GI, Reproductive	Fever, Neurological, Syncope

Part 3
Applications

General

Topic 33

Fever

Temperature control (thermoregulation) is part of a homeostatic mechanism that keeps the human body at optimum operating temperature essential for virtually all its biochemical processes and therefore metabolic processes in the body. This vital role in thermoregulation is managed by the hypothalamic-pituitary-thyroid axis.

The average core body temperature is 37° Celsius. Defined officially as a body temperature above 38° Celsius, fever or pyrexia is the clinical hallmark of infection and inflammation and is a part of the body's natural immune response to infection and tissue injury. When the body's temperature rises a few degrees above the norm and remains transient, it is generally not a cause for alarm. In fact, fever is a manifestation of the immune function being enhanced to contain the growth of invading micro-organisms. It may therefore not be a good idea to bring a fever down too soon since it is a healthy sign that the body is effectively combating an infection.

However, if the body temperature continued to climb above 39° Celsius or remained elevated for an extended period of time albeit a low-grade fever, it becomes a cause for concern and treatment should be initiated.

Regardless of being intermittent or otherwise, when fever persists for weeks of which routine investigation failed to identify a root cause, such a condition could be indicative of some deep-seated disorders relating to chronic systemic inflammation like autoimmune diseases or even cancers. Fever of Unknown Origin is also a major concern for those who are aging or immuno-compromised and should never be treated lightly.

From a TCM perspective...

Fever can be caused by exogenous pathogens or endogenous factors. Based on presenting symptom of higher body temperature, fever caused by exogenous pathogens is akin to fever caused by infection from invading micro-organisms. Oftentimes, fever caused by exogenous pathogens can be further aggravated by the presence of dampness that impedes the dissipation of heat. The goals of treatment for fever caused by exogenous pathogens are to dissipate body heat 清热解毒, detoxification/clearing of the bowels 清腑泻下 and preserve/replenish body fluids 养阴益气.

Persistent low-grade fever is caused by the repressed or stifled flow of blood, fluid, and Qi relating to organ injuries; such injuries may be caused by excesses or deficiencies resulting in Yin-Yang imbalance. There are five general situations where continuing repressed flow is insidiously transformed into heat 久郁化火 that consumes Yin elements in the body. These are Qi repression 气郁, food stagnation 食积, phlegm occlusion 痰滞, dampness retention 湿阻 and blood stasis 血瘀. The general principle of treatment for fever caused by endogenous factors is, therefore, to address the cause of organ injuries and restore the normal flow of blood, Qi, and fluids.

Gua Sha Protocol for Treatment or Symptomatic Relief

a. Shoulder Sweep
b. Governor Vessel Dredge
c. Para-Vertebral Dredge
d. Superior Bladder Meridian Dredge
e. Trapezius Sweep
f. Acupoint Scrapping of L5 尺泽 and PC3 曲泽 at the antecubital fossa region of both arms for rapid heat dissipation
g. Acupoint Scrapping of BL39 委阳, BL40 委中 and KI10 阴谷 at the popliteal region of both legs for rapid heat dissipation
h. Acupoint 'press-and-hold' for LI4 合谷 and LI11 曲池 on both arms

Execution — Detoxification press-stroke for high temperature, moderation press-stroke for a low-grade fever. Acupoint scrapping lines should run about one cm above and below the prescribed acupoint. Acupoints marked for application of 'press-and-hold' technique in each prescription form a set, each set to be repeated three times. 'Press-and-hold' maneuver should be attempted 10 times for each prescribed acupoint within each set. Light skin lubricant to be applied to facilitate sweat evaporation. Observation of *Sha* appearance is preferable especially for fever with high temperature.

Other Considerations — *Gua Sha* provides a means to rapidly bring down elevated body temperature. Subsequent to relief, it is imperative to identify the cause of the fever. Unabated high temperature or recurring low-grade temperature after repeated *Gua Sha* treatment is referral case for medical consultation. Hyperpyrexia, a fever with a temperature above 40° Celsius, is a medical emergency.

Glossary

Phlegm is an endogenous pathological factor in TCM and has a narrow and broad connotation. In its narrow definition, synonymous with contemporary medical description, phlegm refers to the thick viscous substance secreted by mucous membranes of the respiratory passages. In a broader context, phlegm is a by-product of metabolic disorder and can be any substance arising from the concentration of body fluids. Dampness is the genesis of phlegm formation.

Dampness arises when body fluid in its finest form is not duly transported and distributed by Nutritive Qi 营气 but somehow retained by a weak 'Spleen' system. When dampness coalesces, it forms water 湿聚为水 that rises superficially to the cutaneous region and manifests as edema. When the Triple Energizer failed to properly distribute water, water accumulates to form a clear but viscous liquid 水停成饮 retained within the torso area that leads to multifarious ailments. When such viscous liquid is further concentrated over time, it forms a turbid sticky substance called phlegm 饮凝成痰. Thus, phlegm can be retained in any organ/viscus and can flow in random directions into meridians and collaterals, giving rise to phlegm syndrome appearing in almost all diseases.

Topic 34

Hyperthermia/Heat Stroke

Fever is a development of high temperature due to a resetting of the hypothalamic thermoregulatory set point caused by endogenous pyrogens released from host macrophages or endothelial cells under an infectious scenario. Another form of high temperature that differs from fever is hyperthermia when high temperature is developed without resetting the hypothalamic thermoregulatory set point.

Under normal circumstances, the body maintains its core temperature according to the temperature of its surrounding environment and sweating is one of the body's important cooling mechanisms. Hyperthermia is elevated body temperature resulting from failed thermoregulation when a body generates or absorbs more heat than it dissipates.

Intense or prolonged exposure to high temperature and humidity without relief or adequate fluid intake can cause various types of heat-related illness. As the body attempts to cool itself under extreme or prolonged heat, blood rushes to the surface of the skin resulting in less blood reaching the brain, other vital organs and muscles thus interfering both physical strength and mental capacity. In severe cases of extreme temperature elevation, it becomes a medical emergency requiring immediate treatment to prevent disability or death.

Hyperthermia normally occurs in three stages. In the mildest form, heat cramp leads to painful muscle spasms that occur during or after intense exercise, heavy exertion or hard physical labor and sweating in high heat. Heavy sweating causes the loss of minerals, like magnesium, that are essential for the smooth functioning of musculature. Treatment at this stage requires no more than relief and replenishment — discontinue the activity, relocate casualty to a conducive environment, alleviate painful spasm and provide a cold isotonic drink.

Heat exhaustion is a more severe stage of hyperthermia and often time manifests concurrently with heat cramp. It occurs in conditions of extreme heat and excessive sweating without adequate fluid and salt replacement or when activities are blatantly continued after heat cramp is alleviated. Symptoms of heat exhaustion include muscle spasm, paresthesia, nausea, vomiting, headache, fatigue, weakness, anxiety, fainting, and elevated temperature. Treatment for heat exhaustion is similar to heat cramp except in event that relief and replenishment did not alleviate the symptoms, restitution becomes mandatory by way of intravenous fluids administration.

Heat exhaustion, if left untreated, can progress to heatstroke. Heatstroke occurs when the body's thermoregulatory system is overwhelmed by excessive heat and malfunctions, leading to a decrease in the body's ability to perspire and thus dissipate heat. Aside from having symptoms of heat exhaustion, heatstroke has the added signs of high fever, rapid pulse and altered mental state like confusion, agitation, stupor and if left untreated may lead to convulsion, seizure, comatose and death.

People who cannot adapt adequately and swiftly to changes in environmental heat (children/elderly), people who generate more heat and less perspiration during activity (overweight/obese), chronic alcoholics, the immuno-compromised, people on low-sodium diet (heart, lung or kidney ailments) and those taking certain medication like antihistamines and antipsychotic may be particularly susceptible to heat exhaustion.

Similarly, individuals with certain medical conditions that decrease the body's ability to sweat, e.g. Scleroderma or cystic fibrosis and those operating under high humidity that interferes with free sweat evaporation may be at greater risk of developing heat stroke.

From a TCM perspective...

Heatstroke is the result of Yang-based summer-heat pathogenetic invasion. This heat rapidly consumes the body's Yin components, like blood and fluids, leading to the corresponding damage of the Yang-based Qi. As sweat is deemed to be the fluid associated with the heart system, the blood circulation is the first to be compromised which in turn cascades to organ damage of various magnitudes and intensities.

Heatstroke, in its most severe form, is a life-threatening emergency and requires immediate medical attention. Notwithstanding, *Gua Sha* could be applied as an intervention for heat-related illnesses in facilitating recovery or containing the situation when the casualty is still mentally lucid.

Gua Sha Protocol for Treatment or Symptomatic Relief

Move casualty to a cool place. Check casualty's state of mental alertness. Remove unnecessary clothing and drench skin with cold water. Place wet towels under armpits, behind the neck, back and on the groin area. Refresh wet towels when warm. Offer cool isotonic drink if alert and able to drink.

a. Shoulder Sweep
b. Governor Vessel Dredge
c. Para-Vertebral Dredge
d. Superior-Bladder Meridian Dredge
e. Trapezius Sweep
f. Sternal Sweep
g. Ventral Intercostal Space Sweep
h. Umbilical-Pubic Sweep — central line only
i. Acupoint Scrapping of L5 尺泽 and PC3 曲泽 at the antecubital fossa region of both arms
j. Acupoint Scrapping of BL39 委阳, BL40 委中 and KI10 阴谷 at the popliteal region of both legs
k. Acupoint 'press-and-hold' for PC6 内关, LI4 合谷 and LI11 曲池 on both arms

Execution — Detoxification press-stroke. Acupoint press-stroke lines should run about one cm above and below the prescribed acupoint. Acupoints marked for application of 'press-and-hold' technique in each prescription form a set, each set to be repeated three times. 'Press-and-hold' maneuver should be attempted 10 times for each prescribed acupoint within each set. Cold water may be used as skin lubricant to facilitate sweat evaporation. Observation of *Sha* appearance is preferable, especially with high temperature. Avoid nipple regions during Ventral Intercostal Space Dredge.

Other Considerations — *Gua Sha* provides a means to rapidly reduce elevated body temperature. Operator be mindful that hyperthermia could be a medical emergency, alert to any signs of deterioration during treatment and ever ready to relinquish casualty to emergency medical assistance. In the event that the casualty loses consciousness during *Gua Sha* therapy with deteriorating vital signs, Basic Life Support Procedure (CPR+AED) should be performed until the arrival of the Emergency Medical Team.

Cardio-Vascular

Topic 35

Angina

Angina is a coronary heart disease with chest pain or discomfort generally described as "heavy, tight or squeezing situated precordial or retrosternal and may radiate to the jaw, neck and/or arm". It occurs when the heart's arteries are narrowed or obstructed and the heart muscle receives an inadequate supply of blood or ischemia.

Classical angina pectoris is precipitated by physical exertion especially after meals or in cold weather and aggravated by emotional stress. The discomfort is usually predictable and manageable, with the angina stabilize and reversible. The pain disappears when the cardiac demand is normalized or decreased. Variants of angina pectoris include angina decubitus that occurs when the person is lying down and nocturnal angina while the patient is recumbent at night. These variants are induced by higher myocardial oxygen demand with increased venous return during recumbency.

Unlike the aforementioned anginas, Prinzmetal angina is not caused by occlusion but coronary artery spasms. It can, therefore, occur without provocation, usually at rest after midnight and more frequently in women.

Heart disease in men is often caused by occlusion in coronary arteries i.e. Obstructive coronary artery disease. However, a good half of women with anginal symptoms and treated with cardiac catheterization did not suffer from arterial obstruction. Instead, heart disease in women develops more frequently within the very small arteries that branch off the coronary arteries. This is generally referred to as microvascular disease and occurs particularly in younger women. Microvascular angina is caused by spasms within the walls of small arterial vessels causing reduced blood flow to the heart muscle. Symptoms of microvascular angina differ from those of typical angina in that the chest pain is more severe and lasts longer, often beyond 30 minutes, and with shortness of breath.

Stable angina is normally relieved with rest, sublingual Glyceryl Trinitrate (GTN) or both. GTN relaxes the coronary arteries and other blood vessels thereby reducing venous return and easing the heart's workload. Relaxing the coronary arteries also increase the heart's blood supply. Prophylactic therapy ranges from beta-blockers to calcium channel blockers administered orally.

Unstable angina, often caused by reduced blood flow to the heart muscles, presents itself unexpectedly and even without exertion. The pain or discomfort is not resolved with rest or by medication. It generally lasts longer than stable angina and may get progressively worse leading to myocardial infarction (MI). Prinzmetal angina is also an unstable form of angina. Unstable angina should be treated as a medical emergency.

From a TCM perspective...

Angina is caused by Heart's Yang and Qi deficiency, phlegm occlusion, blood stasis or exposure to cold weather. Like in all ailments, the predominant principle of therapy is symptomatic relief during the acute phase before following up with prophylactic treatment that addresses the root cause of the ailment when the situation stabilizes 急则治其标, 缓则治其本.

Gua Sha Protocol for Treatment or Symptomatic Relief

Gua Sha may be used to alleviate angina either symptomatically during the abrupt onset or treat the condition prophylactically to minimize recurrence. During abrupt onset, administration of prescribed emergency medication should be the first line of treatment. The patient should be rested in a comfortable position in a well-ventilated space and GTN administered sublingually. Unless angina is stable, arrangement should be made to convey the patient to the Emergency Unit of a hospital immediately.

To expedite recovery or alleviate patient's discomfort while awaiting medical transfer, the following may be performed:

a. Sternal Sweep
b. Ventral Intercostal Space Sweep
c. Trapezius Sweep from T1 to T9 region
d. Superior Bladder Meridian Dredge from T1 to T9 region
e. Acupoint 'press-and-hold' for BL14 厥阴俞 and BL15 心俞 bilaterally
f. Acupoint 'press-and-hold' for PC6 内关, HT7 神门, LI4 合谷 and LI11 曲池 on both arms

   Prophylactically, the following should be included to boost the circulation of Qi:

g. Governor Vessel Dredge
h. Para-Vertebral Dredge
i. Acupoint 'press-and-hold' for ST36 足三里, ST40 丰隆, SP6 三阴交, KI3 太溪, LR3 太冲 on both legs

Execution — Detoxification press-stroke during abrupt onset, tonification press-stroke prophylactically. Acupoints marked for application of 'press-and-hold' technique in each prescription form a set, each set to be repeated three times. 'Press-and-hold' maneuver should be attempted 10 times for each prescribed acupoint within each set. Use of skin lubricant with herbs having anti-inflammatory, anti-embolism, analgesic and Qi invigorating properties preferred. Observation of *Sha* appearance is not mandatory especially during abrupt onset.

Other Considerations — *Gua Sha* may provide quick relief to discomfort brought upon by angina. Operator be mindful that unstable angina and even stable angina, in its most severe form, is a medical emergency. Operator be alert to any signs of deterioration during treatment and ever ready to relinquish casualty to emergency medical assistance. In the event that the casualty loses consciousness during *Gua Sha* therapy with deteriorating vital signs, Basic Life Support Procedure (CPR+AED) should be performed until the arrival of the Emergency Medical Team.

Topic 36

Cardiac Arrhythmia

The heart pumps blood to the lungs and the rest of the body by a sequence of highly synchronized contractions of its four chambers that give rise to a heartbeat. When heartbeat becomes irregular, blood cannot circulate effectively and vital organs including the brain suffer, leading to damage and may even shut down.

Arrhythmias differ from normal heartbeats in speed or rhythm. Arrhythmia refers to changes in the normal sequence of heart electrical impulses. The electrical impulses may happen too fast, too slowly or erratically — causing the heart to beat faster (tachycardia), slower (bradycardia) or erratically.

The heart has four chambers, two upper chambers termed right and left atrium and two lower chambers termed right and left ventricle. Normal electrical sequence begins in the right atrium (Sino-Atrial node), spreads throughout the atria to the atrioventricular (AV) node. From the AV node, electrical impulses travel down a group of specialized fibers called the His-Purkinje system to all parts of the ventricles. This sets the pace for heartbeat.

Arrhythmias are therefore divided into two categories: ventricular and supraventricular. Ventricular arrhythmias occur in the ventricles or lower chambers of the heart. Supraventricular arrhythmias occur in the area above the ventricles, usually in the atria or upper chambers of the heart.

When arrhythmias are so brief that the overall heart rate or rhythm is not significantly affected, they can be relatively harmless.

But longer duration arrhythmias that cause the heart rate to be too slow or too fast or the heart rhythm to be erratic that could pose health problems or be life-threatening.

Bradycardia is a very slow heart rate of fewer than 60 beats per minute due to electrical impulses that cause heart chamber contraction not being not effectively transmitted to the heart's lower chambers (the ventricles) or the impulses are being originated from heart cells other than the Sino-Atrial (SA) node that malfunctions.

Tachycardia is a very fast heart rate in excess of 100 beats per minute. Those originating from the ventricles are called ventricular tachycardia and if originated from the atria or at the gateway to the lower chambers, supraventricular tachycardia.

Ventricular tachycardia occurs when impulses from the SA node are obstructed from reaching the ventricles resulting in other areas along the lower electrical pathway assuming the pace-making role. As the path for ventricular impulses is short-circuited, heart rhythm quickens and may cause shortness of breath, dizziness, or fainting (syncope).

When several impulses begin concurrently from different locations in the ventricles, the ventricles quiver and ventricular fibrillation occur. This is the most serious, chaotic and damaging arrhythmia with no mechanical or pumping effect. Medical attention is imminent. Cardiopulmonary resuscitation (CPR) should be started soonest and cardioversion or defibrillation necessary to arrest the situation.

A less worrying type of ventricular arrhythmia is a premature ventricular contraction (PVC) when the ventricles contract too soon and out of sequence with the normal heartbeat. Triggered by caffeine and some over-the-counter cough and cold medicines, it is generally self-limiting and therefore not a cause for alarm. It often does not require treatment unless the patient has a history of heart disease.

Supraventricular arrhythmias are generally not as serious as ventricular arrhythmias; often time self-limiting and do not require treatment. Notwithstanding, frequent episodes can weaken the cardiac muscle over time and should, therefore, be addressed with medical intervention to prevent further complications. Like PVCs, atrial arrhythmias can be triggered by a number of stimulants including tobacco, alcohol, caffeine, and cough and cold medication. The disorder may also stem from rheumatic heart disease (scarring) or hyperthyroidism. Supraventricular arrhythmias can cause heart palpitation, very fast pulse, chest tightness and shortness of breath.

Supraventricular Tachycardia (SVT) or Paroxysmal Supraventricular Tachycardia (PSVT) is a type of "short-circuit" arrhythmia that may occur at any age and commonly among patients who have no other types of heart disease. Commonly misdiagnosed as a panic attack, PSVT is typically described as a rapid or racing but regular heartbeat of about 230 beats per minute that starts and stops abruptly. With the exception of some patients with the Wolff-Parkinson-White (WPW) syndrome, PSVT is generally not life-threatening.

SVT or PVST occurs either from atrioventricular nodal re-entrant tachycardia (AVNRT) or from an accessory pathway (AVRT: atrioventricular reciprocating tachycardia) as in WPW syndrome. In AVNRT, a small extra pathway exists in or near the AV node. If an electrical impulse enters this pathway, it starts to travel in a circular pattern causing the heart to abruptly beat faster but regular.

WPW syndrome is a congenital condition in which there is an extra accessory pathway between the atria and the ventricles. The impulses travel along the extra pathway (short circuit) as well as the normal AV-HIS Purkinje system, very quickly in a circular pattern, causing abnormal heartbeat. People with this syndrome may feel dizzy, have chest palpitations or episodes of fainting. WPW syndrome is a common cause of tachycardia among infants and children. Under rare circumstances, WPW syndrome can develop an extremely rapid heart rhythm abnormality that may be life-threatening.

Like ventricular fibrillation, atrial fibrillation happens when the upper chambers of the heart (atria) experience chaotic electrical signals resulting in rapid unproductive contractions with no mechanical effect and little output. Reduced cardiac output causes blood to accumulate in the heart's upper chambers, leading to the formation of blood clumps or clots. Stroke occurs when a blood clot traveling from the heart blocks a smaller artery in the brain (cerebral artery). Atrial fibrillation is, therefore, a main cause of stroke, especially among the elderly, and consequently, patients with atrial fibrillation need antiplatelet therapy.

A strong pulse in the neck, a racing heartbeat or discomfort in the chest, weakness, shortness of breath, fainting, sweaty and dizziness are symptoms of an onset of atrial fibrillation.

From a TCM perspective...

Arrhythmia is caused by Yang and Qi deficiency in the Heart and Kidney systems, phlegm occlusion or blood stasis. Acupoints from the Heart, Pericardium and Kidney meridians should be selected to restore Yang energy, improve circulation and regulate heartbeats, and from the Spleen and Stomach meridian to stimulate metabolism and manage phlegm build-up.

Gua Sha Protocol for Treatment or Symptomatic Relief

In arrhythmia emergencies, rapid and correct diagnosis is essential for appropriate therapy. *Gua Sha* may therefore not be used to alleviate arrhythmia symptomatically during abrupt onset as the situation may be so complex that reading clinical symptoms or performing mere physical examination alone would not correctly identify the root cause. The root cause can only be revealed by specialist analysis of 12-lead electrocardiogram graphs.

Having said that, not all arrhythmias need acute intervention including some conditions that might look dramatic but still perfuse the brain. In these situations, the appropriate strategy could well be to support oxygen-enriched ventilation and observing the development while arranging for casualty conveyance to the Emergency Room.

Casualty conscious level is perhaps the most appropriate indicator of perfusion. While the casualty remains conscious, there is an opportunity to help make the patient more relaxed in the hope that the condition may improve when the stress level is down-regulated.

The patient should be rested in a comfortable position in a well-ventilated quiet space where an AED is easily accessible. GTN is contraindicated even though the risk of GTN-induced hypotension is low.

To expedite recovery or alleviate patient's discomfort while awaiting medical transfer, the following may be performed:

a. Sternal Sweep
b. Ventral Intercostal Space Sweep
c. Superior Bladder Meridian Dredge (T1-T9 region)
d. Para-Vertebral Dredge (T1-T9)
e. Trapezius Sweep
f. Umbilical-Pubic Sweep — central line only
g. Acupoint 'press-and-hold' for BL14 厥阴俞 and BL15 心俞 bilaterally on the torso
h. Acupoint 'press-and-hold' for PC6 内关 and HT7 神门 on both arms
i. Acupoint 'press-and-hold' for KI3 太溪 on both legs

   Prophylactically, the following should be included to boost the circulation of Qi:

j. Governor Vessel Dredge
k. Superior Bladder Meridian Dredge
l. Acupoint 'press-and-hold' for SP6 三阴交, ST36 足三里 and ST40 丰隆 on both legs

Execution — Detoxification press-stroke during abrupt onset, tonification press-stroke prophylactically. Acupoints marked for application of 'press-and-hold' technique in each prescription form a set, each set to be repeated three times. 'Press-and-hold' maneuver should be attempted 10 times for each prescribed acupoint within each set. Use of skin lubricant with herbs having anti-inflammatory, anti-embolism, analgesic and Qi invigorating properties preferred. Observation of *Sha* appearance is not mandatory especially during abrupt onset.

Other Considerations — *Gua Sha* may provide relief to the discomfort brought upon by arrhythmia. Operator be mindful that arrhythmia is fundamentally is a medical emergency. Operator be alert to any signs of deterioration during treatment and should have made prior arrangement for the transport of the patient to the Emergency Room before commencing treatment. In the event that the casualty loses consciousness during *Gua Sha* therapy with deteriorating vital signs, Basic Life Support Procedure (CPR+AED) should be performed until the arrival of the Emergency Medical Team.

Topic 37

Hypertension

Blood circulates around the body, transporting nutrient and removing waste, by virtue of the driving force of the heart. The same driving force exerts pressure on blood vessels and has two attributes — systolic pressure being the maximum pressure exerted to the cardiovascular system when the heart is pumping while diastolic pressure is the minimum pressure exerted to the circulatory system when the heart relaxes.

The Singapore Ministry of Health Clinical Practice Guidelines stipulate hypertension or high blood pressure (HBP) as a chronic medical condition with resting blood pressure consistently manifesting these readings: 140-149/90-99mmHg (Stage 1), 160-179/100-109mmHg (Stage 2) and exceeding 180/110mmHg (Stage 3). Blood pressure in excess of 180/120 is deemed to be a case of hypertensive crisis and is a medical emergency that requires intravenous administration of sodium nitroprusside.

Hypertension may also be classified as either primary of which there is no single identifiable cause but may be attributed to genes, diet, and lifestyle or secondary when hypertension is caused by another disease. Primary hypertension is by far the most common type. Hypertension can become resistant to treatment when there are multiple underlying medical conditions or contributing factors or when the condition is not responsive to treatment of a combination of three antihypertensive drugs including a diuretic.

Pulmonary hypertension is yet a different condition from regular or systemic hypertension. In systemic hypertension, blood pressure throughout the body is elevated and can be simply measured with a blood pressure monitor. In pulmonary hypertension, the circulation to the lungs is compromised by narrowed or damaged blood vessels such that the right side of the heart must pump harder leading to increased blood pressure that may be measured by cardiac catheterization.

Hypertension is a 'silent killer' because it is almost always asymptomatic and is capable of damaging many organs permanently. In its severe form, hypertension is characterized by an occipital headache at awakening, tinnitus, blurred vision and insomnia. Uncontrolled high blood pressure leads to serious complications like heart attack, stroke, blindness, and chronic kidney failure.

Contemporary medicine tackles hypertension with lifestyle changes and by reducing water content from the body/blood volume (diuretics), delivering a slower, less forceful heartbeat (beta-adrenergic blocking agents), relaxing the contraction of heart and blood vessels (calcium channel blockers), reducing brain signals that increase heart rate (central agonists), relaxing overall body muscles (alpha-adrenergic antagonists), dilating blood vessels (ACE inhibitors and Angiotensin II receptor blockers), etc. Like all drugs, antihypertensive drugs come with side-effects, e.g. extended use of hydrochlorothiazide, a diuretic, with strong sunlight exposure is associated with the increased risk of lip cancer[1] and non-melanoma (basal cell) skin cancer[2] due to its photosensitizing effect.

From a TCM perspective...

Hypertension is caused by hyperactivity of the Liver system, Yin deficiencies in the Liver and Kidney systems and Phlegm syndrome originating from the Spleen-Stomach system. Cholesterol and triglycerides are also a form of phlegm that obstructs blood circulation.

Treatment should, therefore, be directed at the Liver system to suppress Liver Yang, at the Liver and Kidney systems to restore and rebalance their Yin level and reinforce the Spleen-Stomach system to raise the general metabolic level and manage the production of phlegm.

Gua Sha Protocol for Treatment or Symptomatic Relief

Hypertension, but not a hypertensive crisis, is a good candidate for *Gua Sha* therapy. Because there is a tendency in mainstream medical treatment to mobilize more than one drug concurrently, Gua Sha as an external intervention will not run afoul with the therapeutic regimen but instead reinforce the effect of mainstream medicine as adjuvant therapy.

a. Four Spirit Extension
b. Occipital-Cervical Sweep
c. Shoulder Sweep
d. Sternal Sweep
e. Ventral-Intercostal Space Sweep
f. Superior Bladder Meridian Dredge (T1-T9 region)
g. Acupoint 'press-and-hold' for ST36 足三里, ST40 丰隆, LR3 太冲, SP6 三阴交, GB31 风市 and KI3 太溪 on both legs
h. Acupoint 'press-and-hold' for PC6 内关, ST4 合谷 and LI11 曲池 on both arms

   In urgent cases, while waiting for the arrival of Emergency Services, the operator may attempt to alleviate the discomfort of the casualty by applying 'press-and-hold' to acupoints PC6 内关, ST4 合谷 and HT7 神门 on the arms, LR2 行间 and LR3 太冲 on the legs, GB20 风池 and GV16 风府 on the head.

Execution — Moderation press-stroke during an emergency situation, tonification press-stroke prophylactically. Acupoints marked for application of 'press-and-hold' technique in each prescription form a set, each set to be repeated three times.

'Press-and-hold' maneuver should be attempted 10 times for each prescribed acupoint within each set. Use of skin lubricant with herbs having anti-inflammatory, anti-embolism, analgesic and Qi invigorating properties preferred. Observation of *Sha* appearance is not mandatory.

References

1. Pedersen SA, Gaist D, *et al.* Hydrochlorothiazide use and risk of nonmelanoma skin cancer: a nationwide case-control study from Denmark. *J. Am. Acad. Dermatol.* **78**(4): 673–681.e9 (Apr 2018).
2. Pottegård A, Hallas J, Olesen M, *et al.* Hydrochlorothiazide use is strongly associated with risk of lip cancer. *J. Intern. Med.* **282**(4): 322–331 (Oct 2017).

Endocrinological

Topic 38

Diabetes Mellitus

The term *Diabetes Mellitus,* comprising the Greek word *diabetes* meaning siphon or to pass through and the Latin word *mellitus* meaning honeyed or sweet, succinctly features the defining characteristic of the disease — excessive sugar in the blood (hyperglycemia) as well as urine (glycosuria) of the patient.

The simplest form of sugar is glucose. Glucose is an important source of energy for the body, especially the brain. But persistent high blood sugar levels lead to macrovascular disease (coronary artery disease, peripheral vascular disease, and stroke) and microvascular damage (retinopathy, nephropathy, and neuropathy).

Diabetes, a chronic and usually irreversible[1] disease, is caused by either relative insulin deficiency or insulin resistance or both. Unlike pre-diabetes that is asymptomatic and generally reversible, diabetes brings long-term damage to the heart, kidney, and vascular system. Insulin is a hormone secreted by the pancreas that controls the amount of glucose in the blood.

Type 1 diabetes mellitus (T1DM) is attributed to a genetic-linked autoimmune process that attacks and destroys the beta cells of the pancreas resulting in progressively diminishing insulin production with the passage of time. With reduced insulin, sugar builds up in the blood instead of being used by cells as an energy form. T1DM is associated with the rapid requirement for insulin and risk of ketoacidosis.

T1DM generally develops in childhood or adolescence but can develop insidiously during adulthood. A recent article revealed that genetic susceptibility to T1DM can present itself throughout the first six decades of life, long after the age once thought.[2]

Latent Autoimmune Diabetes in Adults (LADA) describes people with apparent type 2 diabetes who appear to have immune-mediated loss of pancreatic beta cells. A form of T1DM, LADA is often misdiagnosed as T2DM because it develops over a longer period of time than T1DM.

Type 2 diabetes mellitus (T2DM) is associated with insulin resistance or insulin insensitivity that prevents normal uptake of glucose by cells but allows the sugar to remain in the blood and yet induces excessive insulin production. Over time the extra demand on the pancreas leads to burn out of pancreatic beta cells. Proper management of blood sugar levels through medication, lifestyle change and diet would defer the eventual need for insulin therapy.

The third type of diabetes, gestational diabetes, is a temporary condition that usually occurs during the second trimester of pregnancy. Increased hormones produced by the placenta cause a build-up of blood glucose. Elevated blood glucose levels during pregnancy can lead to high blood pressure, frequent urinary infections and pre-eclampsia. Having gestational diabetes may increase the risk of developing diabetes for both mother and child.

There is yet another Type 3 diabetes mellitus (T3DM), a 'brain diabetes', better known as Alzheimer disease (AD). AD is actually a neuroendocrine disorder that resembles type 2 diabetes mellitus. Reduced expression of insulin and neuronal insulin receptors are found in the brain of AD patients that progressively leads to a breakdown of the insulin-signaling pathway, manifesting in insulin resistance. This, in turn, affects brain metabolism and cognitive functions observed in AD patients. By the same corollary, people having insulin resistance, particularly those with T2DM, have at least 50% increased risk of suffering from AD.

Early symptoms of untreated diabetes are associated with elevated blood sugar levels and loss of glucose in the urine. A large amount of glucose in the blood is excreted by the kidneys through urine causing increased output (frequent urination or polyuria) and dehydration. Dehydration causes increased thirst (polydipsia) and water consumption.

A relative or absolute insulin deficiency precipitates frequent gluconeogenesis that eventually leads to weight loss.[3] This weight loss occurs despite an increase in appetite (polyphagia). Untreated diabetic patients may suffer from fatigue, nausea, and vomiting. High blood glucose weakens immune defenses and increases susceptibility to infections (such as infections of the bladder, skin, and vaginal areas) in people with untreated or poorly-controlled diabetes. Fluctuations in blood glucose levels can lead to blurred vision. Extremely elevated glucose levels can lead to lethargy and coma.

From a TCM perspective...

Diabetes Mellitus is generally characterized by polydipsia (thirst), polyphagia (hunger), polyuria (frequent urination) and emaciation. The disorder comprises of three pathological categories — upper, middle and lower wasting-thirst 消渴 syndrome. The upper wasting-thirst 上消 syndrome is attributed to the accumulation of heat in the Lungs rapidly consuming body fluids leading to thirst. Middle wasting-thirst 中消 syndrome is characterized by unbridled Stomach fire manifesting as excessive appetite and constant hunger while lower wasting-thirst 下消 syndrome is associated with yin deficiency in the Kidney resulting in excessive urination. In reality, all these syndromes exist concurrently though there may be some apparent dominance in symptoms for every case. Such dominance in symptoms is indicative of the relative yin deficiency in the Lung, Stomach or Kidney systems and therefore provide a basis for personalization in treatment. By and large, the general principles of treatment would be to clear the Lung's heat and moisten the Lungs, clear the Stomach's heat and cultivate Stomach's Yin, and revitalize the Kidney's Yin; all to be performed in varying magnitudes while re-invigorating the 'spleen' to rid stagnation of phlegm and dampness.

Gua Sha Protocol for Adjuvant Treatment

a. Occipital-Cervical Sweep
b. Superior Bladder Meridian Dredge (T1-L4)
c. Trapezius Sweep
d. Epigastric-Umbilicus Sweep
e. Umbilicus-Pubic Sweep
f. Sacral V Dredge
g. Acupoint 'press-and-hold' for SP6 三阴交, SP8 地机, ST36 足三里, ST44 内庭, KI3 太溪, KI7 复溜 and LR3 太冲 on both legs
h. Acupoint 'press-and-hold' for LI4 合谷, LI11 曲池, PC6 内关 and LU10 鱼际 on both arms
i. Acupoint 'press-and-hold' for EX B5 胰俞 bilaterally on the back.

   A word of caution is there appear to be a confusion in the Extra Point Naming Reference of EX B5. EX B5 is known to be assigned to another acupoint 下极俞 located medially on the lower border of the spinous process of L3. Acupoint EX B5 mentioned under this topic, however, refers to an Extra Point 胰俞 located bilaterally on the Bladder Meridian under the spinous process of T8 and between BL17 膈俞 and BL18 肝俞. It functions to soothe the liver and gallbladder 疏肝利胆, promote blood circulation 活血化淤, nourish the pancreas and 'spleen' 养胰健脾 and pacify the gastro-intestinal system 调和肠胃.

Execution — Moderation press-stroke recommended. Acupoints marked for application of 'press-and-hold' technique in each prescription form a set, each set to be repeated three times. 'Press-and-hold' maneuver should be attempted 10 times for each prescribed acupoint within each set. Use of skin lubricant with herbs having Qi invigorating properties preferred. Observation of *Sha* appearance is not mandatory.

Other Considerations — *Gua Sha* does not purport to replace any mainstream medical treatment for diabetes including lifestyle changes and diet advisories. *Gua Sha* can be an effective adjuvant therapy that helps promote the general well-being of a diabetic patient, assist in but not disrupt the body in managing its blood sugar levels.

Gua Sha is also contraindicated for patients with healing issues.

More importantly, *Gua Sha* should not be attempted in situations of diabetic emergencies that could manifest themselves as a hyperosmolar hyperglycemic state (HHS) or severe hypoglycemia. HHS occurs when blood sugar levels become dangerously high and hypoglycemia occurs when blood sugar levels are abnormally low. In any case, these situations are medical emergencies beyond the expertise of a *Gua Sha* practitioner. Take heed.

References

1. Ang GY. Reversibility of diabetes mellitus: narrative review of the evidence. *World J. Diabetes* **9**(7): 127–131 (July 15, 2018).
2. Thomas NJ, Jones SE, Weedon MN, *et al.* Frequency and phenotype of type 1 diabetes in the first six decades of life: a cross-sectional, genetically stratified survival analysis from UK Biobank. *Lancet Diabetes Endocrinol.* **6**: 122–129 (Feb 2018).
3. Basu R, Chandramouli V, *et al.* Obesity and type 2 diabetes impair insulin-induced suppression of glycogenolysis as well as gluconeogenesis. *Diabetes* **54**(7): 1942–1948 (July 2005).

Topic 39

Hyperlipidemia

Hyperlipidemia is an extremely common condition in those who keep a sedentary but stressful lifestyle, follow a high-fat diet and are overweight. It is a generic term that refers to any of several acquired or genetic disorders that result in a high level of lipids (fats, cholesterol, and triglycerides) circulating in the blood. Accordingly, hyperlipidemias are classified by the elevated lipid type — hypercholesterolemia, hypertriglyceridemia or combined hyperlipidemia when both cholesterol and triglycerides levels are elevated. Elevated levels of *Lipoprotein(a)* may also be classified as a form of hyperlipidemia. *High Lipoprotein(a)* is the strongest, single, inherited risk factor for aortic stenosis or narrowing of the aorta, early coronary artery disease (CAD) and stroke even when other cholesterol numbers appear normal.

Hypercholesterolemia, also called high cholesterol, is the presence of high levels of cholesterol in the blood plasma. Cholesterol is an essential lipid used in the construction of animal cell membranes and also serves as the precursor of steroid hormones and bile acids. Because cholesterol is so important, 80% of the body's requirement is produced by the liver and intestines with the remainder coming from diet.

Hypertriglyceridemia, like hypercholesterolemia, denotes high blood levels of triglycerides, the most abundant fatty acid in most organisms.

Cholesterol and triglycerides are insoluble in water and must be packaged for transport within the blood plasma by lipoproteins. There are five main classes of lipoproteins based on size and density. The higher the ratio of protein to lipid content the higher the density and these lipoproteins can also morph from one form into another. The largest but least dense lipoprotein is chylomicron, followed by very-low-density lipoprotein (VLDL) that morphs into intermediate-density lipoprotein (IDL) that in turn morphs into low-density lipoprotein (LDL) as the particle progressively yields up its triglyceride component. At LDL level, the molecule becomes smaller but very rich in cholesterol and is associated with the build-up of artery-clogging plaque, hence the name "bad" cholesterol. In contrast, high-density lipoprotein (HDL) is "good" cholesterol because they remove cholesterol from circulation and from artery walls and return it to the liver for excretion. Thus, higher levels of HDL cholesterol are protective.

Hyperlipidemia is often detected through blood screening as elevated serum lipid levels are generally asymptomatic except when pancreatitis is present or as manifestations of atherosclerosis leading to ischemia such as angina, heart attack, stroke, gangrene, calf pain during walking, etc.

The presence of xanthomas or xanthomata is the hallmark of hyperlipidemia. Xanthoma tendinosum are nodules of fatty deposits found in the tendons of the hands, feet, and heel. Xanthoma striatum palma is characterized by yellowish plaques involving the palmar creases and flexural surfaces of the fingers. Xanthoma tuberosum are deposits located over joints while Xanthoma planum are plaques spread diffusely over large areas of the body. Xanthelasma palpebrarum, yellowish collection of cholesterol around the eyelids, may be associated with familial hypercholesterolemia.

Hyperlipidemia is a metabolic disease and usually chronic which means that the first-line treatment should be exercise, weight loss, a low-fat diet and, if applicable, diabetes management. Usually, an anti-cholesterol medication (statins) and in hypertriglyceridemia with niacin added. An adverse side effect leading to a suspension of statin treatment is intolerable muscle and joint aches. Aside from its hepatotoxicity (especially in sustained-release preparation), niacin causes flushing, itching, nausea, diarrhea, and rashes.

From a TCM perspective...

Lipids are considered to be a type of phlegm and the 'Spleen' system is deemed to be the source of phlegm 脾为生痰之源. It is also instructional to note that the function of the 'Spleen' system in the transport and transformation of body nutrients is very much akin to that of modern science gastro-intestinal functions. In TCM, the Stomach and the 'Spleen' systems also form an exterior-interior dyad that reciprocates each other's functions and in the treatment of diseased Spleen-Stomach system, it is vital to moderate an overpowering Liver (wood) system that may overwhelm an already weakened 'Spleen' (earth) system 肝木克脾土. The acupoints along Stomach, Spleen and Liver meridians are therefore selected to dispel dampness and reduce phlegm formation since these meridians are direct pathways to their respective organ-systems. Four Spirit Extension also facilitates the ascent of Yang energy that effectively dispels dampness.

Gua Sha Protocol for Adjuvant Therapy

Gua Sha can be applied both as a form of adjuvant therapy to reinforce first-line treatment or when there is a desire to wean off first-line treatment.

a. Four Spirit Extension
b. Shoulder Sweep
c. Superior Bladder Meridian Dredge
d. Sternal Sweep
e. Acupoint 'press-and-hold' for ST36 足三里, ST40 丰隆, SP6 三阴交, SP9 阴陵泉 and LR3 太冲 on both legs
f. Acupoint 'press-and-hold' for PC6 内关 and LI11 曲池 on both arms

Execution — Moderation press-stroke recommended. Acupoints marked for application of 'press-and-hold' technique in each prescription form a set, each set to be repeated three times. 'Press-and-hold' maneuver should be attempted 10 times for each prescribed acupoint within each set. Use of skin lubricant with herbs having Qi invigorating properties preferred. Observation of *Sha* appearance is not mandatory.

Topic 40

Obesity

Obesity is perhaps the most common and visible manifestation of a metabolic disorder. For its close association with chronic inflammation, insulin resistance, and lipotoxicity, obesity is also an independent predictor for diabetes, hypertension, lipoprotein abnormalities, vascular disorders and chronic kidney disease (CKD). Obesity is even associated with sub-fertility, sleep apnea and cancers.

Overall obesity is traditionally determined 'in the field' by a Body Mass Index (BMI) score in excess of 30. For Asians, a BMI of 27.5 would be considered obese. In obesity, fat distribution or where fat is amassed and deposited poses relative risks to the individual. Abdominal fats are deemed more detrimental and threatening than fats accumulated at the buttocks. In this regard, waist circumference would, therefore, be the more relevant anthropometric measurement and should be used in conjunction with BMI to identify increased disease risk.

Central Obesity is determined by waist circumference in excess of 89 cm for women and 102 cm for men. The Ministry of Health Singapore Guidelines for Obesity 2016 recommends that cutoffs of 80 and 90 cm, respectively, may be more appropriate for Asians based on an Asian-Pacific consensus.

Net caloric uptake, the daily food calorie intake less daily energy expenditure, is usually the cause of simple obesity. Avoidance of calorie-dense food and sedentary lifestyle is, therefore, a common prescription for containment of simple obesity.

The number of adipocytes or fat cells in the body, however, is apparently determined at childhood. This number remains constant throughout adulthood even when the individual is subject to significant weight reduction regimes. It is further observed that neither adipocyte death nor renewal rate is altered during the onset of obesity, suggesting a tight regulation of adipocyte number throughout adulthood. Given that the adipocyte count for an individual is constant, fat mass can only expand by increasing the average adipocyte volume resulting in fat-engorged fully differentiated adipocytes.[1] In this regard, caloric restriction has limited effect as an intervention strategy for obesity.

Endocrinal abnormalities are also associated with obesity. Hypothyroidism, Cushing's syndrome, and growth hormone deficiency generally cause suppressed metabolic levels that predispose the individual to fat accumulation. Some disorders, like Cushing's syndrome, can even regulate the distribution of fat deposits in the body.

Although the causal relationship between obesity and sleep deprivation has yet to be fully established, global cross-sectional studies have demonstrated a consistent increased risk of obesity amongst children and adults who suffered sustained short sleep.[2] Chronic sleep deprivation is associated with reduced serum leptin and elevated serum ghrelin, the two opposing metabolic hormones central to appetite regulation.[3] Leptin is an adipocyte-derived hormone that suppresses appetite, while ghrelin the 'hunger hormone' is a gastrointestinal derived peptide that stimulates appetite and promotes fat storage. This combination of reduced leptin and increased ghrelin invariably stimulates greater food intake, and in the absence of increased energy expenditure, resulting in weight gain and higher BMI reading.

Recent studies suggest that gut microbiota plays a significant role in the development of obesity and its attendant disorders. In fact, the composition of gut flora is found to differ significantly between lean and obese humans. Gut bacterial flora of obese humans present fewer Bacteroidetes and relatively more Firmicutes than that of their lean counterparts,[4] suggesting that difference in microbiota composition could be key in caloric extraction from ingested dietary substances, regulation of energy expenditure, storage of unexpended calories in host adipose tissue, alterations in gut permeability leading to metabolic endotoxemia, systemic inflammation and insulin resistance.[5]

The consumption of broad-spectrum antibiotics is known to disrupt the population and alter the composition of intestinal microbiota and the use of systemic antibiotics among children has been associated with obesity later in life. Studies showed that children who have received in excess of three antibiotic treatments during their first two years of life have a relative increased risk of obesity of up to 50% compared to those not exposed. Macrolides appear to be the antibiotics most often associated with higher risk compared with other antibiotics.[6]

Finally, extended consumption of certain prescribed medication could well be linked to rapid weight gain and therefore obesity. Diabetic drugs (insulin, thiazolidinediones, sulfonylureas), antipsychotics (haloperidol, clozapine, lithium), anticonvulsants (valproate and carbamazepine), anti-depressants (amitriptyline, paroxetine, sertraline), anti-hypertensive drugs (beta-blockers), steroids (prednisone, contraceptives) are some medicines that have demonstrated adverse effects of weight gain.

From a TCM perspective...

Obesity or the undesirable accumulation of fat is associated with the disruption of the natural flow of vital energy or Qi. Qi is the driving force behind blood circulation and fluid distribution within the body that proper functioning of all organs is predicated. When the flow of Qi is impeded, blood stasis and dampness ensue. Dampness is the genesis of phlegm formation.

Phlegm is an endogenous pathological factor in TCM and has a narrow and broad connotation. In its narrow definition, phlegm refers to the thick viscous substance secreted by mucous membranes of the respiratory passages. In a broader context, phlegm is a by-product of metabolic disorder and can be any substance arising from the undesirable concentration of body fluids. Fat is, therefore, a class of phlegm.

Dampness arises when body fluid, derived from ingested dietary substances and in its finest form, is not duly transported and distributed by Nutritive Qi 营气 but somehow retained by a weakened 'Spleen' system. Invigorating the Spleen (Earth 土) system and promoting the Kidney Yang (Fire 火) is, therefore, an intervention frequently used when dampness is identified as a cause of obesity. An adjuvant intervention is a moderation of Liver (Wood 木) system to provide relief for the recovery of a weakened 'Spleen' system.

When dampness coalesces, it forms water 湿聚为水 that rises superficially to the cutaneous region and manifests as water retention or even edema. When the Triple Energizer failed to properly distribute water, water accumulates to form a clear but viscous liquid 水停成饮 retained within the torso area that leads to multifarious ailments. The Triple Energizer provides a vital fluid channel connecting the Lung system, Spleen/Stomach system, and the Kidney system. Improving the function of Triple Energizer will undoubtedly help rid the body of fluid retention, in metabolic waste excretion and thus dampness.

When such retained viscous liquid is further concentrated over time, it forms a turbid sticky substance called phlegm 饮凝成痰. Thus, phlegm can be retained in organs and viscera and can flow in random directions into meridians and collaterals, giving rise to phlegm syndrome appearing in almost all diseases, including obesity and metabolic syndrome.

Gua Sha Protocol for Treatment

a. Occipital-Cervical Sweep
b. Sternal Sweep
c. Superior Bladder Meridian Dredge (T8-L4 region)
d. Epigastric-Umbilicus Sweep
e. Umbilicus-Pubic Sweep

f. Stomach Meridian Dredge (ST34-ST40) on both legs with emphasis on ST34 梁丘, ST36 足三里, ST37 上巨虚, ST39 下巨虚 to ST40 丰隆 using acupoint 'press-and-hold' technique
g. Spleen Meridian Dredging (SP6-SP9) on both legs with emphasis on SP6 三阴交, SP8 地机 to SP9 阴陵泉 using acupoint 'press-and-hold' technique
h. Acupoint 'press-and-hold' for LU7 列缺, PC6 内关 and LI11 曲池 on both arms

Execution — Moderation press-stroke recommended. Acupoint scrapping lines should run about one cm above and below the prescribed acupoint. Acupoints marked for application of 'press-and-hold' technique in each prescription form a set, each set to be repeated three times. 'Press-and-hold' maneuver should be attempted 10 times for each prescribed acupoint within each set. Use of skin lubricant with herbs having Qi invigorating properties preferred. Observation of *Sha* appearance is not mandatory.

Other Considerations — Obesity can be a very complex disorder especially in advanced stages where prescription weight-loss medication failed and bariatric surgery is recommended.

Gua Sha does not purport to replace any mainstream medical treatment for obesity including lifestyle changes and diet advisories. Notwithstanding, dieting and exercise may have a limited weight loss effect on people with Qi deficiency due to a depressed metabolic rate. When the Spleen/Stomach system, primarily responsible for nutrient acquisition and energy regulation, is extremely weak, normal meals will burden the system into starting a vicious cycle of food stagnation, dampness build-up, and phlegm production. This view is in line with contemporary medicine's concept that extreme dieting/calorie restriction will depress metabolic rate and thus not help in weight management.

Gua Sha is, therefore, an excellent therapy to complement either mainstream or TCM treatment for obesity by promoting Qi circulation in the body that in turn improves nutritive absorption and energy balance as well as flush out accumulated toxins that hindered metabolism. It is also an appropriate solution for the overweight.

References

1. Spalding KL, Arner E, *et al.* Dynamics of fat cell turnover in humans. *Nature* **453**: 783–787 (June 5, 2008).
2. Cappuccio FP, *et al.* Meta-analysis of short sleep duration and obesity in children and adults. *Sleep* **31**(5): 619–626 (May 2008).
3. Taheri S, *et al.* Short sleep duration is associated with reduced leptin, elevated ghrelin and increased body mass ndex. *PLoS Med.* **1**(3): 210–217 (Dec 2004).
4. DiBaise JK, Zhang H, Crowell MD. Gut microbiota and its possible relationship with obesity. *Mayo Clin. Proc.* **83**(4): 460–469 (Apr 2008).
5. Shen J, Obin MS, Zhao L. The gut microbiota, obesity and insulin resistance. *Mol. Aspects Med.* **34**(1): 39–58 (Feb 2013).
6. Antibiotics: repeated treatments before the age of two could be a factor in obesity. *Prescrire Int.* **27**(194): 155–157 (June 2018).

Gastro-Intestinal

Topic 41

Cholecystitis

Disorders of the biliary tract are commonly caused by gallstones often developed from biliary sludge, a thick mucous material of particulate solids or sediments precipitated from bile. Sludge conditions are asymptomatic and often self-limiting. Notwithstanding, sludge can slowly consolidate into gallstones in the gallbladder which remain largely asymptomatic until they migrate into the biliary tract.

Smaller gallstones may pass spontaneously out of the bile duct on their own without symptom. However, when a stone is trapped and obstruct the bile duct (choledocholithiasis), medical intervention may be necessary otherwise inflammation, bacterial infection (cholangitis) and even organ damage may occur.

Migrated gallstones that obstruct the cystic duct transiently cause biliary colic, a characteristic pain located in the right upper quadrant of the abdomen that may radiate to the back or even down the arm. Episodes are abrupt with a rapidly escalating pain level that plateau and remain constant for hours before tapering off to a dull ache. The episode, which usually lasts less than 12 hours, is often severe enough to warrant medical relief from the emergency department. Other presenting symptoms include mild right upper quadrant or epigastric tenderness, nausea and vomiting. Unless gallbladder inflammation (cholecystitis) sets in, fever and chills are usually absent.

Once manifested, biliary colic is usually recurring but rarely develop into complications.

Acute cholecystitis is a common complication when stones from the gallbladder (cholelithiasis) obstruct the cystic duct resulting in gallbladder inflammation. Aside from the common symptoms of severe and sudden pain in the right upper abdominal quadrant that spreads to the right shoulder or back with nausea and vomiting, low-grade fever is usually presented due to inflammation and gallbladder distention. The episode is therefore of longer duration and the pain more severe in intensity than biliary colic, resulting in restrictive breathing and involuntary guarding. In more severe obstructions, signs of jaundice and lack of bowel movement (ileus) may appear. Left untreated and when infection sets in, pus builds up in the gallbladder (empyema) leading to tissue death (necrosis) and perforation.

Treatment consists of symptomatic relief and supportive management (hydration, complete bowel rest, analgesics and antibiotics) during the attack and, when desirous, removal of the gallbladder (cholecystectomy) as a permanent solution. Fortunately, most episodes of acute cholecystitis will resolve spontaneously within a week even without treatment.

Acalculous cholecystitis is cholecystitis without stones. Patients with acute acalculous cholecystitis may present with fever, sepsis, peritonitis, and shock. The onset is usually without a history or physical examination finding consistent with acute cholecystitis. With a high mortality rate, this is a rare complication and a medical emergency not within the scope of *Gua Sha* therapy.

Chronic cholecystitis is the consequence of repeated episodes of acute cholecystitis. Intermittent obstruction of the cystic duct by gallstones causes biliary colic but not necessarily overt gallbladder inflammation. Although the extent of inflammation does not correlate with the intensity or frequency of biliary colic, bile stasis triggers the release of enzymes that mediate inflammatory response and cause mucosal damage to the gallbladder.

If the acute inflammation is resolved but infiltrate of chronic inflammatory cells continued to recur, the gallbladder becomes fibrotic, contracted and fail to concentrate bile or empty normally — features of chronic cholecystitis. Extensive calcification or encrustation of gallbladder wall due to fibrosis is called porcelain gallbladder. Porcelain gallbladder has been associated with a moderate risk of gallbladder malignancies, possibly because both conditions are related to chronic inflammation.

Chronic cholecystitis is always suspected in patients with recurrent biliary colic with cholelithiasis.

From a TCM perspective...

Biliary disorders like cholelithiasis are caused by skewed dietary and lifestyle habits. Excessive consumption of high-fat diet and extended exposure to emotional stress or trauma are detrimental to the Spleen/Stomach and Liver/Gallbladder systems respectively resulting in dampness being engendered internally. When part of this entrapped dampness transformed into heat, this heat binds with the remaining dampness, forming damp-heat 湿热 which obstructs the Qi mechanism 气机 and consequently the free circulation of Qi and blood. The inhibited flow of the qi and blood results in Qi stagnation and blood stasis giving rise to intercostal and abdominal pains, while inhibition of the Qi mechanism results in nausea and vomiting.

Emotional distress over an extended period of time causes repression of liver Qi that could result in liver hyperactivity and heat. A hyperactive Liver system may singularly overwhelm the Spleen/Stomach system to disrupt the normal transformation and transportation of nutrients to set off the phlegm production cycle.

Entrapped dampness coalesced to form phlegm within the Spleen/Stomach and Liver/Gallbladder systems. With the passage of time, phlegm in the Liver/Gallbladder forms biliary sludge that further consolidates into gallstones.

Thus, treatment for biliary disorders is focussed towards restoring the normal functions of the Spleen/Stomach and Liver/Gallbladder systems. Another therapeutic goal is internal heat dissipation which is served by the Large Intestine Meridian.

Gua Sha Protocol for Adjuvant Treatment or Symptomatic Relief

a. Para-Vertebral Dredge
b. Trapezius Sweep
c. Superior Bladder Meridian Dredge
d. Ventral Intercostal Space Sweep (right side only)
e. Epigastric-Umbilicus Sweep
f. Acupoint 'press-and-hold' for GB34 阳陵泉, EX-LE6 胆囊, SP6 三阴交, ST36 足三里 and LR3 太冲 on both legs
g. Acupoint 'press-and-hold' for LI4 合谷, LI11 曲池 and PC6 内关 on both arms

Execution — Moderation press-stroke recommended. Acupoint scrapping lines should run about one cm above and below the prescribed acupoint. Acupoints marked for application of 'press-and-hold' technique in each prescription form a set, each set to be repeated three times. 'Press-and-hold' maneuver should be attempted 10 times for each prescribed acupoint within each set. Use of skin lubricant with herbs having Qi invigorating properties preferred. Observation of *Sha* appearance is not mandatory.

Topic 42

Constipation

Constipation is a common gastrointestinal disorder experienced by almost everyone at some point in time of life. It is a symptom rather than a disease and refers to the reduction in the frequency of bowel motions or increased difficulty and straining during defecation. There is, however, no strict definition of constipation as normal bowel function varies widely between individuals. As such, the basis of determining constipation should be the observed change in bowel function of the individual. Notwithstanding, constipation may be clinically diagnosed as the passage of stools less than three times a week or repeated difficulty and pain during the passage of stools. Other accompanying symptoms include flatulence, abdominal and intestinal discomfort.

Reduced frequency of bowel motions implies slower waste movement through the colon. This delay allows excessive absorption of water from the waste by the colonic mucosa, causing feces to be compacted which in turn prevent the bowel walls to contract adequately (peristalsis). Consequently, the feces turn dry and hard, making it difficult to propel and painful to evacuate.

In the alleviation of constipation, it is important to ascertain the extensive underlying causes or predispositions that disrupt normal nutritive absorption, stool formation and evacuation of feces. These include a poor diet with inadequate fiber and fluid content, decreased physical mobility, pregnancy, emotional distress, bowel obstruction (adhesion, tumors), hypothyroidism, consumption of certain anti-hypertensives, anti-depressants, opioids, and even iron supplements.

Elderly people are therefore predisposed to constipation by virtue of many of these underlying factors. If constipation goes unnoticed some severe side effects can occur; such as hemorrhoids and damage or tearing of the anus. Unless persistently recurring, constipation is seldom indicative of a serious underlying condition.

Management and treatment of constipation are often directed at addressing the underlying cause(s) by making dietary and lifestyle adjustments and using laxatives on a short-term basis for symptomatic relief. The use of laxatives on an extended basis is not encouraged as it may lead to serious dysfunction of bowel motility such as intestinal paralysis, cathartic colon,[2] lazy or laxative gut. Colonic irrigation should be avoided altogether.

From a TCM perspective...

Although constipation is primarily due to the transient failing of the large intestine in its transport function, it is intimately related to the functions of other visceral organs, especially the lung, the spleen, and the kidney.

Constipation generally exists in two different states — excess-state and deficient-state constipation. Excess-state constipation is commonly due to Qi stagnation, cold accumulation, and pathogenic heat. Deficient-state constipation is caused by a deficiency in blood and vital fluids of the body.

Heat affects the hydration-lubrication mechanism of the Large Intestine system and hampers its evacuation function. Heat-induced constipation is usually caused by an excessively skewed diet that is overtly acrid, spicy or greasy that overburdens the gastro-enteric system. Another source of heat that afflicts the large intestine is lingering heat from an illness of exogenous heat origin, especially of the respiratory system. Since the Lung and Large Intestine systems are intimately related as an exterior-interior dyad in TCM, such residual heat is reflected when it is transmitted downward to the colon 余热下移大肠.

On the contrary, over-indulgence with cold and raw foods or excessive use of bitter and cold herbs may also cause constipation when the warm Yang energy is subdued, resulting in the retention of Yin-coldness within the intestinal tracts and stalling normal function of Qi.

Excess-state constipation could also arise from extended or extreme emotional distress as well as inadequate physical activity. In both of these situations, the pathogenic effect is similar in that the free circulation of Qi or vital energy is being impeded. Grief is known to cause Qi dissipation and hinders lung Qi function 悲则气消. Pensiveness and worry stagnate Qi flow 思则气结 忧则气郁, preventing the normal nutritive distribution of the Spleen system.

Similarly, physical inactivity taxes the Spleen system leading to the Qi mechanism being compromised 久卧伤气 and followed by reduced intestinal peristalsis before progressing to atrophy of core muscles that facilitate defecation 久坐伤肉.[1]

Deficient-state constipation may be explained as a general physiological underperformance that causes a delay in the evacuation of normal stools. Stools are usually not compacted and dehydrated. Due to a deficiency in Qi, blood and body fluids, peristalsis is reduced leading to extended stool transit duration. This condition is common in people suffering or in convalescence from severe or wasting ailments, post-partum ladies and the elderly with a weak constitution. Occasionally, constipation could also be the aftermath of acute and severe emesis 吐下之余，定无完气.

Diuretic 利尿 or diaphoretic 发汗 herbs induce excessive urination and perspiration respectively. Extended use of such herbs without timely fluid replenishment may deplete body fluids and cause Qi-Yin deficiency when Qi departs in the course of excessive perspiration 气随汗脱 or severe fluid excretion 气随津脱. Often time, fluid deficiency leads to inadequate blood volume which is another cause of deficient-state constipation.

Gua Sha Protocol for Treatment and Symptomatic Relief

a. Para-Vertebral Dredge (T1-L4)
b. Abdominal Spiral Sweep

c. Epigastric-Umbilicus Sweep
d. Umbilicus-Pubic Sweep
e. Sacral V Dredge
f. Spleen Meridian Dredging (SP4-SP9) on both legs with emphasis on SP4 公孙, SP6 三阴交 and SP9 阴陵泉 using acupoint 'press-and-hold' technique
g. Stomach Meridian Dredging (ST36-ST37) on both legs with emphasis on ST36 足三里 and ST37 上巨虚 using acupoint 'press-and-hold' technique
h. Acupoint 'press-and-hold' for GB34 阳陵泉 on both legs
i. Acupoint 'press-and-hold' for TE6 支沟 on both hands
j. Acupoint 'press-and-hold' for SP14 腹结 bilaterally

Execution — In absence of a proper diagnosis, moderation press-stroke recommended. Acupoint scrapping lines should run about one cm above and below the prescribed acupoint. Acupoints marked for application of 'press-and-hold' technique in each prescription form a set, each set to be repeated three times. 'Press-and-hold' maneuver should be attempted 10 times for each prescribed acupoint within each set. Use of skin lubricant with herbs having Qi invigorating properties preferred. Observation of *Sha* appearance is not mandatory.

Other Considerations — *Gua Sha* is an effective therapeutic response for constipation when the symptom is induced by either excess or deficiency; in which case a proper diagnosis should be undertaken and the appropriate press-stroke be performed.

After *Gua Sha* therapy, the patient may raise the thighs closed to the chest with some supporting when seated on the bowl or, in the alternative, adopt a squatting position during defecation. In so doing, the anorectal angle would be moderated to facilitate fecal evacuation. This position is especially useful for Qi deficient type constipation.

More importantly, the practitioner should ensure that the constipation was not caused by physical obstruction but triggered by some physiological disorder. Untreated, intestinal obstruction can be a serious, life-threatening complication when necrosis or tissue death sets in. Necrosis can result in intestinal wall perforation, leading to fecal peritonitis, sepsis and possibly multiple organ failure.

So long as *Gua Sha* does not cause undue delay in seeking appropriate treatment, it may introduce little added risk into a situation of intestinal obstruction or adhesion. It can, however, cause added agony to the patient when *Gua Sha* raises the internal pressure for fecal evacuation.

Glossary

Cathartic colon is caused by prolonged laxative abuse in excess of three times per week for at least a year. The chronic use of stimulant laxative resulted in the anatomic and physiologic change in the colon characterized by loss of haustral folds, suggestive of neuronal injury or damage to colonic longitudinal musculature caused by these agents. Bloating, a feeling of fullness, abdominal pain, and incomplete fecal evacuation are general symptoms of the disorder.

References

1. *Huang Di's Internal Classics.* Chapter 23: Wide Promulgation of the Five Qi 《黄帝内经》《素问·宣明五气》"五劳所伤".
2. Joo JS, Ehrenpreis ED, *et al.* Alterations in colonic anatomy induced by chronic stimulant laxatives: the cathartic colon revisited. *J. Clin. Gastroenterol.* **26**(4): 283–286 (June 1998).

Topic 43

Emesis/Vomiting

Emesis or Vomiting is a forceful retrograde expulsion of gastric contents. Emesis often initiated by a sense of nausea; though nausea could well occur on its own without proceeding to emesis. Nausea is then followed swiftly by retching or an involuntary effort to vomit before the actual act of emesis.

During emesis, stomach relaxation is achieved by the *a priori* nausea, while retching musters up the abdominal muscles and the diaphragm to contract simultaneously so as to forcefully expel the contents from the gastrointestinal system via the mouth.

Emesis has been reckoned as a physiological defense mechanism that protects the body from ingested 'noxious' substances by expulsion rather than allowing them to be retained and absorbed by the guts. The term noxious need not necessarily mean 'toxic' as it could mean anything that is 'situationally' objectionable to the body as in a case of throwing up after overeating. Rather a broader interpretation should be ascribed to emesis as a mechanism that helps relieve the gastro-enteric system of any form of undue load or stress.

Emesis is a symptom and not a medical condition per se. As a symptom, it is commonly associated with gastrointestinal lining irritation, infections, vestibular disorders, adverse endocrine and body chemical changes, increased intracranial pressure, oncological therapy, and post-operative reaction.

Repeated vomiting that contains food particles and occurs after each meal is indicative of gastric motility disorders, pyloric stenosis or obstruction in the small bowel. Vomitus containing blood or coffee ground-like material is associated with bleeding from a source proximal to the upper GI tract or swallowed blood from an oropharyngeal or pulmonary origin. Feculent vomitus suggests a gastrocolic fistula or a fistula between the colon and duodenum. Intestinal obstruction with bacterial degradation of contents may also be associated with feculent vomitus.

Projectile vomiting is characteristic of gastric obstruction or increased intracranial pressure. Early morning nausea and vomiting is associated with pregnancy, the most punishing form being *hyperemesis gravidarum.* Adverse reactions to medications are among the commonest causes of nausea or emesis; the symptoms may be acute or chronic, constant or intermittent.

Emesis can present as a single episode or be recurring. Recurrent vomiting is usually reflective of some underlying medical conditions. Frequent emesis without any underlying medical condition may be representative of cyclic vomiting syndrome, a condition of unknown origin, characterized by vomiting for up to a week and mainly affecting people in their childhood. Frequent vomiting may cause esophagitis and a weakened lower esophageal sphincter.

Severe emesis, particularly protracted or forceful vomiting, can cause tears of the proximal stomach mucosa (Mallory–Weiss tear) and, occasionally, esophageal rupture. These lesions may be due to herniation of the cardia through the diaphragm during vomiting.

Emesis is initiated by a stimulus to either the integrative vomiting center (VC), a central control in the medulla oblongata near the respiratory center, or the chemoreceptor trigger zone (CTZ) in the area postrema on the floor of the fourth ventricle. The CTZ, however, does not initiate vomiting when activated but instead relays the stimulus to the VC which produces the actual act of emesis. These coordination centers can be stimulated through multiple pathways.

Management and treatment of nausea and emesis entail the identification of chemical transmitters that trigger the vomiting reflex and apply the appropriate antiemetic medication to block the reflex pathway. Common antiemetics include dopamine antagonists (metoclopramide), 5HT3 antagonists (ondansetron) and anticholinergics (hyoscine). Aprepitant (substance P/neurokinin 1 antagonist) is often prescribed to prevent nausea and vomiting caused by chemotherapy (CINV) or surgery.

From a TCM perspective...

The stomach, located in the Middle Energizer 中焦, is primarily responsible for receiving food and fluids, and its Qi flows typically downward. The harmonious descent of the stomach Qi depends on the function of the Spleen in its normal nutritive transformation and transportation 升清运化 and the regulatory function of the Liver that ensures uninterrupted operation of the overall Qi mechanism 疏泄条达. When either or both of these organs underperformed, the result is loss of stomach homeostasis 胃失和降. On the contrary, the stomach-Qi can also be compromised by a hyperactive liver that causes disharmony between the stomach and liver systems 肝气犯胃 leading to vomiting.

Emesis is therefore caused by impaired homeostasis of the stomach, the abnormal rising of the stomach-Qi in retrograde fashion 气逆于上 and propelling the ingested food upward. Thus, the point of initiation for vomiting may lie with the stomach but the etiological root of emesis should be traced beyond the stomach to the liver, gallbladder, and spleen.

Emesis is a symptom that relates to either an excess-state or a deficient-state underlying cause. In an excess-state situation, vomiting may be due to invasion by exogenous pathogens, excessively skewed diet, phlegm accumulation or Qi stagnation. Deficiency in spleen/stomach Qi, Yin, and Yang are the principal causes of deficient-state emesis. By and large, emesis could initially be the manifestation of an excess-state syndrome but, when left untreated, may evolve into a chronic deficient-state when the spleen and stomach are impaired. Notwithstanding, an impaired spleen/stomach system when assaulted by exogenous factors will manifest a combined excess and deficient state syndrome.

Emesis initiated by excess-state underlying causes is generally abrupt and forceful with copious vomitus and may occur spontaneously after a meal.

Vomiting induced by deficient-state underlying causes tends to be less vigorous, recurring but less predictable. The build-up to emesis is always less dramatic though often accompanied by nausea and retching with a limited amount of vomitus.

TCM shares the view that vomiting is a physiological defense mechanism that limits exposure of the body to noxious elements by evacuation and thus contains the magnitude of the injury. This is documented in the 'Synopsis of Prescriptions of the Golden Chamber 金匮要略' as early as AD 200 with specific advice not to subdue the expulsion of gastric content in a situation when vomitus is purulent 夫呕家有痈脓， 不可治呕，脓尽自愈[1] or high in alcoholic content 酒疸，心中热，欲呕者，吐之愈.[2]

Careful evaluation of the patient's situation is thus necessary for the treatment of emesis in that intervention is only desirable when vomiting remains unabated in spite noxious substances have been completely expelled.

The key to treatment for emesis lies in harmonizing the stomach and suppressing the retrograde qi flow. This can be achieved by eliminating exogenous pathogen when emesis is caused by external factors and may include allowing emesis to run its course. When food stagnation is the reason, a quick fix would be to relieve food retention by expulsion before promoting digestion in the longer term. In the event that the liver is hyperactive, it is essential to relax the liver prior to addressing other issues. In deficient-state emesis, the therapeutic strategy would be to warm the middle energizer and strengthen the spleen when Yang energy is lacking and nourish the stomach Yin to promote repair of the protective mucosa when stomach-yin is depleted.

Gua Sha Protocol for Treatment and Symptomatic Relief

Gua Sha should not be performed during emesis. It can be executed only when emesis ceases momentarily or between episodes of emesis for control of the symptom.

a. Occipital-Cervical Sweep
b. Abdominal Spiral Sweep

c. Epigastric-Umbilicus Sweep
d. Umbilicus-Pubic Sweep
e. Para-Vertebral Sweep (T7-T12)
f. Superior Bladder Meridian Dredge (T7-T12)
g. Acupoint 'press-and-hold' for ST36 足三里, LR3 太冲 and SP4 公孙 on both legs
h. Acupoint 'press-and-hold' for PC6 内关 and HT7 神门 on both arms

Execution — Detoxification press-stroke for excess-state emesis and tonification press-stroke for deficient-state emesis. In absence of a proper diagnosis, moderation press-stroke recommended. Acupoints marked for application of 'press-and-hold' technique in each prescription form a set, each set to be repeated three times. 'Press-and-hold' maneuver should be attempted 10 times for each prescribed acupoint within each set. Use of skin lubricant with herbs having Qi invigorating properties preferred. Observation of *Sha* appearance is not mandatory.

Other Considerations — Emesis often leads to dehydration, fatigue and in a severe protracted instance may result in loss of acid-base balance and electrolyte depletion. Save for a situation where expulsion of noxious substance is desirous, symptomatic relief should be sought for severe and protracted emesis. It is also important to correct for electrolyte, fluid, and/or nutrient deficiencies.

Glossary

Pyloric stenosis — anatomic obstruction of the gastric pylorus such as by scarring or malignancy.

Gastrocolic Fistula (GCF) — is formed by infiltration of a tumor from the serosa of one viscus into the wall of another viscus, followed by lumen-to-lumen necrosis and resulting in the movement of some stomach contents directly into the colon, bypassing the normal digestive pathway and disrupting the normal digestive process. The fistula results in the reflux of fecal material from the colon into the stomach.

References

1. Zhang Zhongjing 张仲景 (AD 150–219). *Synopsis of Prescriptions of the Golden Chamber*, Chapter 17.
2. Zhang Zhongjing 张仲景 (AD 150–219). *Synopsis of Prescriptions of the Golden Chamber*, Chapter 15.

TOPIC 44

Gastritis — Acute and Chronic

Gastritis is the irritation, inflammation, and damage of the stomach's protective lining known as gastric mucosa. The mucosa is multi-functional as in, aside from producing strong hydrochloric acid to break down food and an enzyme called pepsin to digest protein, it secretes an insoluble mucus that protectively coats the entire stomach lining to prevent the acidic digestive juice from dissolving the stomach tissue. This delicate balance is controlled by three different glands in the gastric mucosa — the cardiac glands, fundic (oxyntic) glands and pyloric glands.

When the stomach lining is inflamed, it secretes less acid and fewer enzymes, giving rise to reduced digestive capacity. At the same time, the mucosa also produces less mucus and other substances that protect the stomach lining from the corrosive nature of own strong acidic digestive juice.

Gastritis should be differentiated from gastroenteritis. As gastritis only affects the stomach, symptoms may include nausea and vomiting. Whereas gastroenteritis affects both the stomach and the intestines, often leading to diarrhea in addition to nausea or vomiting.

Gastritis is not considered as a single disease but rather a condition with numerous causes. Contrary to popular belief, gastritis is usually asymptomatic. However, when symptoms manifest, pain or discomfort is felt in the upper part of the abdomen (epigastrium).

There are two forms of gastritis, acute and chronic.

Acute gastritis refers to the abrupt onset of severe stomach lining inflammation of short duration. Severely distressing but transient pain may be experienced in cycles during an episode. Other symptoms include nausea, vomiting, bloating, loss of appetite and weight loss.

Acute gastritis can be further classified into two sub-types: erosive (e.g. superficial erosions, deep erosions, hemorrhagic erosions) and non-erosive (generally caused by *Helicobacter pylori*). Erosive gastritis is characterized by acute erosions of small shallow lesions or deep bleeding ulcers in the mucosa. In severe erosive gastritis, symptoms could include black tarry stool and vomitus containing blood or coffee ground-like material. The more common non-erosive gastritis causes inflammation in the stomach lining without erosions or ulcers.

Excessive exposure to acute irritants that overwhelm the protective mucosa of the stomach is the cause of acute gastritis. Irritants include aspirin or other NSAIDs (non-steroidal anti-inflammatory drugs), poisons (including strong alcohol and tobacco) and infections, including early stages of *Helicobacter pylori* infection. The inflammation usually extinguishes itself when the source of irritation is removed.

Chronic gastritis is marked by persistent, low-grade inflammation that progressively damages the stomach lining over a long duration, possibly a lifetime, if left untreated. The presence of inflammatory cells, including lymphocytes, in the mucosa is indicative of an immune response. The gastric mucosa becomes thinner as the normal cells are destroyed with progressive severity. Mucosal changes may progress to a stage called metaplasia, with an increased risk of gastric cancer.

In the vast majority of cases, chronic gastritis is asymptomatic until when the damage to the mucosa is so severe that the stomach loses its ability to produce gastric acid and intrinsic factor. Only then may the patient experience digestive upsets and possibly symptoms of pernicious anemia.

Infection by *Helicobacter pylori* is the most common cause of chronic gastritis. Other causes of chronic gastritis may include an auto-immune disease (sarcoidosis), specific infections (HIV/AIDS), Crohn's disease and gastric surgeries (gastrectomy, gastric bypass) that increase bile reflux.

The goals of gastritis treatment are to provide rapid relief by eliminating the source of irritation that causes mucosal inflammation in the first instance followed by reduction of the stomach acid volume to relief pain and promote mucosal healing and, if necessary, address the underlying cause(s) for the longer term.

Elimination of the source of irritation could be as simple as avoiding the use of NSAIDs, abstinence from alcohol or even adopting a less stressful lifestyle. Gastric juice can also be a source of irritation and its neutralization by antacids provides rapid relief of gastritis pain.

Reduction of stomach acid volume is usually achieved by administration of proton pump inhibitors (omeprazole, esomeprazole) and histamine H2-receptor antagonists (ranitidine, famotidine). However, long-term use of proton pump inhibitors is associated with an increased risk of osteoporotic-related fractures, *Clostridium difficile* infection, community-acquired pneumonia, vitamin B12 deficiency, kidney disease, and dementia.[1] H2 blockers have adverse effects like central nervous system symptoms (mental confusion, headache, depression) and rare cases of thrombocytopenia.[2] Long term usage of some antacids may cause diarrhea or constipation, altered calcium metabolism, magnesium build-up, and even kidney issues.

Addressing underlying cause is essential in the treatment of gastritis, acute or otherwise. When an infection is noted, eliminating the causative infection (usually *H. pylori*) with antibiotics is mandatory to prevent 'disease' progression, but the stomach mucosa rarely returns to normal. Vitamin B12 deficiency is treated by intermittent injections.

From a TCM perspective …

Gastritis is a disorder of the stomach with the associated pain located at the epigastrium 上中下脘. The disease is often caused by the invasion of an exogenous cold pathogen, indiscriminate ingestion, and emotional distress, resulting in Qi stagnation, phlegm accumulation, and blood stasis. These causative factors may operate singularly or in concert to initiate an onset. The disorder lies mainly with the stomach but is closely related to liver Qi stagnation 肝气郁, spleen weakness as well as the gallbladder malfunctioning. The symptoms of gastritis include, but not limited to, loss of appetite, nausea, and vomiting, and gastric reflux. Etiology for gastritis is the loss of stomach homeostasis 胃失和降, obstruction of Qi mechanism 气机不利 and lack of nutritive support to the stomach 胃失濡养.

The pathogenesis of this condition is relatively simple. The onset of acute gastritis is an excess-state syndrome, caused mainly by invasion of an exogenous cold pathogen that leads to food stagnation 饮食停滞, liver Qi stagnation, stomach Qi stagnation, obstruction of Qi mechanism, spleen/stomach damp heat and blood stasis. Pain, in TCM context, is caused by flow obstruction 不通则痛, including the stagnation of ingested food, Qi, and fluids, and blood stasis. This string of development could also be initiated by emotional stress causing liver Qi stagnation, bypassing pathogenic invasion stage.

Repeat assaults by acute gastritis could inflict injury to the stomach, transforming the condition from an excess-state to deficient-state syndrome or chronic gastritis. In a deficient-state, chronic gastritis would manifest symptoms of stomach Yin-deficiency 胃阴虚 and gastroparesis 脾胃虚寒.

The treatment of acute gastritis is predicated on the overarching principle of regulating Qi 理气 to restore stomach homeostasis 和胃 thereby achieving pain relief. This is based on the basic TCM tenet that unblocking obstruction to Qi circulation is key to pain relief 通则不痛. The Qi mechanism may be obstructed in many instances — by cold consolidation 寒凝, phlegm accumulation, food stagnation, blood stasis, and damp-heat. Warming the stomach to dispel cold, resolving phlegm accumulation, improving digestion, promoting blood circulation and clearing heat are various options to unblock obstructed Qi. In the application of these options, however, one should be mindful of Ye Tianshi's 叶天士 admonition "to avoid extremity but adopt moderation 忌刚用柔".

In deficient-state chronic gastritis, the rule of thumb is to reinforce the vital energy, re-build the constituent and promote strength with the aim to eliminate pathogenic factors. Warming the Qi and nourishing the yin to benefit the stomach is an indispensable therapeutic strategy for this condition.

Gua Sha Protocol for Adjuvant Therapy and Symptomatic Relief

Treatment for gastritis requires reducing inflammation of the stomach mucosa. Neutralization of the irritant is more effective when the intervention is exercised close to the source of irritation. In this regard, consumed medication, mainstream or otherwise, may be preferred over external intervention. Notwithstanding, *Gua Sha* can still provide symptomatic relief and may be used in conjunction with any other forms of treatment.

a. Trapezius Sweep
b. Para-Vertebral Sweep (T1-T12)
c. Superior Bladder Meridian Dredge (T1-T12)
d. Epigastric-Umbilicus Sweep
e. Umbilicus-Pubic Sweep
f. Acupoint 'press-and-hold' for SP4 公孙, SP6 三阴交 and ST36 足三里 on both legs
g. Additional for Acute Gastritis — Acupoint 'press-and-hold' for PC6 内关 on both arms
h. Additional for Chronic Gastritis — Acupoint 'press-and-hold' for LR3 太冲 on both legs

Execution — Moderation press-stroke recommended. Acupoints marked for application of 'press-and-hold' technique in each prescription form a set, each set to be repeated three times.

'Press-and-hold' maneuver should be attempted 10 times for each prescribed acupoint within each set. Use of skin lubricant with herbs having Qi invigorating properties preferred. Observation of *Sha* appearance is not mandatory.

Other Considerations — Recurrent gastritis should be tested for *H. pylori* infection.

> **Glossary**
>
> Gastroparesis is a disorder that occurs when the stomach takes too long to empty food.

References

1. Maes ML, *et al.* Adverse effects of proton-pump inhibitor use in older adults: a review of the evidence. *Ther. Adv. Drug Saf.* **8**(9): 273–297 (Sep 2017).
2. Sax MJ. Clinically important adverse effects and drug interactions with H2-receptor antagonists: An update *Pharmacotherapy* **7**(6 Pt 2): 110S–115S (1987).

TOPIC 45

Gastro-Esophageal Reflux Disease

Gastro-Esophageal Reflux Disease (GERD) occurs when two medical conditions coexist — acid reflux caused by a retrograde flow of acidic stomach contents into the esophagus and a lower esophageal sphincter (LES) malfunction.

Reflux, however, does not necessarily lead to GERD symptoms or histologic changes and can occur among healthy individuals especially obese people and pregnant ladies in their late trimesters. This is known as physiologic gastroesophageal reflux.

The LES is a 4-cm ring of strong muscle that acts as a one-way valve between the esophagus and the stomach. When the LES relaxes abnormally or malfunctions and does not close perfectly, stomach contents well up into the esophagus under pressure of the gastric distention, motility and emptying. The severity of GERD depends on the severity of LES dysfunction as well as the type and amount of gastric content being brought up from the stomach and the neutralizing effect of saliva.

A hiatal hernia may weaken the LES and therefore increases the risk for GERD. Hiatal hernia occurs when the upper part of the stomach moves up into the chest through the diaphragmatic hiatus. The diaphragm is the muscle separating the abdomen from the chest and the opening in the diaphragm helps support the lower end of the esophagus. Hiatal hernia is usually asymptomatic but predisposes the individual to acid reflux as it may allow stomach contents to reflux more easily into the esophagus.

Acid reflux or heartburn is the most prominent symptom of GERD but sporadic episodes of acid reflux do not count towards GERD. GERD is usually experienced as a persistent, at least twice a week mild heartburn or a weekly moderate to severe heartburn. Heartburn is the burning sensation in the chest that often radiates towards the throat, caused by retrograde stomach contents touching the lining of the esophagus. This constant acidic backwash irritates the sensitive esophageal lining causing it to become inflamed and scarred. Lying down or bending over may instigate heartburn. In this regard, night-time reflux is more damaging than if it occurred during the day as the individual may not be aware of the reflux and took no step to neutralize the condition while asleep.

The symptoms of GERD are often so classic and characteristic that it can be identified in a clinical diagnosis, i.e. clinicians can confidently make a diagnosis based on symptoms alone.

Aside from food regurgitation and sensation of a lump or tightness in the throat, GERD sufferers may also experience other symptoms depending on how far the acidic content is carried into and up the esophagus. When refluxed gastric acid is aspirated, it may cause dry coughing, persistent sore throat, morning hoarseness, voice changes, sinusitis, asthma or even pneumonia. Dysphagia (difficulty in swallowing), a sensation of food stuck in the throat, burning chest pain or nausea could be signs of disease progression including erosive esophagitis, esophageal ulceration or even esophageal cancer that is usually preceded by Barrett's esophagus, a condition that manifest by a histological change in the esophageal lining.

The treatment of GERD takes three forms: surgery, medical therapy and holistic therapy, including dietary and lifestyle changes and the intake of specific herbal supplements. The surgical option is a major consideration as it may aggravate certain existing conditions such as stricture and motility disorders. Medical treatment of GERD includes Proton Primer Inhibitors, H2 blockers, and antacids. These pharmaceuticals are very similar to those prescribed for gastritis. While acid reflux may be alleviated temporarily by taking any or all of these prescription medications, the reader should be mindful of the adverse effects when used on a protracted basis. (please refer to Gastritis topic).

In most cases, GERD can be relieved with over-the-counter medication and through diet and lifestyle changes. Avoidance of certain foods like chocolate, peppermint, greasy and spicy food, alcohols and those that irritate damaged esophageal lining and weaken the LES is often recommended to reduce the incidence of GERD episodes. Smoking is found to have a role in weakening or relaxing the LES. Along with dietary changes, practicing disciplined eating habits like portion size control, regular meals and not eating hours before bedtime may reduce reflux. Losing weight, avoid lying down or bending over after meals can also be part of the holistic regimen to minimize recurrence.

From a TCM perspective...

Retrograde flow of gastric content is caused by loss of gastric homeostasis 胃失和降 that may be aggravated by the invasion of external pathogens, especially from damp-heat. This is first mentioned in 'Plain Questions 素問' that acidic reflux and diarrhea are caused by entrapped heat.

In terms of flavor-organ connection, acidity 酸 is associated with the liver. Liver belongs to the wood element under the Five Element 五行 Theory and the growth and development of the liver-wood need to be cultivated by the middle earth 中土 or the 'Spleen' 脾. Dampness of the middle earth causes the liver wood Qi 肝木 to not rise, and the entrapped liver Qi is transformed into heat. In addition, the damp-heat in the middle energizer 中焦湿热 will also disrupt the normal functions of the stomach, giving rise to acid reflux.

Thus, GERD may originate from dysfunctional stomach and esophagus but is closely related to the proper functioning of the liver, gallbladder, and spleen. If the relationships and functions of these organs are not harmoniously coordinated as in having hepatobiliary stagnation 肝胆疏泄不利 and/or spleen weakness, homeostasis of the stomach shall be impinged and GERD results. This, therefore, becomes the basis of GERD treatment. In the final analysis, TCM reckons the disorder as an intra-systemic interruption that shall be fixed by addressing not only the dysfunctional organ system but the larger system holistically.

Gua Sha Protocol for Adjuvant Therapy and Symptomatic Relief

a. Sternal Sweep
b. Epigastric-Umbilicus Sweep
c. Superior Bladder Meridian Dredge (T7-T12)
d. Acupoint 'press-and-hold' for ST36 足三里, ST40 丰隆, SP8 地机, GB34 阳陵泉 on both legs

Execution — Moderation press-stroke recommended. Acupoints marked for application of 'press-and-hold' technique in each prescription form a set, each set to be repeated three times. 'Press-and-hold' maneuver should be attempted 10 times for each prescribed acupoint within each set. Use of skin lubricant with herbs having Qi invigorating properties preferred. Observation of *Sha* appearance is not mandatory.

Other considerations — Apart from deploying *Gua Sha* therapy in relieving GERD symptomatically, individuals suffering from the disorder are advised to sleep on the left side of the body and preferably with the head of the bed raised.

Glossary

Barrett's esophagus is a condition of irreversible histological changes found in the esophagus. Though a significant precursor (100 times more likely to develop) to esophageal cancer, fewer than 1% progressed to malignancy.

Erosive Esophagitis is the inflammation and swelling of the esophagus.

Esophageal stricture is the gradual narrowing of the esophagus that can lead to swallowing difficulties.

Topic 46

Globus Pharyngeus/Globus Hystericus

Globus Hystericus is an age-old yet common disorder of indeterminate origin first identified by Hippocrates some 2000 years ago. Patients commonly describe it as a sensation of a lump, retained food bolus or tightness in the throat accentuated by an urge to swallow and the discomfort does not impede but disappears completely during eating or drinking. Statistically, the condition is slightly biased towards afflicting the female gender; in the proportions of men and women at 35% and 53% respectively.[1]

The name Globus Hystericus assumed a psychological component associated with the disorder; which is not erroneous as up to 95% of individuals with Globus Hystericus reported symptom onset or exacerbation during periods of high emotional intensity and the discomfort disappeared with some form of emotional release (e.g. after crying).[1,2]

The disorder was however renamed Globus Pharyngeus and more recently being defined as (i) a persistent or intermittent non-painful sensation of a lump or foreign body in the throat for at least 12 weeks, (ii) occurrence of the sensation between meals, (iii) absence of dysphagia and odynophagia, (iv) absence of pathological gastroesophageal reflux (GERD), (v) absence of histopathology-based esophageal motility disorders.[3]

As pain is often indicative of a localized structural disorder, the lack of pain in Globus Pharyngeus makes it distinctly a functional disorder unrelated to any anatomical abnormality. But the etiology of Globus Pharyngeus remains uncertain and indeterminate.

Many factors, including cricopharyngeal spasm, lingual tonsil, cervical osteophytosis, hiatus hernia, gastroesophageal reflux, sinusitis, postnasal drip, goiter, foreign body, anxiety, and hypopharyngeal cancer, have been postulated to cause the Globus symptoms but at time of writing, none has been proven conclusively.

Among the suggested factors, the closest association drawn however was that half the individuals with Globus sensation are reported to have proximal acid exposure secondary to GERD. Clinicians are therefore led to postulate that Globus sensation is associated with acid reflux in the esophagus stimulating a vagal reflex to produce the sensation or, in the alternative, when the refluxate passes into the larynx, the mucosa of the larynx could be damaged leading to a similar sensation. But this inference is not fully supported by clinical outcomes in that proton pump inhibitor (PPI) therapy, the gold standard of treatment for GERD, often delivers disappointing results.[4]

Although the etiology of Globus Pharyngeus relating to laryngopharyngeal reflux (LPR) remains controversial, the *de facto* therapeutic strategy for individuals suffering from Globus sensation suspicious of GERD is still aggressive treatment with PPI twice daily for at least three months.[5] Lest the *de facto* treatment yields little improvement, Rikkunshito, a traditional Japanese herbal concoction widely used to treat GERD and dyspepsia, could improve Globus sensation in patients with PPI-resistant LPR.[6] Rikkunshito's effective components that stimulate gastric emptying are akin to a combined TCM prescription of 半夏泻心汤 and 半夏厚朴汤 used for the same purpose.

To date, Globus Pharyngeus is known to be a multifactorial disease with no single effective treatment despite its common clinical symptom. With symptoms persisting up to three years in 75% of patients, prospects for prompt symptomatic relief can be remote. Given the benign nature of the condition, the likelihood of long-term symptom persistence, and the absence of effective pharmacotherapy, the mainstay of present treatment rests with explanation and reassurance.[3]

From a TCM perspective...

Globus Hystericus/Pharyngeus 梅核气 is known since the ancient times and is well documented in the Internal Classic 内经, the Treatise on Febrile and Miscellaneous Diseases 伤寒杂病论 and the Treatise on Causes and Symptoms of Diseases 诸病源候论. The clinical manifestations recorded is a subjective sensation of a plum-pit like foreign body being stuck in the throat that can neither be spat out nor swallowed but does not impede eating and has no positive localized findings.

The etiology of Globus Hystericus is due to dysfunction of the spleen in transformation and transportation of nutrients leading to the Qi stagnation, dampness accumulation, and phlegm formation in this order. It is further observed the onset of Globus Hystericus is generally instigated by significant and unresolved emotional incidents that compromise the spleen function 忧思伤脾 whilst causing the liver function to be suppressed, ensuing in liver Qi stagnation 肝气郁结. What then follows is Liver Qi retrogrades 肝气上逆, rising up to and accumulating at the pharynx. At this initial stage, the Globus sensation would only be mild discomfort.

Protracted liver Qi stagnation may, in turn, aggravate the condition of a dysfunctional spleen 肝木侮土, 乘脾犯胃 causing the general Qi mechanism to be occluded, resulting in dampness accumulation and formation of phlegm 津聚为痰; the phlegm blending inextricably with the rising liver Qi 痰气交阻 to coalesce and accumulate at the pharynx. Now that the rising liver Qi is presented with some tangible pathogenic by-product, the Globus sensation would be more pronounced.

The principle of the treatment, therefore, is to regulate the liver Qi, fortify the spleen function and resolve the accumulated phlegm. This is achieved through selected acupoints from the Liver, Spleen, Stomach, Kidney meridians and Conception Vessel. In particular, it would be instructional to note that the combination of LI4 合谷 and LR3 太冲 termed the four-gate point selection 四关穴 has an excellent effect on Qi and blood regulation/decongestion.

Gua Sha Protocol for Treatment and Symptomatic Relief

a. Occipital-Cervical Sweep
b. Sternal Sweep with emphasis on CV17 膻中 and CV22 天突 using acupoint 'press-and-hold' technique
c. Clavicular Sweep
d. Shoulder Sweep
e. Trapezius Sweep
f. Acupoint 'press-and-hold' for LI4 合谷, PC6 内关, HT7 神门, LU7 列缺 on both hands
g. Acupoint 'press-and-hold' for ST36 足三里, ST40 丰隆, SP6 三阴交, KI3 太溪, KI6 照海, LR3 太冲 for both legs

Execution — Unless TCM diagnosis suggests otherwise, moderation press-stroke recommended. Acupoints marked for application of 'press-and-hold' technique in each prescription form a set, each set to be repeated three times. 'Press-and-hold' maneuver should be attempted 10 times for each prescribed acupoint within each set. Use of skin lubricant that invigorates Qi and dispels blood stasis preferred. Observation of Sha appearance not mandatory.

Glossary

Dysphagia refers to difficulty or discomfort in swallowing whereas Odynophagia refers to pain during swallowing. Dysphagia can manifest without Odynophagia (dysfunction without pain) and Odynophagia may also occur without dysphagia (pain without dysfunction) or both conditions may occur concurrently.

Rikkunshito comprises of 8 ingredients: Glycyrrhizae radix 甘草(4.7%), Zingiberis rhizoma 干姜(2.3%), Ginseng radix 人参(18.6%), Pinelliae tuber 半夏(18.6%) Hoelen or Poria 茯苓(18.6%), Atractylodis lanceae rhizoma 苍术(18.6%), Zizyphi fructus 枸杞子(9.3%) and Aurantii nobilis pericarpium 枳壳(9.3%). Its effective components are akin to the combined TCM prescription of 半夏泻心汤 and 半夏厚朴汤 used for the same purpose.

References

1. Thompson WG, Heaton KW. Heartburn and Globus in apparently healthy people. *Can. Med. Assoc. J.* **126**: 46–48 (1982).

2. Moser G, *et al.* Globus sensation: pharyngoesophageal function, psychometric and psychiatric findings, and follow-up in 88 patients. *Arch. Intern. Med.* **158**(12): 1365–1373 (1998).
3. Galmiche JP, Clouse RE, B´alint A, *et al.* Functional esophageal disorders. *Gastroenterology* **130**(5): 1459–1465 (2006).
4. Manabe N, Tsutsui H, Kusunoki H, *et al.* Pathophysiology and treatment of patients with globus sensation — from the viewpoint of esophageal motility dysfunction. *J. Smooth Muscle Res.* **50**: 66–77 (2014).
5. Lee BE, Kim GH. Globus pharyngeus: a review of its etiology, diagnosis and treatment. *World J. Gastroenterol.* **18**(20): 2462–2471 (May 28, 2012).
6. Tokashiki R, Okamoto I, Funato N, *et al.* Rikkunshito improves globus sensation in patients with proton-pump inhibitor-refractory laryngopharyngeal reflux. *World J. Gastroenterol.* **19**(31): 5118–5124 (Aug 21, 2013).

Topic 47

Rectal Prolapse

Rectal prolapse is a condition in which part or all of the wall of the rectum loses its normal attachments inside the body, allowing it to slide out of place and through the anus, thereby exposing the inside walls outwards. There are three types of rectal prolapse.

Partial prolapse or mucosal prolapse is when the lining or mucous membrane of the rectum slides out of place and remains outside of the anus. This may happen while exerting during a difficult bowel movement. The protrusion may be physically returned to its place after a bowel movement.

In a complete prolapse, the entire wall of the rectum slides out of place and usually outside of the anus. Initially, this may occur only during bowel movements but left untreated it may eventually slide out every time an upright posture (standing or walking) is adopted. In severe cases, the prolapsed tissue could remain outside the body permanently.

In internal prolapse or intussusception, part of the wall of the large intestine (colon) or rectum may slide into or over another part, like a Chinese sleeve. The rectum, however, remains inside of the anus. Intussusception rarely afflicts adults but when happens it is usually related to some other intestinal issue like polyps or tumor. More common in children though, the cause of intussusception is usually unknown.

The progression in rectal prolapse tends to be gradual, with the prolapse initially descending during bowel movement before returning to its normal position. As the prolapse worsens, the individual may feel heaviness and obstruction in the anus until the prolapse is pushed back manually. In severe cases, a section of the large intestine may descend from its normal position when the tissues holding it in place stretched out. Anatomically, the anorectal flexure is a sharp bend where the rectum meets the anal canal with a purpose of preventing fecal incontinence. With rectal prolapse, this bend and other curves in the rectum may straighten, making it difficult to maintain stool from leaking out.

Another reason for fecal incontinence is when the prolapse descends beyond the anal sphincter, a muscular structure that aids bowel continence. The internal anal sphincter involuntarily contracts to prevent leakage of flatus or feces and a prolapse beyond this sphincter allows stools and mucus to pass uncontrollably.

Pudendal nerve injury is also presented in many prolapse cases. The pudendal nerve contributes to anal sphincter control and its damage can result from direct trauma (birthing injury), back injury or even surgery. An anal sphincter that is constantly stretched by the prolapse itself becomes incompetent and is a risk factor for fecal incontinence.

On the contrary, constipation may also be presented with prolapse as a result of the bunching up of the rectum, creating a blockage that is aggravated with straining, generalized pelvic floor coordination issues and problems with colonic peristalsis that increase the transit rate of stools. For this reason, individuals with rectal prolapse may experience both bouts of constipation and incontinence.

Other symptoms of rectal prolapse often include frequent urges to defecate and a feeling of not being able to completely evacuate bowels, the passage of small stools, anal pain, itching, and irritation. With the passage of time, prolapsed rectal mucosa becomes thickened, ulcerated and causes significant bleeding. Rarely does a prolapse becomes stuck or "incarcerated" outside the anus; a situation that could warrant surgery. Often time, rectal prolapse may be confused with significant hemorrhoid disease.

While rectal prolapse may be uncomfortable, embarrassing and has a significant negative impact on the individual's quality of life, it is rarely life-threatening. Although surgery is not always required, the definitive treatment of and permanent solution for serious rectal prolapse is surgery. Untreated rectal prolapse, however, does not develop into cancer.

Individuals duly diagnosed with rectal prolapse may choose to passively observe its development. Choosing to do nothing may however cause the prolapse to aggravate over time and recur more easily and frequently. Delayed treatment, without having a prolapse repaired, increases the likelihood of permanent fecal incontinence. As the anal sphincter is repeatedly stretched out, it becomes progressively incompetent and raises the chance of nerve damage. Notwithstanding, when the prolapse is small or the individual's physical condition is not conducive for surgery, the use of supportive garments may be useful in reducing the incidence of prolapse and therefore deferring its progression.

From a TCM perspective...

Organ prolapse, in general, is caused by the collapse or sinking of the Qi in the Middle Energizer 中焦气陷, where the significant organs are the spleen and stomach. This can be frequently observed in malnutritional children having insufficient Qi and blood, in the elderly with declining Qi and blood or deficiency of Qi in the Middle Energizer, in women exhausted by childbirth resulting in a deficiency of Qi and blood, and in those suffering from chronic diarrhea, habitual constipation, and chronic cough.

In TCM the spleen system dominates the state of musculature 脾主肌肉. In its normal state, the Spleen Qi rises upwards, constantly nourishes and provides support to the musculature. As all internal organs within the body cavity are secured in their normal positions by smooth muscles, weakness in these smooth muscles will cause the organs to be gradually displaced downwards under the influence of gravity.

TCM, therefore, treats any organ prolapse organs with the same therapeutic principle — elevating the Qi of Middle Energizer by tonifying the spleen and promoting Qi and Yang energy. Elevating spleen Qi can, therefore, lift prolapsed organs. Beside elevating 升提 Qi, there is also a need to reinforce 固涩 the ascending Qi for sustained therapeutic efficacy.

Gua Sha Protocol for Adjuvant Therapy and Symptomatic Relief

a. Four Spirit Extension
b. Sternal Sweep
c. Ventral Intercostal Space Sweep
d. Umbilicus-Pubic Sweep
e. Back Rejuvenation Dredge
f. Sacral V Dredge
g. Acupoint 'press-and-hold' for ST36 足三里, BL57 承山 on both legs
h. Acupoint 'press-and-hold' for LI11 曲池, TE6 支沟 on both hands

Execution — Moderation press-stroke recommended. Acupoints marked for application of 'press-and-hold' technique in each prescription form a set, each set to be repeated three times. 'Press-and-hold' maneuver should be attempted 10 times for each prescribed acupoint within each set. Use of skin lubricant with herbs having Qi invigorating properties preferred. Observation of *Sha* appearance is not mandatory.

Other considerations — there is minimal risk in attempting to restore a prolapsed rectum but one should not force the situation if it does not return to its normal place. Avoid constipation by appropriate hydration and maintaining a diet containing adequate fiber. Often, dietary modification is adequate in bringing about an improvement or even reverse a prolapse of the lining of the rectum (partial prolapse). Avoid straining during bowel movement and, if necessary, use a laxative or stool softener. Retrain and reinforce the pelvic musculature by performing Kegel exercise regularly.

Gynecological

Topic 48

Amenorrhea/Absence of Menstruation

Amenorrhea, the absence of menstrual bleeding, is normal in prepubertal, pregnant, and post-menopausal females. In females of reproductive age, amenorrhea is often a symptom of another health problem, potential or otherwise, and can happen for many reasons. There are two different types of amenorrhea.

Primary amenorrhea is the failure of menarche (first menstrual bleeding) in the absence of puberty by age 13 or with development of normal growth and secondary sexual characteristics by age 16.

Secondary amenorrhea is defined as the cessation of menses sometime after menarche has occurred. Because a menstrual cycle in excess of 90 days is statistically abnormal in a reproductive female, individuals should be evaluated for secondary amenorrhea if menses have been absent for more than three months or three typical cycles.

Although some variation in menstruation is acceptable for women of childbearing age, menstrual periods that extend regularly beyond 35 days should be diagnosed as oligomenorrhea. A consensus is yet to be reached by the medical community regarding the point at which oligomenorrhea may be recognized as amenorrhea.

For most reproductive female, menstruation is a fairly regular and predictable event spanning between 21 to 35 days from the first day of the period to the first day of the following period. This occurs when the lining of the uterus, the endometrium, has primed itself for a possible pregnancy by becoming thicker and richer in blood vessels. However, when an egg released by the ovary remains unfertilized, the endometrium that did not receive implantation is sloughed, accompanied by bleeding in preparation for another cycle. The bleeding or menses usually lasts for three to eight days.

A menstrual cycle can be divided into three physiologic phases: follicular, ovulatory, and luteal with each phase being associated with distinct hormonal secretion.

The follicular phase spans 13 days, from the first day of menses, is characterized by the release of follicle-stimulating hormone (FSH) by the pituitary glands, which is in turn triggered by gonadotropin-releasing hormone (GnRH) released by the hypothalamus. FSH causes the ovary to produce a single matured egg from maturing follicles and in the process also delivers high levels of estrogen that stimulate and proliferate uterine endometrial growth (after menstruation is over). The production of estrogen peaks just before the end of the follicular phase but commences declining at ovulation. The presence of estrogen further stimulates the production of GnRH causing the pituitary gland to secrete luteinizing hormone (LH). The surges in LH and FSH cause the egg to be released from the follicle.

The ovulation phase happens on about Day 14 with the release of the matured egg resulting from the onset of LH and FSH surges over the previous day. LH and FSH levels however peak and then decline during the ovulation phase. The released egg from the follicle enters the fallopian tube where fertilization may take place. Once the egg is released, the follicle seals up and becomes the corpus luteum that produces estrogen and progesterone. The matured egg, however, disintegrates after about 24 hours, if no fertilization occurred.

In a normal menstrual period, the luteal phase sets in after ovulation from after about Day 14 when the corpus luteum declines in function over a duration of about 11 days. The corpus luteum, however, continues to produce progesterone which prevents the endometrial lining from being shed. If no fertilization occurred, the corpus luteum disintegrates, which causes progesterone levels to drop and signals the endometrial lining to slough, commencing the next menstrual cycle.

From the foregoing, menarche and sustained menstrual cycles require normal functioning of the endocrine Hypothalamus-Pituitary-Gonads (HPG) axis. Any disruption in this HPG axis may result in amenorrhea and identifying the point of dysfunction along this axis or pipeline is critical in determining the pathophysiology of amenorrhea. When part of this system malfunctions, ovulatory dysfunction occurs and menstruation may not occur; resulting in anovulatory amenorrhea. Most amenorrhea, particularly secondary amenorrhea, is anovulatory.

A common cause of amenorrhea, particularly secondary amenorrhea, is functional hypothalamic amenorrhea, characterized by abnormal hypothalamic GnRH secretion, decreased gonadotropin pulsations, depressed FSH and LH concentrations, abnormal follicular development, and low serum estradiol.

There are three types of functional hypothalamic amenorrhea — weight loss-related, exercise-related and stress-related amenorrhea. These conditions can be caused by eating disorders, excessive physical exercise, (competitive athletes) and prolonged mental stress including major psychiatric disorders. A correlation appears to exist between low body fat levels and menstrual abnormalities suggesting that a threshold body fat level must be present for normal functioning of the reproductive system. Endocrine disorders and severe chronic medical conditions may also result in amenorrhea.

Pituitary amenorrhea is characterized by hypogonadotropic hypogonadism that causes loss of LH and FSH. Three etiologies for this condition are genetic diseases that stall gonadotropins production (e.g. Turner syndrome, emochromatosis), hypopituitary states and pituitary tumors.

Hypopituitary states may arise from autoimmune or granulomatous pituitary destruction, traumatic brain injury or pituitary atrophy.

Tumors may constrict the pituitary and prevent normal LH and FSH release. Prolactin-secreting pituitary adenomas (prolactinoma) can compress the pituitary stalk and induce hyperprolactinemia which suppresses LH and FSH, leading to amenorrhea. Prolactinoma is the most common pituitary benign tumor that causes persistent hyperprolactinemia and is frequently noted in secondary amenorrhea.

All told, pituitary dysfunction should be suspected in anyone with a pituitary lesion, granulomatous brain disease, traumatic brain injury, brain surgery or irradiation, congenital craniofacial abnormalities, unexplained gonadal dysfunction, and previous pregnancy-associated hemorrhage.

The gonad or the ovary plays a central role in the production of female sex hormones, estrogen, progesterone, and testosterone. Gonadal dysgenesis is characterized by congenital defective development of germ cells in the gonad during organogenesis, with the gonad's reproductive tissue being replaced with functionless, fibrous tissue (streak gonads). The most common form of gonadal dysgenesis in females is Turner syndrome (45, X). Turner syndrome, with loss of a chromosome, causes depletion of ovarian follicles invariably leads to amenorrhea.

Spontaneous Primary Ovarian Insufficiency (POI) or premature ovarian failure is hypergonadotropic hypogonadism, characterized by oligomenorrhea, estrogen deficiency, and symptoms associated premature menopause such as hot flashes, vaginal dryness, dyspareunia, and insomnia. POI is another condition afflicting woman before the age of 40 that results in amenorrhea.

Polycystic Ovarian Syndrome (PCOS), an endocrine disorder associated with excessive androgen production, is perhaps the most common cause for secondary amenorrhea, but in some cases may be presented as primary amenorrhea.

Sometimes, amenorrhea can occur even under conditions of normal hormonal functioning (ovulatory amenorrhea). Anatomical abnormalities of the female reproductive tract, congenital or otherwise, can prevent the appearance of menses and result in amenorrhea. Developmental abnormalities that cause outflow obstruction, like imperforate hymen and vaginal septum, create perirectal mass by pooling menstrual blood in the vagina (hematocolpos) or accumulation of blood in the uterus (hematometra) often give rise to cyclic pelvic pain common in girls with such disorders.

Congenital anatomic abnormalities cause only primary amenorrhea. All disorders that cause secondary amenorrhea can cause primary amenorrhea. Acquired anatomic abnormalities, such as endometrial scarring/adhesion after instrumentation for postpartum hemorrhage or infection (Asherman syndrome), cause secondary ovulatory amenorrhea.

From a TCM perspective...

Reproductive development in the female is quite similar to the views held by contemporary biomedicine. In the book 'HuangDi's Internal Classics — Plain Questions'[1] the female reproductive development cycle is segmented into distinct periods of seven years. It reads:

At age 7, the Kidney Qi abounds causing the [first] teeth to be substituted and the hair grows long.

At age 14, the *Heavenly Gui* 天癸 arrives, the Conception Vessel 任脉 becomes patent and the Great Thoroughfare Vessel 太冲脉 becomes abound with Qi. The monthly affair [menstruation] appears in due time and thus a woman may bear children.

At age 21, the Qi of the Kidneys reaches its normal level; hence, the wisdom teeth emerge and females reach their full sexual maturity.

At age 28, the sinews and bones are firm and the hair has grown to its full extent. The body and the limbs are in a state of abundance and strength.

At age 35, the Rising Yang Meridian [Stomach Meridian] weakens; the face commences to lose its luster and the hair begin to shed.

At age 42, the three Yang vessel types weaken where they converge at the head, causing the face to parch and the hair to turn white.

At age 49, the Conception Vessel becomes depleted and the Great Thoroughfare Vessel weakened with its contents diminished. Thus, the *Heaven Gui* is exhausted [menopause], the process of menstruation becomes unavailable. Hence, the physical appearance languishes and a woman can no longer bear children.

The factors identified in the above that impact the female reproductive development are Kidney Qi, Heavenly Gui, the Conception

Vessel, Great Thoroughfare Vessel, and the three Yang vessel types, in particular, the Stomach Meridian. Great Thoroughfare Vessel refers to the combination of Penetrating or Thrusting Vessel 冲脉 and the Kidney Meridian 肾经 with both meridians crossing at KI21 幽门. The Penetrating Vessel also made its crossing with the Stomach Meridian at ST30 气冲.

The word 'heavenly' has a congenital connotation and 'gui' is a character from the Five-element 五行 Theory representing Ying water that is closely associated with the Kidney system, in particularly the kidney essence. Above all, the teaching states 'heavenly gui' is the driver of reproductive development and physical growth, an agent of reproductive sustainability in both gender and its progressive depletion reflects physiological aging. In terms of location, it appears that the exhaustion of 'heavenly gui' is concentrated at the head where the Yang meridians converge, commencing with the Stomach Meridian whose physiological condition reflects the abundance of Qi and blood or otherwise. Given its functional description and locational references (head to kidney essence), the 'heavenly gui' closely corresponds to the Hypothalamus-Pituitary-Gonad (HPG) axis.

The functions of the Penetrating Vessel 冲脉 can be summarized as "the sea of the 12 Meridians 十二经之海", "the sea of internal organs 五脏六腑之海" and "the sea of blood 血海". By saying "the sea of the 12 Meridians" it emphasizes the importance of the Vessel in the passage and distribution of Qi among the 12 Meridians. This Vessel, the Governor Vessel (GV) and the Conception Vessel (CV) originate from a deep-seated point 下丹田 posterior to CV6 气海 before branching out from the perineum CV1 会阴. That all Yang meridians in the body converge on the Governor Vessel (GV) 阳脉之海 and all Yin meridians in the body converge on the Conception Vessel (CV) 阴脉之海, the Penetrating Vessel provides a rendezvous for the two meridians, GV and CV, and indirectly for the 12 meridians, at which Qi flow be coordinated and rebalanced throughout the body. By the same corollary, this same network with the Penetrating Vessel in its central role serves to distribute Qi and essence, both innate and acquired, 先天、后天精气 to all vital organs, thus giving this Vessel its appellation "the sea of internal organs".

Because the Penetrating Vessel connects with and regulates both the Kidney (KI) and Stomach (ST) meridians, it ensures the adequacy of blood in the body. In TCM, the Kidney is the foundation of innate strength 先天之本 and the root of nascent Qi 原气之根. The Kidney is also known to store vital essence 肾藏精 that can readily be converted into blood 精化血, a notion that corresponds to the biomedical theory of erythropoiesis.

The Stomach, on the other hand, is the source of acquired strength 后天之本 and the powerhouse of nutrition 水谷之海. The ability of the Penetrating Vessel in coordinating these organs functionally allows it to control the timely and adequate production of blood in the body. For this reason, the Penetrating Vessel is labeled "the sea of blood". Make no mistake that the Penetrating Vessel is not itself a production house for blood but provides the essential signals and messages to the organ-systems to ensure blood supply adequacy.

The appellation "sea of blood" for the Vessel has special significance with reproductive functions. In the 'Annotations to Plain Questions', Wang Bing 王冰 noted that "only when the Penetrating Vessel delivers its role as the Sea of Blood and in concert with the Conception Vessel exerting its dominance over the gonads that conception may occur 冲为血海，任主胞胎，两者相资，故能有子".

From the foregoing, it can be appreciated that fundamental principle in the treatment of female reproductive disorders is in the rectification of blood and Qi deficiencies through tonification and promotion of the Kidney Qi and essence, and making appropriate adjustments to the Penetrating Vessel and the Conception Meridian. Organ-systems are the biochemical factories for Qi and blood; meridians are the messaging pathways that interconnect these organ-systems. It is therefore essential to treat the disorder holistically by involving the relevant systems — kidney, liver, spleen, and stomach.

Gua Sha Protocol for Adjuvant Therapy and Symptomatic Relief

Gua Sha is not a suitable therapy for ovulatory amenorrhea arising out of outflow obstruction that may only be resolved by surgical intervention. *Gua Sha* may also not be appropriate for primary anovulatory amenorrhea where the loss of function is caused by pituitary destruction. It is, however, useful in the relief of secondary amenorrhea.

a. Occipital-Cervical Sweep
b. Back Rejuvenation Sweep with emphasis on BL 20 脾俞 and BL 23 肾俞
c. Sacral V Dredge
d. Umbilicus-Pubic Sweep
e. Spleen Meridian Dredge (SP1-SP10) with emphasis on SP6 三阴交, SP8 地机, SP9 阴陵泉, SP10 血海 using acupoint 'press-and-hold' technique
f. Acupoint 'press-and-hold' for ST29 归来, BL17 膈俞 and BL18 肝俞 bilaterally on the torso
g. Acupoint 'press-and-hold' for ST36 足三里, ST40 丰隆 and LR2 行间 on both legs
h. Acupoint 'press-and-hold' for PC6 内关 on both hands

Execution — Moderation press-stroke recommended. Acupoints marked for application of 'press-and-hold' technique in each prescription form a set, each set to be repeated three times. 'Press-and-hold' maneuver should be attempted 10 times for each prescribed acupoint within each set. Use of skin lubricant with herbs having Qi invigorating, blood tonification and dispersal of blood stasis properties preferred. Observation of Sha appearance is not mandatory.

Other Considerations — Gua Sha practitioner should be mindful that a common cause of amenorrhea is pregnancy. It is therefore prudent and mandatory to obtain a confirmation from the patient before attempting any related procedure.

Glossary

Anovulatory means absence of ovulation.

Estradiol (E2) is one of the three main naturally occurring forms of estrogen in females. The other two are estrone (E1) and estriol (E3).

Hypergonadotropic hypogonadism (HH) is a condition which is characterized by diminished functional activity of the gonads — the testes or the ovaries, due to an impaired response of the gonads to the gonadotropins, follicle-stimulating hormone (FSH) and luteinizing hormone (LH), and in turn a lack of sex steroid production and elevated gonadotropin levels.

Organogenesis [organ genesis = beginning of organ] is the phase of embryonic development that starts at the end of gastrulation and continues until birth.

Dyspareunia is difficult or painful sexual intercourse.

Vessel is another term for and is synonymous with the word Meridian. In this book, the author has made a slight distinction in reserving 'meridian' for naming pathways of the 12 principal meridians and name pathways of the 8 extraordinary meridians as 'vessels'.

Erythropoiesis is the generation of red blood cells (erythrocytes), stimulated by decreased oxygen in circulation detected by the kidneys which then secrete the hormone erythropoietin that acts on bone marrows.

Reference

1. Unshuld P, Tessenow H. Discourse on the true [Qi endowed by] Heaven in high antiquity. *Huang Di Nei Jing Su Wen*, Vol. 1. Berkeley & Los Angeles: University of California Press (2011), pp. 37–44. 《黄帝内经 素问. 上古天真论》

Topic 49

Abnormal Discharge

The vagina is a natural access from outside the body to the uterus and the rest of the internal reproductive system, and in fact into the peritoneum. The vagina is also a dynamic and complex ecosystem which bacterial composition exists in a defined environment of acidity and moisture to form the vaginal microbiome. This environment is sensitive to changes coming from outside of the body and from within.

Fluid secreted by glands inside the vagina and cervix that carry away sloughed epithelial cells and bacteria make up normal vaginal discharge. Secreted under the influence of the female hormones, it helps cleanse the vagina, keep it lubricated as well as free from ascending infection and other germs not part of the microbiome. For this reason, menopausal women normally having minimal vaginal discharge have a higher incidence of infections. Vaginal discharge is not usually noticeable until it exits the vagina.

Vaginal discharge may be evaluated from three attributes — volume, color and consistency, and odor.

In premenopausal women, it is normal to expect about 2 to 5 ml of clear, mucus-like and almost odorless vaginal discharge daily. The volume and consistency of the discharge, however, varies among individuals. The volume may also vary during different phases of the menstrual cycle with mucous production steadily increasing with estrogen levels during the follicular phase, to a peak at ovulation. Consistency also changes throughout the cycle, from thick and sticky during the non-fertile phase to clearer, stretchy and slippery towards ovulation. During the luteal phase, secretion decreases and again becomes thick and sticky in consistency, owing to reducing levels of estrogen and increasing levels of progesterone.

The discharge may become more noticeable in the week before the onset of menstruation, during pregnancy and with the use of contraceptives.

Normal vaginal discharge should be clear but turns milky when exposed to the air. During or after menstruation, the discharge may be brown or bloody due to staining. A normal discharge often has a slight but not unpleasant odor and may cause mild irritation of the vulva.

Having vaginal discharge is a natural part of being a woman in the reproductive age unless it is accompanied by itching, burning, significant color and texture change and/or foul odor, any of which may signify an issue. The natural balance of the vagina can be disrupted by anything that interferes with its normal environment. The microbiome is particularly dynamic, making compositional changes in response to infection, pregnancy, menstruation and even aging and menopause.

Abnormal vaginal discharge is discharge that significantly departs from the individual's norm in terms of volume, color and consistency and odor attributes. Abnormal vaginal discharge is not a disease in itself but rather a symptom of other disorders that may either be infective or non-infective. The infective causes could be non-sexually transmitted, like bacterial vaginosis and candida, or sexual transmitted, like *Neisseria gonorrhea* and *trichomonas vaginalis.* On the contrary, non-infective causes of abnormal vaginal discharge are embedded foreign bodies (e.g. condoms, retained tampons), allergic reaction, fistulae, cervical polyps, cervical ectropion, and genital tract malignancy. Others precipitating factors that predispose one to abnormal discharge could be the protracted use of antibiotic, steroid or contraceptives, use of scented soaps, lotions, and bubble baths, douching, smoking, diabetes, pelvic inflammatory disease, pelvic infection after surgery and vaginal atrophy.

Usually, abnormal vaginal discharge is discovered by observation of color change in the discharge. Brown or blood-stained discharge is associated with irregular menstrual cycles or abnormal vaginal bleeding and less often cervical or endometrial cancer. Yellow, greenish or greyish discharge is usually caused by bacteria infection while yeast infection results in thick white cheesy discharge. Infections are usually accompanied by a strong characteristic unpleasant odor. Other associated symptoms include burning and itching sensation to the genital, abdominal or pelvic pain, urinary incontinence, and bleeding between periods.

From a TCM perspective...

Normal vaginal discharge is a combination of vestibular gland secretions, vaginal mucosal exudate, cervix and endometrial gland secretions to form a raw egg-white like mucus of little amount and a slight odor. It is physiological discharge. Abnormal discharge refers to a condition in which the discharge manifests an unusual color and/or unpleasant odor.

Abnormal discharge is labeled by the different colors and is divided into white discharge 白带, yellow discharge 黄带, red discharge 赤带, green discharge 青带, black discharge 黑带 and mixed-color discharge 五色带. Clinically, white, yellow and red discharges are more common. A green discharge may be purulent. A black discharge may be due to a small amount of old secretion or secretions of genital malignant lesions. Mixed-color discharge is more commonly observed in menopausal women and mostly associated with the secretion of genital malignant lesions. By and large, abnormal discharge is common in various vaginal and cervical inflammations.

Physiological vaginal discharge is the result of the interaction among the Conception Vessel 任脉, the Governor Vessel 督脉, and the Girdle Vessel 带脉. The Conception Vessel regulates the production of all Yin elements, including blood, fluids, and essence. The Governor Vessel regulates all Yang elements, including Qi, warmth, and immunity. The appropriate amount of discharge is regulated by the Girdle Vessel under the influence of the Governor Vessel. Failure to receive adequate Yang influence by the Governor Vessel causes dampness and vaginal discharge to be turbid. Similarly, without due influence from the Conception Vessel, the Girdle Vessel loses its ability to regulate the fluid volume and result in abnormal discharge.

The etiology of abnormal discharge is, therefore, the invasion of dampness upon the Conception Vessel and Girdle Vessel. Dampness may be accumulated internally due to general weakness as aforesaid or caused by the invasion of external pathogens associated with damp-heat.

When dampness is due to poor general health, the etiology is that of deficiency syndrome and invariably relates to Spleen and/or kidney Yang deficiency. Recalling that Liver and Spleen is associated with Wood and Earth elements in the Five-Element Theory, a hyperactivity Liver could injure the Spleen, causing Spleen deficiency that leads to a situation of heat-dampness interlock.

Abnormal discharge associated with deficiency state and with little heat (infection) is characterized by a constant and continuous flow of clear discharge that is odorless or with a slight odor. The texture of discharge could be of normal viscosity for Spleen deficiency but non-viscous and watery when the Kidney Yang is deficient. In the case of Kidney Yin deficiency reflective of low-grade heat 虚热, a more viscous discharge with slight blood staining may be observed.

Invasion by external pathogens associated with damp-heat is consistent with the precipitating factors that cause infective abnormal discharge. The same could be inferred when deficiency transforms into heat 虚郁化热 which essentially a situation of infection under low immunity. In TCM, heat, fire, and toxicity lie on a continuum where extreme heat transforms into fire 热极化火 and intense fire breeds toxins 火极生毒. In conditions where the presence of heat (infection) are more appreciable than dampness, the discharge becomes sticky, purulent and emits a foul odor; the intensity of which corresponds to heat and toxic damage. In less severe cases, the texture of discharge may turn tofu-like as in Yeast infection.

Gua Sha Protocol for Adjuvant Therapy and Symptomatic Relief

Gua Sha is not a suitable therapy for infective abnormal discharge which mainstream medical treatment should be sought without delay. *Gua Sha* therapy may, however, be still deployed in such situations as adjuvant therapy to raise the immunity against the infection as well as for symptomatic relief. Gua Sha is particularly effective in pure deficiency state abnormal discharge.

a. Occipital-Cervical Sweep
b. Back Rejuvenation Dredge
c. Sacral V Dredge
d. Umbilicus-Pubic Sweep
e. Spleen Meridian Dredge (SP1-SP10) with emphasis on SP1 隐白, SP6 三阴交, SP8 地机, SP10 血海 using acupoint 'press-and-hold' technique
f. Acupoint 'press-and-hold' for LR3 太冲 and LR6 照海 for both legs

Execution — Moderation press-stroke recommended. Acupoints marked for application of 'press-and-hold' technique in each prescription form a set, each set to be repeated three times. 'Press-and-hold' maneuver should be attempted 10 times for each prescribed acupoint within each set. Use of skin lubricant with herbs having Qi invigorating properties preferred. Observation of Sha appearance is not mandatory.

Other Considerations — Patient should be advised to engage in genital health practices that discourage the introduction of bacterial infection and those that promote the normally acidic bias pH value of the vaginal ecosystem. Such practices include avoidance of douching, avoidance of hot baths with scented products, wearing cotton instead of synthetic material undergarment, frequent changing of tampons and pads during menses and proper cleansing technique after visiting the washroom. From a dietary perspective, reduced consumption of sugars and alcohols and the repopulation of gut probiotics after the use of antibiotics are recommended.

Glossary

Fistula (pl. fistulae) is an abnormal connection or tunnel between two hollow spaces, technically two epithelialized surfaces, such as blood vessels, intestines or other hollow organs. Fistulae are usually caused by injury or surgery but may result from an infection or inflammation that perforated the surfaces.

Cervical ectropion, also known as cervical erosion and ectopy, is a common condition caused when cells from inside the cervical canal, known as glandular cells (columnar epithelium), are present on the outside surface of the cervix (neck of the womb). The cells on the 'outside' of the cervix are called squamous epithelial cells.

Topic 50

Breast Engorgement

Breast engorgement is painful congestion of the breasts with milk usually occurring within the first week post-partum when the breasts begin to produce milk. It is the outcome of a dynamic adaptation process between milk supply and demand that leads to an input-output issue. Primary engorgement occurs during the first few days after birth when the mother's body is making adjustments to the production of milk that the baby demands. Secondary engorgement occurs later when the mother is not feeding as frequently as she used to, or the baby withdrew less milk from the breasts. Augmentation mammoplasty has also lately been identified as a cause of breast engorgement when women who have had such operations start to breastfeed.

This condition is characterized by the painful swelling of the breasts associated with the sudden and rapid increase in milk volume, vascular congestion, and edema during the first week after birth. This initial physiological engorgement results in the build-up of milk and overfilling of the breasts, causing lymphatic and vascular congestion and edema of the glandular breast tissue. Swelling may occur in the areolae or the periphery of the breasts or both. The breasts become distended and tender with the nipples progressively taut and flattened. In cases when the breast is severely engorged, the nipple is likely to retract into the areola. Engorgement may affect breasts singularly or bilaterally. Some women experience loss of appetite, fatigue, weakness and even a low-grade fever and chills.

Although ineffective milk removal is a common cause, engorgement resulting from overfilling of breast milk should be differentiated from non-infectious mastitis, an inflammatory condition due to milk duct blockage.

Several approaches for the treatment of breast engorgement for breastfeeding women have been investigated and found to be effective: warm compresses before breastfeeding, cold therapy, cabbage leaf application, breast massage, milk expression, and analgesic oral medications. Of late, Gua *Sha* therapy is also included in the repertoire of effective interventions for the management of breast engorgement. This is an interesting development as, together with cabbage leaf application, it appears that mainstream medicine has started to see merit in alternative and complementary medicine.

Green cabbage leaf application has been used frequently as an effective intervention in reducing moderate to severe breast engorgement for postnatal mothers without side effects.[1,2] Duly cleansed green cabbage leaves may be used chilled or at room temperature between feedings as a twenty-minute compress per session. The intervention should stop once the engorgement is relieved since it also appears to decrease milk supply. Botanically, cabbage belongs to the *Brassicaceae* family, has both antibiotic and anti-irritant properties. Cabbage is known to contain sinigrin (allyl isothiocyanate) rapine, mustard oil, magnesium, oxalates, and sulfur heterosides. The natural mixture of these components seems to promote vasodilatation of tiny blood vessels, allowing the body to reabsorb fluids trapped in the breasts and reduce local tissue congestion. Squeezing out milk should be avoided after treatment as the action tends to increase milk supply and sustain the distension.

Gua Sha therapy has also been applied as an effective intervention for breast engorgement issues at primary care setting.[3] In Asian societies, exposure to cold immediately after post-partum is a major cultural prohibition; which makes cold compression and green cabbage leaf applications less favored interventions. If engorgement is predicated on vascular congestion and edema, then *Gua Sha* therapy that promotes blood circulation and improves the dissemination of fluids is a viable solution that effectively resolves fluid retention (edema) and blood stasis.

Gua-Sha therapy is found to be statistically significant in being more efficacious in lowering body and breast temperatures and relieving engorgement, pain, and discomfort than conventional massage and heat therapies. The lowering of body and breast temperatures strongly correlates to the relief of engorgement symptoms.

In Germany, *Gua Sha* therapy was found to stimulate surface skin and microcirculation[4] by extending blood vessels, improving partial blood circulation and metabolism, which facilitate the evacuation of heat and toxins. Another observation is that *Gua-Sha* relieves pain by relaxing tight muscles and promoting blood circulation. Gentle stroking that stimulates the areola despatch nerve impulses to the hypothalamus that in turn stimulates the pituitary to secrete oxytocin which decreases anxiety and facilitates milk ejection.

From a TCM perspective...

Nipples are served by the Liver meridian whereas the breasts are served by the Stomach meridian. Any disorder of the breast is therefore directly reflective of the dysfunction in these meridians. The Spleen meridian, however, is collaterally connected to the Stomach meridian and so is the Kidney meridian that has a branch entering the Liver. Invariably, dysfunction in these meridians has an effect on the normal functioning of the breast. Notwithstanding, the Penetrating Vessel 冲脉 and Conception Vessel 任脉 that exert a pervasive influence on a women's gynecological well-being need to be revitalized and rebalanced when engorgement occurs. The etiology of breast engorgement is Qi stagnation and blood stasis so that the general therapeutic principle is to regulate Qi and dispel blood stasis.

Gua Sha Protocol for Treatment and Symptomatic Relief

That breast engorgement is a distention that stretches the skin thin, extreme caution must be exercised to ensure that the stroke pressure does not aggravate the discomfort already encountered by the patient. There is, therefore, a need for constant communication with the patient to ensure that the stroke pressure is tolerable. By and large, light press-stroke relaxes the flesh but with increased intensity, the tissue may react to oppose the external force. Thus, light short strokes are recommended to remedy breast engorgement such that only mild skin redness and elevation be observed.

Depending on the patient's inclination, light press-strokes may be applied radially around the entire breast and in the direction of the nipples to stimulate microcirculation (refer [e] hereinafter). Treatment time should preferably be before feeding time when the breasts can be severely distended. Intervention time should also be limited to about 5 minutes per mammary gland.

a. Shoulder Sweep
b. Sternal Sweep with emphasis on CV17 膻中 using acupoint 'press-and-hold' technique
c. Clavicular Sweep
d. Acupoint 'press-and-hold' for SI11 天宗, ST16 膺窗, ST18 乳根, SP17 食窦 on torso bilaterally
e. Additional short light press strokes for ST16, ST18, and SP17 radially in the direction towards the nipples
f. Acupoint 'press-and-hold' for ST36 足三里 on both legs

Execution — Moderation press-stroke recommended. Acupoints marked for application of 'press-and-hold' technique in each prescription form a set, each set to be repeated three times. 'Press-and-hold' maneuver should be attempted 10 times for each prescribed acupoint within each set. No or light skin lubricant be applied but to avoid areola areas and nipples. Observation of Sha appearance is not mandatory.

Other Considerations — Patient should be advised that the key to managing breast engorgement is promoting the frequent and effective ejection of milk from the breast. Post-partum women should breastfeed or express with a pump at least 8 to 12 times a day within a three-hour interval between feeds. Heat therapy before feeding helps stimulate milk flow. Cooling the engorged breast provides temporary pain relief. The patient should seek medical attention if engorgement symptoms did not clear within two days or if flu-like symptoms developed or deterioration is presented, since engorgement may lead to mastitis.

Supplementary Notes — Mastitis

Mastitis is a condition of a woman's breast tissue becoming painful and inflamed that is most common in breastfeeding women in the initial post-partum months. Mastitis occurring during breastfeeding is referred to as lactation mastitis or puerperal mastitis while mastitis of non-breastfeeding women is of a type called periductal mastitis. On rare occasion, mastitis affects men as granulomatous mastitis.

The main cause of mastitis is milk entrapped in the breast after failing to completely discharge during feeding and causing the milk ducts to become obstructed, infected and inflamed. Another potential avenue for infection is bacteria entering the breast through a broken skin surface of the nipple while feeding. Milk stored within the breast then provides an excellent environment for bacteria cultivation and proliferation.

Mastitis usually affects one breast at a time with symptoms developing rapidly. Symptoms of mastitis indicative of infective inflammation include:

- Erythema (redness), swelling, tenderness, burning sensation and pain on the affected breast area; the pain could be continuously or while breastfeeding
- Thickening of breast tissue, a breast lump or area of hardness on the breast
- Nipple discharge that may contain blood streaks
- General flu-like symptoms such as aches, a high temperature, chills and fatigue

Mastitis not treated in a timely manner can result in the accumulation of pus at the inflamed location that develops into an abscess which requires surgical intervention. Whilst it is essential to engage antibiotics to rapidly resolve the infection, *Gua Sha* can effectively alleviate the blocked Qi, blood and milk in the breasts. The integrative treatment will rapidly reduce the engorgement and inflammation and further minimize the incidence of recurrence while providing significant symptomatic relief.

Gua Sha Protocol for Symptomatic Relief

a. Sternal Sweep
b. Epigastric-Umbilicus Sweep
c. Umbilicus-Pubic Sweep
d. Shoulder Sweep
e. Trapezius Sweep
f. Acupoint Scrapping of LU5 尺泽 and PC3 曲泽 at the antecubital fossa region of both arms for rapid heat dissipation
g. Acupoint 'press-and-hold' for LI4 合谷, LI11 曲池 and PC6 内关 on both hands
h. Acupoint 'press-and-hold' for SP6 三阴交, ST36 足三里 and LR3 太冲 on both legs
i. Acupoint 'press-and-hold' for ST18 乳根 and SI11 天宗 bilaterally on the torso

Execution — Moderation press-stroke recommended. Acupoint scrapping lines should run about one cm above and below the prescribed acupoint. Acupoints marked for application of 'press-and-hold' technique in each prescription form a set, each set to be repeated three times. 'Press-and-hold' maneuver should be attempted 10 times for each prescribed acupoint within each set. No or light skin lubricant be applied but to avoid areola areas and nipples. Observation of Sha appearance is not mandatory.

References

1. Lim A-R, Song J-A, Hur M-H. Cabbage compression early breast care on breast engorgement in primiparous women after cesarean birth: a controlled clinical trial. *Int. J. Clin. Exp. Med.* **8**(11): 21335–21342 (2015).

2. Wong BB, Koh S, Hegney DG, *et al.* The effectiveness of cabbage leaf application (treatment) on pain and hardness in breast engorgement and its effect on the duration of breastfeeding. *JBI. Libr. Syst. Rev.* **10**(20): 1185–1213 (2012).
3. Chiu JY, Gau ML, Kuo SY, *et al.* Effects of *Gua-Sha* therapy on breast engorgement: a randomized controlled trial. J. Nurs. Res. 18(1): 1–10 (2010).
4. Nielsen A, Knoblauch NT, *et al.* The effect of Gua-Sha treatment on the microcirculation of surface tissue: a pilot study in healthy subjects. *J. Sci. Healing* **3**(5): 456–466 (2007).

TOPIC 51

Dysmenorrhea/Painful Menstruation

Dysmenorrhea is the medical term for menstrual cramps, which are caused by uterine contractions. It is normal to have mild cramps during a menstrual period when the uterine muscles contract to expel blood but when the intensity of pain becomes debilitating and psychologically taxing, it develops into a medical condition that warrants attention, though not life-threatening.

Menstrual cramps are not the same as Premenstrual Syndrome (PMS). PMS is a combination of emotional and physical factors including symptoms such as fatigue, irritability, mood swings, breast soreness, food cravings and bloating which occur during the luteal phase of the menstrual cycle, varying between 2 and 12 days before the onset of menses, before resolving within the first 24 hours of flow. On the other hand, Dysmenorrhea refers to the intense pain and cramping women experience before, during and after menstruation.

Dysmenorrhea can be divided into 2 broad categories:

— primary that refers to common menstrual cramps occurring in the absence of pelvic pathology, and
— secondary resulting from identifiable organic diseases or disorders in the reproductive organs.

Primary dysmenorrhea is menstrual pain that is not symptomatic of an underlying gynecologic disorder but related to the normal menstrual process. The spasms are caused by contraction of the uterine muscles triggered by prostaglandin F2α (PGF2α), a potent myometrial stimulant and vasoconstrictor, in the secretory endometrium. The pain results from the excessive release of these hormones when the endometrium is sloughing off during period, leading to extended uterine contraction and decreased blood flow and therefore oxygen supply to the myometrium of the uterus. In women suffering from dysmenorrhea, elevated prostaglandin levels were found in the endometrial fluid that correlated with the degree of pain. The level of prostaglandins, however, decreases as menstruation continues and so does the endometrial sloughing. Pain usually decreases as the level of prostaglandins decreases.

Increase in endometrial prostaglandins occurs from the follicular phase to the luteal phase, with a further increase occurring during menstruation. The upsurge in prostaglandins in the endometrium in the late luteal phase following a fall in progesterone results in increased myometrial tone and excessive uterine contraction. When primary dysmenorrhea is not responsive to treatment of prostaglandin antagonists, it is suspected that the presence of leukotrienes heightened the sensitivity of pain in uterine fibers. Vasopressin, a pituitary hormone, may also be involved in myometrial hypersensitivity, reduced uterine blood flow, and pain in primary dysmenorrhea. The more severe pain in primary dysmenorrhea seems to be the result of a combined effect of vasopressin and PGF2α.[1]

Primary dysmenorrhea often begins in women after late adolescence who have started menstrual periods. Menstrual cramps, though recurrent, could become less painful with maturity and may stop entirely after pregnancy. The main symptom of dysmenorrhea is sharp spasmodic or dull congestive pain that occurs in the lower abdomen hips, lower back or thighs during menstruation. Pain may range from mild to severe and, in severe episodes, accompanied by nausea, vomiting, headache, bloating, fatigue and even diarrhea or constipation. High levels of prostaglandins could cause nausea, dizziness, and diarrhea. Blood clots from the endometrial shedding could be expelled during menstruation.

Aggravating factors of primary dysmenorrhea include a retroverted uterus (uterus that tilts backward), longer and early menarche, heavier or irregular menstrual periods, obesity, sedentary lifestyle, psychological or social stress, smoking, alcohol consumption and family history of dysmenorrhea.

Secondary dysmenorrhea is generally related to a disorder in the reproductive system. It usually begins later in life than primary dysmenorrhea, affecting women during adulthood. Unlike primary dysmenorrhea, clinical features of secondary dysmenorrhea appear to more severe over time, begins earlier in the menstrual cycle, and often last longer and may even not subside after menstruation. Elevated prostaglandins may play a role in secondary dysmenorrhea, but by definition, concomitant pelvic pathology must be present. The pain is not typically accompanied by nausea, vomiting, fatigue, or diarrhea.

Secondary dysmenorrhea is often indicated by menstrual cramps after previous relatively painless cycles, heavy menstrual flow or irregular bleeding, pelvic abnormality, history of infertility, vaginal discharge, dyspareunia (painful coitus) and poor response to NSAID or oral contraceptive treatment.

Secondary dysmenorrhea may be caused by a number of conditions, including:

- Endometriosis — a condition in which the endometrial tissue is found outside of the uterus. Endometriosis tissue breaks down and bleeds in response to hormonal changes especially in conjunction with the menstrual cycle, causing pain and adhesion where bleeding occurs.
- Adenomyosis — a condition where endometrial tissue grows into the muscle of the uterus.
- Cervical stenosis or occlusion — narrowing or complete closure of the opening to the uterus.
- Congenital malformations (e.g. bicornuate uterus or subsceptate uterus, transverse vaginal septum).

- Pelvic congestion syndrome — a chronic condition that occurs when varicose veins form below the abdomen within the pelvic region.
- Lesions — fibroid, cyst, benign tumor and polyp on the outside, inside or within the wall of the uterus.
- Intrauterine adhesion — Asherman's Syndrome or scarring of the uterine cavity due to trauma caused by surgical procedures, extended use of IUD or even infection of the endometrium.
- Pelvic inflammatory disease — an infection caused by bacteria that starts in the uterus and can spread to other reproductive organs.

By and large, primary dysmenorrhea is treated by providing symptomatic relief as well as inhibiting the underlying processes that cause symptoms. Medication prescribed may include NSAIDs that target at reducing the levels of prostaglandins as well as oral contraceptives containing estrogen and progestin. Muscle relaxants are also often prescribed with NSAIDs to hasten relief. Vitamin B1 or magnesium supplements that ease muscular spasm may also be helpful. Lifestyle change may also be recommended as a longer-term solution to alleviate symptoms. When relief is not forthcoming from medication, especially in secondary dysmenorrhea, surgical options may be sought.

From a TCM perspective...

Dysmenorrhea is divided into two major categories by virtue of TCM syndrome differentiation 中医辨证: excess syndrome 实证 and deficiency syndrome 虚证. Generally, so long as the menstrual blood commences its timely discharge, abdominal pain shall be alleviated or may not even appear.

This disorder is closely related to the cyclical physiological changes of the Penetrating Vessel 冲脉 and the uterus. The pathogenesis lies in the uterine dwelling of external pernicious influence 外邪 or the deficiency of blood as well as the rapid physiological changes pertaining to the Penetrating Vessel 冲脉, Conception Vessel 任脉, and the Governor Vessel 督脉 before and after the menstrual period. This causes the blood supply to the uterus to circulate poorly that in turn leads to a condition of stagnation-mediated pain 不通则痛 or loss of the nutrient supply to the uterus that translates to deficiency-mediated pain 不荣则痛. Relative to the organ-system, dysmenorrhea is closely associated with the disorder of the Spleen, Kidney, and Liver.

By observing the time of pain occurrence, pain location, nature of pain and patient's preference for or against pressure on pain location, dysmenorrhea can be further classified as cold or heaty type, deficiency or excess type and Qi or blood-related. As a rule of thumb, pain occurring prior to and during menstruation, of severe nature that guards against the application of pressure is deemed to be excess type; pain occurring after menstruation, of mild and nagging nature that favors massage for relief are generally the deficiency type. Pain that favors heat application is cold-related whereas pain that intensifies with heat therapy is heaty type. Pain that is sharp relative to a feeling of distention is related to blood stasis and likewise, pain that is dull akin to distention is related to Qi stagnation. Pain located bilaterally at the iliac region is associated with the Liver while pain located in the lumbar region is associated with the kidneys.

Common classifications of dysmenorrhea include kidney Qi deficiency, Qi and blood deficiency, Qi stagnation and blood stasis, cold-mediated blood coagulation and damp-heat accumulation.

Stagnation of Qi and Blood that disrupt or obstruct the flow in meridians shall cause pain with inflammation during menstruation. The fundamental therapeutic principle of TCM in the treatment of dysmenorrhea is, therefore, to alleviate pain by invigorating Qi and dispelling blood stasis to improve blood circulation for excess syndrome or in the alternative nourish liver and kidney, regulate menstruation cycle and relieve pain for deficiency syndrome. When exogenous and pernicious influence is also a contributing factor to dysmenorrhea, it is essential to remove the influence. Cold entrapped in the uterus causing blood stasis should be eliminated by warming the affected meridians to restore the Yang energy and dispel blood stasis 温经散寒, 化瘀止痛. Damp-heat, a combined pernicious influence, when present must be cleared in priority to other issues.

Gua Sha Protocol for Adjuvant Therapy and Symptomatic Relief

Blood circulation ameliorates inflamed tissues. As blood circulation increased in inflamed areas, pro-inflammatory responses are down-regulated. *Gua Sha* can improve blood circulation significantly especially when the appropriate acupoints are selected for dysmenorrhea.

a. Para-Vertebral Dredge (T7-L2)
b. Superior Bladder Meridian Dredge
c. Epigastric-Umbilicus Sweep
d. Umbilicus-Pubic Sweep
e. Sacral V Dredge
f. Spleen Meridian Dredge (SP4-SP10) on both legs with emphasis on SP4 公孙, SP6 三阴交, SP8 地机, SP10 血海 using acupoint 'press-and-hold' technique
g. Liver Meridian Dredge (LR2-LR5) on both legs with emphasis on LR2 行间, LR3 太冲, LR5 蠡沟 using acupoint 'press-and-hold' technique
h. Acupoint 'press-and-hold' for LI4 合谷, HT7 神门 on both arms
i. Acupoint 'press-and-hold' for KI12 大赫, EX CA1 子宫 bilaterally on the torso

Execution — Moderation press-stroke recommended. Acupoints marked for application of 'press-and-hold' technique in each prescription form a set, each set to be repeated three times. 'Press-and-hold' maneuver should be attempted 10 times for each prescribed acupoint within each set. Unless TCM diagnosis suggests otherwise, light skin lubricant that invigorates Qi preferred. Observation of Sha appearance is not mandatory.

Reference

1. Strömberg P, Akerlund M, *et al.* Vasopressin and prostaglandins in premenstrual pain and primary dysmenorrhea. *Acta Obstet. Gynecol. Scand.* **63**(6): 533–538 (1984).

TOPIC 52

Lactation Incompetence

Milk production depends on normal lactation ability, adequate breast stimulation, and regular, complete breast drainage.

Mammogenesis, the development of the female breasts to its functional state, begins at birth. The reproductive hormones act directly on the mammary gland, whereas the metabolic hormones act indirectly by altering the endocrine response and nutrient flux to the mammary gland. Before puberty, the breasts are immature and small but upon reaching adolescence the ducts and gland buds begin to develop under the influence of estrogen and progesterone. Ductal growth is primarily regulated by estrogen and growth hormone, and alveolar development requires progesterone, prolactin, and possibly placental lactogen. It is however only during gestation that the ductile proliferation and lobular-alveolar development occurs. Placental lactogens and prolactin, together with increased levels of estrogen and progesterone, stimulate this physical breast growth so that the breasts contain more glandular epithelial cells than stroma tissue but suppress and defer the production of milk.

Lactogenesis begins during mid-pregnancy with the initiation of milk synthesis. During pregnancy, the high levels of circulating progesterone inhibit the secretory process of the mammary gland. Lactation begins around parturition with the secretion of milk being triggered by the expulsion of the placenta and decline of progesterone and upregulation of prolactin. Elevated levels of prolactin, cortisol, insulin, growth and parathyroid hormones are essential at this stage to facilitate mobilization of nutrients and minerals in the milk production.

Galactokinesis is the process of milk ejection outside the breast by virtue of the suckling mechanism of the baby and the contractile action which expresses milk from the alveoli into the ducts. This contraction is brought about by the operation of oxytocin released from the posterior pituitary lobe during nipple stimulation. However, this milk ejection reflex may be inhibited by breast engorgement.

Galactopoiesis is the ongoing production of milk that is dependent on frequent, effective nipple stimulation; complete drainage or emptying of the breast; and an intact hypothalamic-pituitary-prolactin (HPP) axis. The active process of lactation is mainly controlled by prolactin and oxytocin levels.

Between feeds, milk passes via passive diffusion from the glands to collect in the lactiferous ducts. This foremilk, that is low in fat and protein but high in lactose, may then pool in large quantities to cause the breasts to become full and taut before the next feed. When the nipple and lactiferous sinuses are directly stimulated, afferent nerve pathways to the anterior pituitary trigger surges of prolactin, which result in the production of hindmilk that has higher fat and protein content. The quantity of milk decreases though but the quality and fat concentration improve throughout the feed. If the breasts are not drained adequately, the pressure in the ducts builds up and slowly reduces the amount of milk formed. Complete drainage is a major stimulus to ongoing milk production.

Adequate lactation therefore depends on the proper functioning of four vital processes — mammogenesis, lactogenesis, galactokinesis and galactopoiesis, the development of which is influenced by a complex hormonal milieu including reproductive hormones (estrogen, progesterone, placental lactogen, prolactin and oxytocin) and metabolic hormones (glucocorticoids, insulin, growth hormone and thyroid).

Factors that impede successful mammogenesis may include genetically predetermined phenomena, inadequate breast tissue receptors, or an inadequate hormonal milieu. Maternal health factors that interfere with lactational ability include breast surgery, such as reduction and augmentation mammoplasty. Other causes of primary inability to lactate are severe illness such as anemia, postpartum hemorrhage with Sheehan's syndrome, polycystic ovarian syndrome (PCOS), infection, smoking or hypertension.

Insufficient lactation may also be due to a retained placenta and delayed breastfeeding.

Lactogenesis may be hampered if remnants of the placenta are inadvertently retained in the uterus causing high progesterone levels to sustain and inhibiting milk production.

Delayed breastfeeding is a common but legitimate occurrence when mother and child are separated due to infant protective isolation or maternal post-partum issues. Studies pertaining to delayed breastfeeding as a predisposing factor to reduced lactogenesis demonstrate that the duration of lactation correlates inversely with the time of first breastfeeding. This implies that early initiation of effective breast stimulation is critical to establishing adequate lactation.

Inadequate breast drainage is the main predisposing factor to impaired galactopoiesis.

Galactagogues or lactogogues are medications or supplements for promoting the maintenance or augmentation of maternal lactation. The most widely used prescribed medications are the common anti-emetics, metoclopramide and domperidone, that increase hypothalamic prolactin levels. Being dopamine antagonists, these drugs cause extrapyramidal side effects, which may include tremor, bradykinesia (slow movements), and other dystonic reactions; though domperidone that does not readily cross the blood-brain barrier is less likely to produce the neurological side effects.

Herbs and natural supplements traditionally and frequently used for increasing milk production include fenugreek (*Trigonella foenumgraecum*), moringa (*Moringa oleifera*), shatavari (*Asparagus racemosus*), fennel (*Foeniculum vulgare*) and milk thistle (*Silybum marianum*).

From a TCM perspective...

There are two broad categories of lactation incompetence — an excess situation when blood and Qi are adequate but somehow obstructed or impeded, or a deficiency situation when blood is lacking and Qi function is weak. In both situations, the flow of blood and Qi is compromised. If obstruction is the cause, it should be dispelled to ease blood stasis and/or Qi stagnation. If blood and Qi, especially the primordial Qi 元气, are functionally weak, this should be addressed by nourishment/tonification. This is because milk production is predicated on the transformation of blood and Qi regulated by the Penetrating Vessel 冲脉 and Conception Vessel 任脉.

In excess situation, it is observed that the breasts are distended and painful, and expression is generally difficult due to milk's viscous texture. Etiology for excess type lactation incompetence is usually stagnation of the Liver Qi. In a deficiency type lactation incompetence, the converse is manifested where the breasts are soft and not distended, expression of milk does not hurt and both quantity and quality of milk are poor. The common cause for deficiency situation is blood and Qi debility. There is however yet another clinical form usually manifested by obese post-partum women where the breasts are full but not distended and with little milk production. This is due to obstruction by phlegm and turbidity.

According to Fu Qingzhu's Obstetrics and Gynecology,[1] the production of milk is predicated fundamentally on the resilience of Yang-Ming/Stomach system that is associated with the Earth element in the Five-Element Theory. Healthy post-partum women though may have lost blood during delivery, the robust Yang-Ming Stomach Qi can still sustain the function of the stomach and in collaboration with the Wood-Liver Qi, shall commence lactation. The process of lactation is conditional upon the interplay of the Stomach and Liver Qi as opposed to mere blood circulation. For milk production is determined primarily by the functional condition of Qi and not that of blood. Lactation would commence days after post-partum, engorging the breasts. Notwithstanding that Qi stagnation is the cause for failing to express milk, regulating the Liver Qi would spontaneously open the Yang-Ming or stomach Qi channel and therefore appropriately address lactation incompetence.

《傅青主女科》: 乳汁之化，原属阳明，然阳明属土，壮妇产后，虽云亡血，而阳明之气实未尽衰，必得肝木之气以相通，始能化成乳汁，未可全责之阳明也。盖乳汁之化，全在气而不在血。今产后数日，宜其有乳，而两乳胀满作痛，是欲化乳而不可得，非气郁而何?…治法宜大疏其肝木之气，而阳明之气血自通，而乳亦通也

In the final analysis, lactation relies on efficient transformation 气化 of blood and primordial Qi. Primordial Qi is the combination of the innate Qi and the acquired Qi. The source of innate Qi is the kidney and the continuing supply of acquired Qi is via the stomach and lungs. In layperson parlance, it means that lactation requires inherent maternal health (innate Qi), adequate nutrition (acquired Qi) and hormonal balance (harmony between Liver-Wood and Stomach-Earth). Hormonal imbalance caused by a hyperactive liver will prevent proper nutritive absorption 木郁克土，脾失健运 and thus lactation incompetence.

Gua Sha Protocol for Adjuvant Therapy and Symptomatic Relief

a. Occipital-Cervical Sweep
b. Sternal Sweep
c. Ventral Intercostal Space Sweep
d. Trapezius Sweep
e. Superior Bladder Meridian Dredge (T1-T12)
f. Umbilicus-Pubic Sweep
g. Acupoint 'press-and-hold' for SP6 三阴交, ST36 足三里, LR3 太冲, KI1 涌泉 on both legs
h. Acupoint 'press-and-hold' for PC6 内关, SI1 少泽 on both hands
i. Acupoint 'press-and-hold' for SP18 天溪, ST18 乳根 on the torso bilaterally

Execution — Moderation press-stroke recommended. Acupoints marked for application of 'press-and-hold' technique in each prescription form a set, each set to be repeated three times. 'Press-and-hold' maneuver should be attempted 10 times for each prescribed acupoint within each set. Use of light skin lubricant preferred. Observation of Sha appearance is not mandatory.

Glossary

Sheehan's syndrome is hypopituitarism or decrease in pituitary function occasioned by ischemic necrosis due to blood loss and hypovolemic shock during and after childbirth. This permanent injury is also known as postpartum pituitary gland necrosis requires appropriate life-long hormone replacement therapy.

Reference

1. *Fu Qingzhu's Obstetrics and Gynecology* 傅青主女科 (1827).

Topic 53

Menorrhagia/Heavy Menstruation

Menorrhagia or excessive menstrual bleeding is a common clinical problem that can adversely affect the quality of life for women. It is also one of the most significant causes of ill health in women and therefore a common complaint in contemporary gynecology.

In a normal menstrual cycle, the duration is between 21 and 35 days during which bleeding lasts an average of 7 days with flow volume between 25 and 80 ml without significant clots. Clinically menorrhagia is defined, against this norm, as menstruation at regular cycle intervals but with flow volume in excess of 80 ml per cycle and/or with a menstrual bleeding duration that lasts longer than 7 days. This quantification of menstrual blood loss can, however, be challenging as the bleeding volume is a perception and subjective interpretation usually based on patient's observation. Thus, the exact problem definition and therefore objective diagnosis can be made difficult in a clinical setting.

Notwithstanding, few suggestions were made to provide estimates of blood loss during menstruation but these proxies are deemed low in quantitative precision. Solely relying on the number of menstruating days as a gauge is far from accurate as up to 78% and 91% of total blood loss occurred by the second and third day respectively.[1] There is also scant deviation in the distribution of total blood loss between normal menses and menorrhagia.[2] Neither is counting the number of sanitary products used for the duration of the period representative as this statistic can be marred by woman's personal hygiene practices, frequency of attention to menstrual flow and financial resources. Moreover, this measurement is predicated on the assumption of consistency in product absorbency, the volume that is known to the patient.[3] Notwithstanding, what is now adopted as a more objective assessment of menorrhagia is menstrual pictogram that purports to standardize blood loss equivalents visually but requires some training and practice to yield clinically useful information.

A convenient but less than practical definition suggested for menorrhagia may be a menstrual loss that is greater than what is deemed reasonably manageable by the patient. Perhaps a rule of thumb for assessment that bleeding should be considered dysfunctional could be if a change of sanitary product is required after about two hours, having to wake up at night to change sanitary protection or when clot sizes are greater than an inch in diameter.

Etiologies of menorrhagia can be divided into anatomic, endocrinologic and organic categories.

Anatomic etiologies for menorrhagia are usually benign lesions that include endometrial polyps, uterine fibroids, and endometrial hyperplasia.

Uterine fibroids are noncancerous muscle growths within the walls of the uterus while endometrial polyps are abnormal tissue growths within the endometrium, the inner lining of the uterus. The mechanism by which endometrial polyp or fibroid causes menorrhagia is not well understood. It is however postulated that because blood supply required to feed the lesion is greater than normal endometrial supply, this may impede venous return, thereby causing blood pooling in the areas of the lesion. Bleeding ensues when heavy pooling weakens the endometrium surrounding the lesion during menstruation.

The cessation of menstrual bleeding is achieved by endometrial hemostasis via platelet aggregation, fibrin deposition, and thrombus formation. Tissue factor and thrombin (precursor to fibrin) play a key role locally in the cessation of menstrual bleeding through the instigation of the coagulation factors. Uterine fibroids may inhibit muscle contracture, thereby preventing normal uterine attempts at hemostasis. Deficiencies in either of platelets or fibrin (factor Ia) result in menorrhagia for patients with platelet function disorders (thrombocytopenia) or von Willebrand disease.

Fibrinolysis prevents clot organization within the uterine cavity and limits the fibrin deposits in the unshed layer. Formation of thrombus or blood clot is limited to the shedding surface of the endometrium. Following thrombin plug formation, vasoconstriction occurs and contributes to hemostasis.

Endometrial hyperplasia is the abnormal thickening of the lining of the uterus due to an increase in the number of endometrial glands, usually resulting from unopposed estrogen (without progesterone) production. Unopposed estrogen allows the endometrium to proliferate and thicken. The endometrium finally outgrows its blood supply and degenerates. The end result is an asynchronous breakdown of the endometrial lining at different levels. This is also the reason for anovulatory bleeding to be heavier than normal menstrual flow. This disorder most often affects young women who are just beginning to menstruate and older women approaching menopause. Endometrial hyperplasia can lead to endometrial cancer in 1–2% of patients with anovulatory bleeding.

Endocrine causes of menorrhagia include anovulatory cycles, thyroid, and adrenal gland dysfunction, PCOS, obesity and pituitary tumors.

Anovulatory cycle is the most common etiology of heavy uterine bleeding among the adolescent and perimenopausal women; population at the extreme ends of reproductive age. In anovulatory cycles, the menstrual cycle is characterized by irregular intervals without known organic etiology and the absence of ovulation and a luteal phase. In the absence of ovulation, there will be infertility and an insufficient level of progesterone that leads to heavy bleeding. In adolescents, the most common cause is an immature hypothalamus-pituitary-gonads axis. (i.e. the chemical signaling process between the brain and the ovaries). In perimenopausal women, it can be due to the depletion of the ovarian function.

It is well documented that hyperthyroidism is a common cause for menorrhagia but hypothyroidism is a lesser-known but significant cause. Even subclinical cases of hypothyroidism can produce heavy uterine bleeding in patients with unresolved menorrhagia. In these cases, the acid test of causation is whether treatment of the condition corrects the menstrual dysfunction. Menorrhagia disappeared within 3 to 6 months and did not reappear in 1 to 3 years of follow up in all patients with early hypothyroidism to whom L-thyroxine was given.[4]

The hallmarks of PCOS are anovulation, irregular menses, obesity, and hirsutism. Insulin resistance and compensatory hyperinsulinemia are direct consequences of obesity. Androgen synthesis is elevated when an increased amount of progesterone is being converted into aldosterone and at the expense of decreased estrogen output.

In response to gonadotropin-releasing hormone (GnRH) from the hypothalamus, the pituitary gland synthesizes follicle-stimulating hormone (FSH) and luteinizing hormone (LH), which induce the ovaries to produce estrogen and progesterone. Prolactin-producing pituitary tumors cause menorrhagia by disrupting (GnRH) secretion. This leads to decreased LH and FSH levels that cause hypogonadism. Menorrhagia usually manifests during these interim stages until the full clinical presentation of hypogonadism.

Infection of genitourinary origin, coagulation disorders, and organ dysfunction are organic causes for menorrhagia.

Coagulation disorders that can be either inherited or acquired, include von Willebrand disease; prothrombin deficiency (factor II), Hemophilia B (factor IX), V and VII deficiencies; idiopathic thrombocytopenic purpura (ITP); and thrombasthenia. Any of these bleeding disorders may only manifest after menarche when heavy menstrual flow is present.

Organ dysfunction associated with menorrhagia are non-coagulation related disorders and include hepatic or renal dysfunction. With chronic liver disease, the capacity to metabolize hormones is reduced. Delayed clearance of hormones accentuates estrogen stimulation during the follicular phase resulting in the proliferation of the endometrium. Increased endometrial thickness when shed leads to heavy uterine bleeding. Chronic liver disease also indirectly result in coagulation disorders as the production of clotting factors is usually impaired. In chronic renal disease, uremic coagulopathy arising from platelet and factor VIII dysfunctions is the usual cause of menorrhagia.

Treatment regimens are usually targeted at addressing the aspects of the menstrual cycle perceived to be abnormal with respect to cycle length and/or flow volume. The extent of treatment reversibility will always be considered as it may impinge on the issue of procreation.

Baseline treatment directed at regulating hormonal imbalance includes implantation of Levonorgestrel intrauterine system, combined oral contraceptive, and oral progestogen. The restoration of hormonal balance will to some extent regulate blood loss subsequent to treatment.

In less severe cases, NSAIDs are prescribed to reduce the concentration of prostaglandins in endometrial tissue at the onset of menstruation that may contribute to heavy menstrual bleeding. Prostaglandins are postulated to disturb the hemostatic mechanism of the endometrium by disrupting platelet aggregation, various coagulation factors and cause vasodilation. The alternative is the administration of a prostaglandin synthetase inhibitor, naproxen.

When bleeding is massive and unrelenting, treatment with anti-fibrinolytic agents like tranexamic acid or aminocaproic acid is required to slow the breakdown of blood clots and prevent prolonged bleeding. Plasmin is the major enzyme of the human fibrinolytic system that dissolves formed clots by degrading fibrin. Plasmin is produced in the liver as an inactive form, plasminogen. Anti-fibrinolytic operates by blocking the lysine binding sites on plasminogen, preventing it from being converted into plasmin. This medication is non-hormonal in nature and will not affect fertility.

When conservative therapy failed, surgical options may be sought and include endometrial ablation, uterine artery embolization, and radical hysterectomy.

Infrequent episodes of menorrhagia usually do not carry severe risks to women's general health. Women with untreated heavy or prolonged bleeding are at risk of developing iron-deficiency anemia.

From a TCM perspective ...

The etiology of menorrhagia is complicated and involves dysfunction at various levels including Qi and blood, the Penetrating Vessel 冲脉 and Conception Vessel 任脉 and the liver, spleen, and kidney. Empirical methods of treatment for excessive bleeding comprise of plugging the flow 塞流, cleansing the source 澄源, rejuvenation 复旧, hemostasis 止血, dispel blood stasis 消瘀 and nourishing blood 补血, but the overriding principle in the application of these treatment protocols should be to redirect blood back to its appropriate channel 引血归经.

Although all treatment protocols are narrowly directed at inducing bleeding cessation, the overriding principle takes a broader perspective of excessive bleeding and adopts a situational approach to address the root cause, especially for gynecology cases.

Generally, when the menstrual flow is heavy but not unrelenting, the conventional protocols for inducing bleeding cessation may still apply without undue consequences, but in the case of severe menorrhagia, there is bound to be blood stasis and any attempt to merely 'plug the flow' instead of 'redirecting the flow' would invariably accentuate the blood stasis and aggravate bleeding.

Therefore, patients with major bleeding should be treated based on the underlying conditions of the cold or heat, excess or deficiency whilst providing symptomatic relief to stop the bleed.

The second principle of treating menorrhagia is to prevent blood stasis whilst inducing coagulation 治崩防留瘀. This implies avoiding cold medication even though the underlying cause of menorrhagia is heat-related. In such cases, the heat should be cleared to cool the blood instead of neutralizing heat with cold-based therapies that could be counterproductive. This is because blood circulation should flow unimpeded in its normal course. But blood stagnates when it encounters cold and deviates from its normal course under the influence of heat; both deemed unsuitable therapies in redirecting blood back to its appropriate channel. In event that cooling of blood is inevitable, there is a need to temper the therapy with elements to invigorate blood, dispel blood stasis as well as warm the transport mechanism.

The third principle of treating menorrhagia is to address both underlying conditions as well as provide symptomatic relief concurrently. In case the underlying condition relates to Qi deficiency leading up to the loss of uplifting function 气虚下陷, treatment protocol should be tonify Qi to restrain bleeding 补气摄血. When the underlying condition relates to blood deficiency inter-twined with cold 血虚有寒, the appropriate treatment should be warm the meridians to restrain bleeding 温经摄血. Similarly, for menorrhagia caused by blood deficiency with heat symptoms 血虚有热, the appropriate prescription should be to nourish the Yin whilst confining the menstrual loss 养阴摄血. When menorrhagia is caused by heat entrapped in the Liver meridian 肝经郁热, soothing the Liver whilst controlling bleeding is the appropriate response 疏肝敛血. There will also be occasions when dissipating heat 泄火泄热 from the hyperactive heart and liver 心肝火旺 systems may address excessive bleeding.

Gua Sha Protocol for Adjuvant Therapy and Symptomatic Relief

a. Occipital-Cervical Sweep
b. Sternal Sweep
c. Superior Bladder Meridian Dredge
d. Back Rejuvenation Dredge (T11-L4)
e. Umbilicus-Pubic Sweep
f. Sacral V Dredge
g. Acupoint 'press-and-hold' for SP1 隐白, SP6 三阴交, SP10 血海, ST36 足三里, LR1 大敦, LR3 太冲, LR8 曲泉 on both legs
h. Acupoint 'press-and-hold' for SP12 冲门, EX CA1 子宫 on the torso bilaterally

Execution — Unless TCM diagnosis suggests otherwise, moderation press-stroke recommended. Acupoints marked for application of 'press-and-hold' technique in each prescription form a set, each set to be repeated three times. 'Press-and-hold' maneuver should be attempted 10 times for each prescribed acupoint within each set. Use of skin lubricant that invigorates Qi preferred. Observation of Sha appearance is not mandatory.

Other considerations — confirmation of bleeding disorders be obtained from the patient.

Supplementary Notes — Metrorrhagia/Irregular Menstruation

Metrorrhagia or irregular menstruation is abnormal bleeding or spotting that occurs between periods or that is not associated with menstruation. Also known as dysfunctional uterine bleeding (DUB), it is a common pathological condition in women of extreme reproductive age i.e. during the early years of menarche and when close to menopause. The bleeding is usually mild but serious bleeding can occur in some cases.

Although numerous medical conditions may cause metrorrhagia, it is usually not serious and upon identification can be treated effectively. These include cervical infection, hormonal imbalance associated with endocrinal dysfunction or caused by contraceptives, bleeding disorders, endometrial hyperplasia, cervical erosion, ruptured cervical or endometrial polyp, retained fetal debris, ectopic pregnancy, and uterine or vaginal cancer. Irregular bleeding may also occur during pregnancy with the possibility of miscarriage.

In TCM, the vital essence in both the Penetrating Vessel 冲脉 and Conception Vessel 任脉 are exhausted immediately after menstruation and has to be rebuilt over the course of the cycle and between periods. The need to regenerate Yin essence may be performed at the expense of Yang-Qi revitalization. The body, however, remains in a normal state when the Yin and Yang are well regulated.

The Yin collateral can be easily injured with blood overflowing in the form of mild vaginal bleeding if the kidney-Yin is deficient and impacted by the force of Yang-Qi revitalization. Alternatively, entrapped damp-heat in the light of Yang upsurge can cause blood to be misdirected 血热妄行 and resulting in vaginal bleeding. Similarly, blood stasis or slow-moving circulation does not augur well with the rapid Yang energy upsurge and cause vaginal bleeding when blood is forced out of its usual channel 离经之血.

The etiologies of metrorrhagia can, therefore, be categorized into any of these four causes — kidney Yin deficiency 肾阴亏虚, entrapped damp-heat 湿热内蕴, Qi stagnation & blood stasis 气滞血瘀 and spleen Qi deficiency 脾气亏虚.

Gua Sha Protocol for Adjuvant Therapy and Symptomatic Relief

a. Trapezius Sweep
b. Superior Bladder Meridian Dredge
c. Back Rejuvenation Dredge (T11-L4)
d. Sacral V Dredge
e. Epigastric-Umbilicus Sweep
f. Umbilicus-Pubic Sweep
g. Acupoint 'press-and-hold' for SP6 三阴交, SP10 血海, ST36 足三里, LR2 行间, LR4 中封 on both legs
h. Acupoint 'press-and-hold' for EX CA1 子宫 on the torso bilaterally

Execution — Unless TCM diagnosis suggests otherwise, moderation press-stroke recommended. Acupoints marked for application of 'press-and-hold' technique in each prescription form a set, each set to be repeated three times. 'Press-and-hold' maneuver should be attempted 10 times for each prescribed acupoint within each set. Use of skin lubricant that invigorates Qi preferred. Observation of Sha appearance is not mandatory.

Other considerations — Confirmation of non-pregnancy be obtained from the patient.

References

1. Rybo G. Menstrual blood loss in relation to parity and menstrual pattern. *Acta Obstet. Gynecol. Scand.* **45**(Suppl 7): 25–45 (1966).
2. Haynes PJ, Hodgson H, *et al.* Measurement of menstrual blood loss in patients complaining of menorrhagia. *Br. J. Obstet. Gynaecol.* **84**: 763–768 (1977).
3. Grimes DA. Estimating vaginal blood loss. *J. Reprod. Med.* **22**: 1990–1992 (1997).
4. Wilansky DL, Greisman B. Early hypothyroidism in patients with menorrhagia. *Am. J. Obstet. Gynecol.* **160**: 673–677 (1989).

Topic 54

Pelvic Organ Prolapse

Pelvic organ prolapse is a disorder in which a defect in the pelvic floor allows one or more of the pelvic organs to descend from their normal anatomical position. This is caused by injury to the muscles or tissues that support the pelvic organs. These musculatures are known as Delancey's three levels of support. Working downwards towards the orifices:

> Level 1 refers to the cardinal-uterosacral ligament complex providing apical attachment of the uterus and vaginal vault to the bony sacrum. Uterine prolapse occurs when the cardinal-uterosacral ligament complex is damaged or weakened.
>
> Level 2 refers to the arcus tendinous fascia pelvis and the fascia overlying the levator ani muscles that provide support to the middle part of the vagina. Damage usually leads to cystocele and rectocele.
>
> Level 3: The urogenital diaphragm and the perineal body provide support to the lower part of the vagina.

Often time, more than one organ can be affected concurrently and may occur in stages. The severity of prolapse is determined by the distance the organ is displaced from its original position; in mild cases, the organs descended only a short distance, whereas in severe cases the organs may be visible having moved a greater distance out of the body.

Uterine prolapse is caused by the herniation of the uterus into and beyond the vagina resulting from weakening or failure of ligamentous and fascial support. In severe uterine prolapse, the uterus may visibly protrude from the vagina, drawing along with it the anterior and posterior walls of the vagina. Uterine prolapse can occur with bladder prolapse, small intestine prolapse or rectal prolapse.

The severity of uterine prolapse has been quantified by various systems that measure the most distal portion of the prolapse during straining via Valsalva maneuver. In these systems, Stage I is defined as descent of the uterus to any point in the vagina up to 1 cm proximal to (before) the introitus/hymen; Stage II is a descent within 1 cm distal to (after) the introitus/hymen; Stage III is a descent beyond 1 cm distal to the introitus/hymen; and Stage IV as total uterine prolapse or procidentia.

Pelvic organ prolapse can also occur in women who have had a hysterectomy. In such a situation medically known as vaginal vault prolapse, the sutured top of the vagina descends without the uterus and creates a bulge that may protrude outside of the vagina in severe cases. Like uterine prolapse, vaginal vault prolapse is associated with bladder prolapse, small intestine prolapse, or rectal prolapse.

Bladder prolapse (cystocele) occurs when the bladder descends, often in conjunction with uterine prolapse or vaginal vault prolapse, and creates a bulge into the anterior wall of the vagina. Pushing the vagina wall ahead of it, the bulge can protrude outside the vagina in severe cases. Bladder prolapse is a common cause of stress urinary incontinence (involuntary loss of urine while coughing, sneezing, or laughing).

Rectal prolapse (rectocele) occurs when the rectum descends, often in conjunction with uterine prolapse or vaginal vault prolapse, and creates a bulge into the posterior wall of the vagina. In severe cases, the bulge in pushing the vagina wall ahead during the descend can protrude outside the vagina.

Small intestine prolapse (enterocele) occurs when the small intestine descends and creates a bulge via the recto-uterine pouch (Pouch of Douglas) or, in post-hysterectomy cases, into the vaginal vault. Small intestine prolapse may occur with uterine prolapse, bladder prolapse or rectal prolapse.

The etiology of any prolapse, as defined by the displacement of an organ from its normal anatomical position, is the weakening of supporting musculature and tissues. Pelvic organ prolapse is no different.

The primary cause of prolapse is pregnancy and childbirth. A typical adult uterus weighs about 60 grams and during pregnancy, the average weight gained may escalate to 12 kg which makes pregnancy one of the main reasons for prolapse. Gravity acting on the increased weight over a protracted period of time invariably causes muscles to be attenuated. Difficult traumatic labor and increased parity especially with vaginal delivery of large-sized babies accentuate the risk of prolapse due to the extended stretch of the levator ani musculature during childbirth.

Similarly, extreme physical activity that creates high intra-abdominal pressure such as physically strenuous exercise, high-impact exercise, repeated heavy lifting, intense coughing, and frequent straining during bowel evacuation may subject the pelvic musculature to injury due to excessive tissue displacement. In seat-belt related injuries, uterine prolapse can be a rare complication due to a sudden increase in intra-abdominal pressure caused by the trauma and position of the seat belt.[1,2]

Being overweight or obese is another risk factor for pelvic organ prolapse as additional bodyweight creates chronic elevation in intra-abdominal pressure.[3,4]

Collagen is the building block of connective tissues and the source the latter's tensile strength. In one study, genitourinary prolapse in premenopausal women is found to be associated with a reduction of total collagen content and a decrease in collagen solubility. During normal tissue turnover, MMPs are a group of enzymes responsible for the degradation of most extracellular matrix proteins, of which collagen forms a major class. Collagen turnover, as indicated by matrix metalloproteinase (MMP) activity, was up to four times higher in prolapse tissue.[5] Since the women were premenopausal, the increased in collagenolytic activity causing loss of collagen in prolapse tissue suggests that the condition could be congenital. In another study, it was found that premenopausal nulliparous women with genuine stress incontinence had significantly less collagen in their tissues than those in the control group.[6] This hypothesis is further supported by observational work showing a relationship between joint hypermobility and prolapse.[7] Genetic predisposition towards weakness in or dysfunction of connective tissue, e.g. Marfan syndrome, therefore, is a possible risk factor for prolapse.

It is known that estrogen has a marked effect on tendon collagen synthesis as the elevation of estradiol levels appear to influence tendon morphology and biomechanical properties in postmenopausal women compared to women with low estradiol concentration.[8] This implies that lower estrogen level after menopause is a risk factor for prolapse. And so is increasing age.

Clinical presentations of pelvic organ prolapse depend on the stage and severity of the defect. Unless in severe cases, patients are usually asymptomatic even when signs of development are observed. Notwithstanding when the leading edge of the descent is 0.5 cm distal to the introitus (late-stage II), symptoms may be felt. These symptoms are fundamentally relating to urinary voiding, defecation, and sexual dysfunctions and may typically include a sensation of lower abdominal discomfort, vaginal fullness or pressure, and sacral back pain. When the walls of the vagina or the cervix protrude through the vaginal introitus, spotting from ulceration of the protruding cervix or vagina may occur.

Treatment of severe pelvic organ prolapse is a complex subject in the realms of gynecology that require professional assessment. Mild cases of prolapse may be addressed by improving the strength of supporting musculature through prescribed exercise.

From a TCM perspective ...

The etiology of pelvic organ prolapse is Qi deficiency leading to Qi descent 气虚下陷 and therefore an inability to maintain internal organs in their normal anatomical position. Frequent parity or protracted strenuous activity is identified as the cause for Qi deficiency resulting in exhaustion of the eight exceptional meridians

八脉空虚, especially the Penetrating Vessel 冲脉 and Conception Vessel 任脉 which are known to cause most gynecological issues. In the light that prolapse is fundamentally a deficiency-mediated disorder, the appropriate general therapeutic principle to be adopted shall be "replenish the deficiency and counteract the descent 虚者补之，陷者举之".

Ye Tianshi was first to associate the operation of eight exceptional meridians with the liver and kidney functions in clinical practice; and emphasized that hepatic, renal and gonadal related diseases invariably reside with the eight exceptional meridians, a fundamental tenet when ignored would lead to futile treatment. Elaborating on treatment principles, pain radiating upwards from the back is associated with the Governor Vessel and treatment be directed at the kidney; whereas pain that radiates upwards from the abdomen is associated with the Penetrating Vessel and Conception Vessel, and treatment be focussed on the liver or the stomach.[9]

> 叶天士: "奇经八脉,隶于肝肾为多", "肝肾下病, 必留连奇经八脉,不知此旨, 宜乎无功"。 "凡冲气攻痛,从背而上者, 系督脉主病, 治在少阴, 从腹而上者,治在厥阴, 系冲任主病,或填补阳明,此治病之宗旨也。

As such, *Gua Sha* protocol shall encompass the strengthening of Qi as well as reinforcing the function of the kidney system by address deficiencies of the liver, kidney and spleen/stomach systems.

Gua Sha Protocol for Adjuvant Therapy and Symptomatic Relief

a. Four Spirit Extension, Sternal Sweep
b. Ventral Intercostal Space Sweep
c. Umbilicus-Pubic Sweep
d. Back Rejuvenation Dredge
e. Sacral V Dredge
f. Acupoint 'press-and-hold' for ST36 足三里, BL57 承山, SP9 阴陵泉, LR3 太冲 on both legs
g. Acupoint 'press-and-hold' for LI11 曲池, TE6 支沟 on both hands

Execution — Unless TCM diagnosis suggests otherwise, moderation press-stroke recommended. Acupoints marked for application of 'press-and-hold' technique in each prescription form a set, each set to be repeated three times. 'Press-and-hold' maneuver should be attempted 10 times for each prescribed acupoint within each set. Use of skin lubricant that invigorates Qi preferred. Observation of Sha appearance is not mandatory.

Glossary

Hysterectomy — the complete removal of the uterus by surgical means.

Valsalva maneuver — a breathing technique that can be used to help diagnose medical problems and also used to help restore a normal heart rate in an arrhythmic situation. It is performed by moderately forceful attempted exhalation against a closed airway, usually by closing the mouth and pinching the nose shut while pressing out as if blowing up a balloon.

Parity is the number of times a female carries pregnancy to full term.

References

1. Mukalian GG. Traumatic uterine prolapse. *J. Trauma* **42**: 553–554 (1997).
2. Lohiya GS. Uterine prolapse and cystocele after an automobile accident. *Ann. Emerg. Med.* **42**(6): 850–851 (2003).
3. Varela JE, Hinojosa M, Nguyen N. Correlations between intra-abdominal pressure and obesity-related co-morbidities. *Surg. Obes. Relat. Dis.* **5**(5): 524–528 (Sep-Oct 2009).
4. Smit M, Werner MJM, Lansink-Hartgring AO, *et al.* How central obesity influences intra-abdominal pressure: a prospective, observational study in cardiothoracic surgical patients. *Ann. Intensive Care* **6**: 99 (2016).
5. Jackson SR, Avery NC, Tarlton JF, *et al.* Changes in metabolism of collagen in genitourinary prolapse. *Lancet* **347**(9016): 1658–1661 (June 15, 1996).
6. Keane DP, Sims TJ, Abrams P, *et al.* Analysis of collagen status in premenopausal nulliparous women with genuine stress incontinence. *Br. J. Obstet. Gynaecol.* **104**(9): 994–998 (Sep 1997).
7. Veit-Rubin N, Cartwright R, Singh AU. Association between joint hypermobility and pelvic organ prolapse in women: a systematic review and meta-analysis. *Int. Urogynecol J.* **27**(10): 1469–1478 (Oct 2016).
8. Hansen M, Kongsgaard M, Holm L, *et al.* Effect of estrogen on tendon collagen synthesis, tendon structural characteristics, and biomechanical properties in postmenopausal women. *J. Appl. Physiol. (1985)* **106**(4): 1385–1393 (Apr 2009).
9. Ye Gui. *Clinical Practice Guidelines & Medical Cases* 临证指南医案 (1746).

TOPIC 55

Perimenopausal/Menopausal Syndrome

Menopause refers to the cessation of menstrual flow lasting at least 12 months resulting from the cessation of ovarian follicular activity and in the absence of obvious pathologic or physiologic cause. It is associated with a reduction in the normal estrogen levels arising from the progressive decline in ovarian follicular activity. The transition leading up to menopause is called perimenopause and is the intervening period in a woman's life that signals the end of the fertility phase in a woman as a consequence of the body's natural aging process. The duration following the last period which is 12 months without menstruation is called post-menopause.[1]

Perimenopause and menopause are not diseases but are healthy and natural progression in a woman's life. The average age for natural menopause is 51 years. However, when menopause occurs much earlier before the age of 45, it is deemed early menopause and menopause before the age of 40 is known as premature menopause.

The age at natural menopause (ANM) varies with environmental exposure, lifestyle and genetic factors. Smoking, caloric restriction particularly during early childhood, excessive exercise, severe weight loss, nulliparity, and short-length menstrual cycles accelerate ANM. In contrast, irregular menstrual cycles, height, socioeconomic status, parity and giving birth before the age of 25 extend ANM. Nutrition may affect ANM, as in vegetarian diet accelerates ANM by about

2 years; a high intake of fat, cholesterol, and caffeine also accelerate menopause, while moderate alcohol consumption delays it. Notwithstanding, the influence of dietary factors has not been adequately documented due to a relatively small number of studies.[2,3]

Medical treatment can at times induce menopause. Cancer treatments, including chemotherapy, pelvic radiation, and surgery, can cause early menopause. Bilateral oophorectomy (removal of both ovaries) brings about immediate menopause with certainty. Logically, having an ovary-sparing hysterectomy alone (removal of the uterus only) does not cause menopause but terminates menstruation permanently by the elimination of the endometrium. Notwithstanding, Duke University Medical Center reported that having a hysterectomy may express the occurrence of natural menopause by approximately two years. The risk for menopause was highest among women who had one ovary removed along with their uterus, but it remained elevated even when both ovaries are preserved.[4]

The transition from reproductive to non-reproductive years in women undergoing menopause is characterized by increased manifestations of menopausal symptoms that may begin up to 6 years before the final menstrual period (FMP) and continue for a varying number of years after FMP. As the post-menopausal years progress, these symptoms decline correspondingly with the accompanying loss of ovarian response to gonadotropin stimulation.

Because the causes of these symptoms could be multi-dimensional and interwoven with the complex physiological changes during this period of a woman's life, it is difficult to segregate with certainty what is associated with aging or other life changes that dovetailed with menopause. Moreover, the hormonal level for each individual could fluctuate for years before eventually being low enough to present as full-blown menopause and, in different lifestyle settings, give rise to an absence of universal menopause syndrome.[5] Notwithstanding, aside from irregular menstruation, there are four core symptoms identified relating to the likelihood that estrogen being effective in relieving symptoms in menopausal women. These are vasomotor anomalies, vaginal dryness, sleep disturbance, and adverse mood.[6]

The vasomotor symptoms experienced during menopause include hot flashes and night sweat. Ovarian aging and hormonal changes have been consistently linked to these vasomotor symptoms and some urogenital symptoms. Hot flash episodes may last between one and 30 minutes but on average about three minutes and may recur for years in some individuals though most women suffer from them for only a short period of time.

The exact cause of hot flashes is still not well understood but it is theorized that with fluctuations in estrogen level, there could be a resetting and narrowing of the body's thermoregulatory system. Serotonin levels are known to vary in sync with decreased estrogen levels and by operation of negative feedback mechanism, additional serotonin is released due to the upregulation of serotonin receptors in the hypothalamus. This activation, in turn, changes the set point temperature and results in hot flashes.

More than a third of menopausal women are thwarted by moderate to severe symptoms of vaginal dryness resulting in dyspareunia. Vaginal dryness and change in urine pH also cause the urinary tract to be susceptible to infection. Aside from mere lack of natural lubrication, the vaginal tissue could undergo atrophy, leading to narrowing and shortening of the vaginal canal as well as possible uterine prolapse from loss of pelvic muscle tone.

Without appropriate long-term treatment, vulvovaginal atrophy is not self-limiting as it results from urogenital tissues that have estrogen receptors being deprived of the hormone. Fluctuation in estrogen levels during the menopausal transition, followed by sustained low levels after menopause, can render vaginal tissue regeneration less robust resulting from the aforesaid distress.

An effective clinical response to vaginal atrophy and dryness is menopausal hormone therapy, which is the administration of low dose systemic or vaginal estrogen during the menopausal transition. Although the minimum effective dose remains elusive, menopausal hormone therapy is effective and generally safe in alleviating the adverse development associated with vaginal atrophy. Notwithstanding, women receiving this treatment, especially those on conjugated equine estrogens (CEE), may be at increased risk of all types of urinary infection that escalates over time.

Sleep disturbance generally increases with aging and is often aggravated by physiological changes associated with menopause. In fact, sleep efficiency for women in late productive age progressively deteriorates across the menstrual cycle with the decline being most pronounced during the premenstrual week. Sleep quality deterioration is characterized by lower sleep efficiency, shorter sleep time and increased activity during sleep. As much as 25 minutes of sleep per night may be lost during the week preceding menstruation that corresponds to the time when Follicle Stimulating Hormone (FSH), progesterone and estrogen levels decline. Sleep quality degradations may be further aggravated by socio-demographic and lifestyle factors including unfavorable body mass index, financial strain, and smoking.[7]

Further compromise in sleep quality is associated with the rate of hormonal changes associated with the menopausal transition. Association with sleep attributes is much stronger with FSH than with estradiol (estrogen). When the reproductive life of women is partitioned into age-specified epochs defined by significant rates of FSH change, it was noted that the rate of increase is most acute around the time of FMP; a stage reflecting the frequent failures and repeated trials to establish a dominant follicle and subsequent corpus luteum as well as decline in Anti-Müllerian hormone (AMH) and inhibin levels.[8]

Women suffering from sleep disturbance in conjunction with night sweat should be subject to hormone therapy. There are however other non-hormone related factors that might cause nighttime awakening and prescribing treatment for sleep deprivation is therefore complex and multi-dimensional.

Women in menstrual transition are vulnerable to adverse mood swings or even depression. In some instances, anxiety appears to instigate depressive episodes. Previous episodes of depression may also confer increased risk for the development of yet another onset. Depression was once thought to be the outcome of a cascading process in which other menstrual symptoms worked in concert with hot flashes leading to sleep disturbance and consequently causing daytime fatigue that lowers one's resilience to environmental stress before impinging on the quality of life and thus manifesting as depression. Research however demonstrated otherwise, and that depressive symptoms more often precede hot flashes when both symptoms co-exist.[9]

The monoamines, serotonin, and norepinephrine, are neuromodulators that act on various characteristics of the brain function. While norepinephrine is more involved in motivation, energy, interest, and focus, serotonin drives impulsiveness, sexual function, and appetite. The function of these neurotransmitters, however, overlaps in the areas of mood, sleep, stress, and pain. Serotonin is paramount in the feelings of elation and positivity that help protect one against anxiety and depression. Imbalance in serotonin, relative to norepinephrine and dopamine, is a common cause of depression.

Estrogen enhances serotonin function, particularly when serotonin and/or tryptophan the precursor to serotonin, are deficient.[10] Estrogen can alter serotonergic activity by increasing serotonin synthesis, moderating the activity of serotonin 5-HT receptors that mediate both excitatory and inhibitory neurotransmission and downregulating monoamine oxidase (MAO) activity, thereby delaying the degradation of serotonin and norepinephrine in the Central Nervous System. Significant instability and decline in estrogen concentration during menopause are therefore likely to contribute to mood change and depression.

Treatment of a major depressive episode may involve psychotherapy, antidepressants, or a combination thereof and are often tailored to patient preference and severity of depression. Selective serotonin reuptake inhibitors (SSRIs) are the first-line medications used in the treatment of depression. In more complex situations, serotonin and norepinephrine reuptake inhibitors (SNRI) may be prescribed.

Menopause is the period during which serious health problems such as cardiovascular diseases, osteoporosis, and even gynecologic cancers occur with increasing frequency. Understanding the factors which determine menopausal age and making appropriate lifestyle changes that result in sustaining natural estrogen production would, therefore, defer menopause and all its attendant issues.

From a TCM perspective ...

Menopause occurs, as recorded in HuangDi's Internal Classics — Plain Questions, "at age 49 when the Conception Vessel becomes depleted and the Great Thoroughfare Vessel weakened with its contents diminished. Thus, the Heaven Gui is exhausted [menopause], the process of menstruation becomes unavailable. Hence, the physical appearance languishes and a woman can no longer bear children."

> 《黄帝内经 素问·上古天真论》: "女子七七，任脉虚，太冲脉衰少，天癸竭，地道不通，故形坏而无子也"

The age of natural menopause (ANM) is computed based on the physiological life of women from birth to the termination of fertility over a period of seven equal phases of seven years each; with each stage manifesting significant physiological changes. Taken from puberty to menopause, the number of periods would be five [please refer details under earlier topic Amenorrhea]. This model augurs well with STRAW staging model that similarly depicts the reproductive period of a woman from menarche to FMP in five distinct periods.[11]

The etiology of the menopausal transition is a gradual decline of renal Qi, giving rise to disharmony in the body's Yin and Yang that leads to instability in hormonal levels. Another cause is Kidney Yin deficiency resulting in the failure to bridle in the body's Yang elements that set off a wave of changes including but not limited to dysfunction of the heart, liver, spleen and stomach systems and their associated meridians as well as a manifestation of intermittent hot flashes during the menopausal transition.

In kidney Yin deficiency-related perimenopause, the syndrome characteristics are menstrual irregularities, vaginal dryness resulting in dyspareunia, light or absence of vaginal discharge, hot flashes, dizziness, tinnitus, sleep disturbance, night sweating, mood swings and possibly pruritus. When kidney Yin deficiency is exacerbated to the point when the heart system is affected, sleep disturbance, palpitation, mood instability, and cognitive decline become more apparent as the kidney-water is incompetent in restraining the heart-fire 水火不济, 心肾不交, 心火妄动.

When perimenopause is induced by kidney Yang deficiency, the symptoms are expanded to include osteoporosis as manifested by weakness in weight-bearing joints of the lower limbs, edema that is more pronounced in the lower extremities and incontinence; when the spleen Yang becomes compromised in due course 脾肾阳虚, symptoms of diarrhea and low tolerance toward cold would be added to the list.

However, the most common etiology observed in a clinical setting is a hybrid situation where both Yin and Yang are deficient 阴阳两虚型 that give rise to a combined syndrome.

Gua Sha Protocol for Adjuvant Therapy and Symptomatic Relief

a. Four Spirit Extension
b. Lesser Yang Plough
c. Occipital-Cervical Sweep
d. Sternal Sweep
e. Trapezius Sweep
f. Superior Bladder Meridian Dredge
g. Sacral V Dredge
h. Acupoint 'press-and-hold' for SP6 三阴交, ST36 足三里, ST40 丰隆, KI3 太溪, LR3 太冲 for both legs
i. Acupoint 'press-and-hold' for PC6 内关, HT7 神门, LI4 合谷 for both hands

Execution — Unless TCM diagnosis suggests otherwise, moderation press-stroke recommended. Acupoints marked for application of 'press-and-hold' technique in each prescription form a set, each set to be repeated three times. 'Press-and-hold' maneuver should be attempted 10 times for each prescribed acupoint within each set. Use of skin lubricant that invigorates Qi preferred. Observation of Sha appearance is not mandatory.

Glossary

Nulliparity — a medical term for a woman who has never given birth either by choice or for any other reason. The term also applies to women who have given birth to a stillborn baby, or a baby who was otherwise not able to survive outside the womb.

References

1. Sherman S. Defining the menopausal transition. *Am. J. Med.* **118**(12B): 3S–7S (2005).
2. Elias SG, van Noord PA, Peeters PH, *et al.* Caloric restriction reduces age at menopause: the effect of the 1944–1945 Dutch famine. *Menopause* **10**(5): 399–405 (Sep–Oct 2003).
3. Biela U. Determinants of the age at natural menopause. *Przegl Lek.* **59**(3): 165–169 (2002).
4. Moorman PG, Myers ER, *et al.* Effect of hysterectomy with ovarian preservation on ovarian function. *Obstet. Gynecol.* **118**(6): 1271–1279 (Dec 2011).
5. Avis NE, Brockwell S, Colvin A. A universal menopausal syndrome? *Am. J. Med.* **118**(12B): 37S–46S (2005).
6. Santoro N, Epperson CN, Mathews SB. Menopausal symptoms and their management. *Endocrinol. Metab. Clin. North Am.* **44**(3): 497–515 (Sep 2015).
7. Zheng H, Harlow SD, Kravitz HM, *et al.* Actigraphy-defined measures of sleep and movement across the menstrual cycle in midlife menstruating women: Study of Women's Health Across the Nation sleep study. *Menopause* **22**(1): 66–74 (2015).
8. Sowers MF, Zheng H, McConnell D, *et al.* Follicle stimulating hormone and its rate of change in defining menopause transition stages. *J. Clin. Endocrinol. Metab.* **93**(10): 3958–3964 (Oct 2008).
9. Freeman EW, Sammel MD, Lin H. Temporal associations of hot flashes and depression in the transition to menopause *Menopause* **16**(4): 728–734 (2009).
10. Epperson CN, Amin Z, Ruparel K, *et al.* Interactive effects of estrogen and serotonin on brain activation during working memory and affective processing in menopausal women. *Psychoneuroendocrinology* **37**(3): 372–382 (Mar 2012).
11. Soules MR, Sherman S, Parrott E, *et al.* Executive summary: Stages of Reproductive Aging Workshop (STRAW). *Fertil. Steril.* **76**: 874–878 (2001).

Topic 56

Subfertility

Subfertility, which can be classified as primary or secondary, is a failure to conceive after one year of unprotected, regular sexual intercourse. When continuing missed conception occurs to a couple who has no previous history of pregnancies, the state of subfertility is deemed to be primary. Secondary subfertility, however, is the inability to conceive or, when conceived, failed to carry a fetus to a full term even though there had been a record of a successful pregnancy. Though secondary subfertility is influenced by many of the causes of primary subfertility, the probability of successful conception is much higher than in a situation of primary subfertility.

Most couples frustrated by subfertility are not sterile or completely infertile. They merely experienced varying difficulty in getting conceived. Statistically, the conception rate during the first month of attempt is about 30% with the probability of conception declining to about 5% by the end of the first year. The outlook for conception is usually rosy for the first six months as the conception rate on a cumulative basis is closed to 75%; which then continues to climb, albeit at a slow rate, to 90% at the end of the first year of attempt. The probability of unassisted conception, however, declines sharply for the second year, giving a cumulative conception rate of only 5%.

There is a strong association between subfertility and advancing age that applies equally to both genders. The decline in fertility is most remarkable in women with age between the late 30s and early 40s. In comparison with younger counterparts aged 20 to 25 years, women in this age bracket have only 60% cumulative rate of spontaneous conception at first year and 85% by the end of year two. This downward trend is observed even with assisted conception and could be inferred from possible lower ovarian reserve and poorer oocyte quality with the passage of time.

Though less affected by age, a marked declining trend in male fertility was also observed for all periods for men aged over 40 years. With a social inclination in women towards later marriage and thus delay in starting a family, the combined effect of fertility reduction in both genders inevitably exacerbate the depressed probability of conception. This is due to genetic defects in gametes that increase with age for both genders. For female, the rate clearly rises after age 35 and for male, the point of inflection is after age 40.[1]

There also appears to be an inversed relationship between the duration of subfertility and the probability of spontaneous conception. As a rule of thumb, couples who endured unexplained subfertility for more than three years have half the chance of conceiving as compared to counterparts who did not; which implies that treatment for subfertility is time-sensitive.

For effective conception, sperms need to be deposited in the female genital tract before they are impeded by progesterone-induced changes in cervical mucus that occur immediately after ovulation. Coinciding coitus with ovulation therefore greatly improves the probability of conception.

As it stands, the fertile interval for a female is six days with the day of ovulation being last day and the most probable day for conception following coitus being the second day before ovulation when the cervical mucus turns more fluid. This observation holds well for females age between 19 and 34. For women in a higher age bracket of age 35–39, the fertile interval is five days ending on the day of ovulation. The probability of conception during the fertile interval is also influenced by age, with probability for the age bracket 19–26 being a shade more than 0.5 and dropping 0.1 for every higher age bracket. By the time women reached age 35, the peak probability of conception during the fertile interval drops to 0.25.[1]

Body mass is an important indicator of general health that also reflects reproductive capability, especially in women. The relationship between body weight and fertility is an inverted U shape. Extremities in body mass are detrimental to conception and it appears that women with body mass index (BMI) exceeding 30 or less than 20 are less likely to conceive in comparison with their counterparts that hold healthier scores.

The impact of obesity on reproductive function, especially ovulatory disorders, is mainly attributed to endocrine mechanisms in that adipose tissue acting as an endocrine organ increased peripheral aromatization of androgen to estrogen and interfere with neuroendocrine and ovarian functions through disturbance of the hypothalamus-pituitary-ovarian axis. The outcome is anovulation; not mentioning increased risk in miscarriage, poor pregnancy outcomes and compromised fetal well-being. The ovarian reserve and oocyte quality in obese females are also adversely affected by elevated circulating levels of C-reactive protein (CRP) that causes chronic low-grade inflammation. Excess free fatty acids exert a toxic effect on maturing follicular tissue and produce persistent cell damage.[2] As such, the fertility of obese women in assisted conception programs may continue to be impaired if these reasons are not duly addressed.

Fertility and conception also work against women with a BMI < 20 and those who are exercising excessively; due to an increased probability of anovulation. Menstrual dysfunction is common among athletes, such as endurance athletes and dancers, with very low body mass.[3] Being considerably underweight is associated with an increased risk of miscarriage and intrauterine growth retardation.

A recent trend in lifestyle could also work insidiously against fertility, especially in female. In the quest for deferred aging and perhaps youth preservation, it was observed that high levels of the hormone IGF-1 increased the risk of degenerative diseases such as Alzheimer's and retinal degeneration. Reduced IGF-1 signaling promoted by calorie restriction, however, delays aging by reducing insulin secretion combined with enhanced insulin sensitivity which typically declines with aging. Reduced thermogenesis resulting from calorie restriction also diminishes oxidative damage of macromolecules, the likely final common pathway of these effects.[4]

Though a lower IGF-1 level appears to improve health and aging, the downside is it may have a deleterious effect on reproduction. Circulating IGF-1 stimulates growth in all cells, from skeletal muscle and bone to organ tissue and vessel linings with the type of processes that are being initiated depending on the levels of IGF-1. However, very low levels of IGF-1 send the body into a self-preservation mode, switching energy allocation away from the lower priority reproductive functions and devoting resources to maintenance and DNA repair.

From a pathological perspective, major causes of subfertility can be grouped broadly as ovulation disorders, tubal damage, unexplained, other causes such as endometriosis and fibroids and male partner factors (which include disorders of spermatogenesis or obstruction). Tubal infertility is more common in those with secondary subfertility and in populations with a higher prevalence of sexually acquired infections.

The proportion of each type of subfertility varies with different countries, but generally, unexplained etiology always make up the largest segment in any population.

From a TCM perspective ...

There are 5 types of non-conceiving female 五不女 and the descriptions from the ancient medical text[5] refer to the five observed congenital physical deformities of the women's genital namely spiral 螺, lines 紋, drums 鼓, horns 角, veins 脈, which in modern-day context represent longitudinal vaginal septum 螺, vaginal stenosis 紋, hymen atresia or imperforate hymen 鼓, clitoromegaly or clitoral hyperplasia 角 and amenorrhea 脈 respectively. There was no known solution during ancient times to address the congenital structural defects that may today be resolved easily by surgical means.

Although TCM may be less than adequate in the treatment of congenital defects, it has through the ages accumulated invaluable empirical experience and gynecology theories that can effectively manage the issues of acquired pathological infertility. In fact, it was first proposed by Sun Simiao of the Tang Dynasty in his work 'Essential Prescriptions Worth a Thousand Gold — Seeking Offspring' that "for childless mortals, the cause is invariably due to internal injuries and debilitations suffered by the couple arising from *five strains and seven injuries*".

《千金要方·求子》: "凡人無子，當為夫妻俱有五勞七傷、虛羸百病所致"

This statement highlights treating infertility or subfertility require addressing the health of the couple as an integral unit and has significant implications for lifestyle changes.

In TCM, the common etiologies of subfertility are kidney Qi, Yin and/or Yang deficiencies, liver Qi stagnation and blood stasis and phlegm/dampness obstruction; the last etiology usually reflective of people with obesity. The focus of treatment is to warm and promote kidney Qi, nourish the vital essence and blood, regulate the Penetrating Vessel 冲脉 and Conception Vessel 任脉, dispel blood stasis and invigorate Qi to clear phlegm/dampness obstruction.

Contemporary medicine emphasizes on the regulation of various hormones and where necessary surgical intervention to assist conception. TCM, on the other hand, underscores the reinforcement of kidney Qi, Yin and Yang and regulation of liver Qi as proxies to improve the function of the Hypothalamic-Pituitary-Adrenal axis that in turn mediates the Hypothalamic-Pituitary-Gonad axis that impact on fertility and fetal development.[6]

Gua Sha Protocol for Adjuvant Therapy

a. Epigastric-Umbilicus Sweep
b. Umbilicus-Pubic Sweep
c. Sacral V Dredge
d. Back Rejuvenation Dredge

e. Spleen Meridian Dredge (SP6-SP10) with emphasis on SP6 三阴交, SP8 地机, SP10 血海 using acupoint 'press-and-hold' technique
f. Acupoint 'press-and-hold' for ST36 足三里, ST40 丰隆 and LR3 太冲on both legs
g. Acupoint 'press-and-hold' for LI11 曲池, PC6 内关 on both hands
h. Acupoint 'press-and-hold' for EX CA1 子宫 bilaterally on the torso

Execution — Unless TCM diagnosis suggests otherwise, moderation press-stroke recommended. Acupoints marked for application of 'press-and-hold' technique in each prescription form a set, each set to be repeated three times. 'Press-and-hold' maneuver should be attempted 10 times for each prescribed acupoint within each set. Use of skin lubricant that invigorates Qi preferred. Observation of Sha appearance is not mandatory.

Glossary

Five strains and Seven injuries 五劳七傷 are explained in 'HuangDi's Internal Classics — Plain Questions' as follows:

Five strains and their adverse effects are: extended belaboring of the vision exhausts blood 久视伤血, extended recumbency damages Qi 久卧伤气, sitting for extended periods compromises (atrophies) the flesh 久坐伤肉, standing for extended periods degenerates bones 久立伤骨 and walking for extended periods wears out sinews 久行伤筋.

Seven injuries refer to gluttony-induced injuries to the 'Spleen' 大饱伤脾, anger-induced injuries to the liver 大怒气逆伤肝, kidney injuries induced by forced load lifting or sitting on damp ground for protracted period 强力举重久坐湿地伤肾, impairment to the lungs due to exposure to cold and consumption of cold drinks 形寒饮冷伤肺, impairment to the heart due to worries and sorrows 忧愁思慮伤心, impairment to anatomical structure and form associated with exposure to inclement weather 风雨寒暑伤形 and impairment to resilience due to uncontrollable fear 恐惧不节伤志.

References

1. Dunson DB, Colombo B, Baird DD. Changes with age in the level and duration of fertility in the menstrual cycle. *Hum. Reprod.* **17**: 1399–1403 (2002).

2. Silvestris E, de Pergola G, *et al.* Obesity as disruptor of the female fertility. *Reprod. Biol. Endocrinol.* **16**: 22 (2018).
3. Shangold MM. Menstrual irregularity in athletes: basic principles, evaluation, and treatment, *Can J Appl Sport Sci.* 1982 **Jun 7**(2): 68–73
4. Bartke A, Chandrashekar V, Dominici F, *et al.* Insulin-like growth factor 1 (IGF-1) and aging: controversies and new insights. *Biogerontology* 2003 **4**: 1–8
5. Wan Mi Zhai 万全(密斋). *Critical Success Factors for Procreation — On Mate Selection* 《广嗣纪要·择配篇》 1573.
6. Joseph DN, Whirledge S. Stress and the HPA axis: balancing homeostasis and fertility. *Int. J. Mol. Sci.* **18**(10): pii: E2224 (Oct 24, 2017).

Musculoskeletal

TOPIC 57

Cervical Spondylosis

The neck comprises seven small vertebrae, stacked one on top of another and beginning at the base of the skull. Between each pair of vertebrae is a centimeter thick resilient intervertebral disk that prevents adjacent vertebrae from abrasion against each other when the body is subject to shock during motion. More importantly, the intervertebral disk provides healthy clearance or space between the vertebrae for spinal cord nerve roots to freely and laterally emerge through the foramen (openings).

These bony structures, forming part of the spine that protects the spinal cord, are one of the most flexible configurations in the skeletal system. Because of its frequent movement, the neck is also extremely vulnerable to degeneration with the passage of time. Cervical spondylosis, commonly called arthritis of the neck, is the medical term for these age-related, degenerative injuries.

Aging causes the intervertebral disks in the spine to lose height and buckle. They may also lose water content, begin to dry out and weaken. This problem causes settling or collapse of the disk spaces and the loss of disk space height such that the vertebrae press against each other.

Like any joint, the facet joints when subject to pressure begin to degenerate, starting with the smooth protective articular cartilage, resulting in arthritis. Alternatively, the direct abrasion of adjacent vertebrae may elicit the overgrowth of new bone in response to the loss of protective cartilage. Such bone overgrowth or bone spurs (osteophytes) may over time narrow the opening of the foramen causing cervical stenosis and pinching the emerging nerves passing through the opening. Cervical stenosis may result in tingling or paresthesia and even loss of strength in the extremities.

Cervical spondylosis is a consequence of aging. Everyone will, in due course, be affected by this degenerative condition characterized by pain and stiffness in the neck that ranges from mild to severe. The pain is usually aggravated by postural inactivity such as protracted session of surfing the internet. The pain usually responds well to conservative treatment and also improves with rest or lying down.

Other symptoms may include headaches, dizziness or even blackouts when the condition results in compression of blood vessels supplying blood to the brain.

Notwithstanding the above, many people with cervical spondylosis are asymptomatic too.

Diagnosis of cervical spondylosis is usually confirmed with imaging technology. X-ray and Computed Tomography (CT) can reveal defects in vertebral alignment as well as degenerative changes in the cervical spine such as intervertebral disk atrophy and the presence of osteophytes. For soft tissue injury such as herniated intervertebral disk, Magnetic Resonance Imaging (MRI) provides clearer images than X-ray or CT scans.

Treatment of the first choice for cervical spondylosis is usually nonsurgical and therapeutic options include physiotherapy (cervical traction) to take the load off the joints instantly but temporarily, muscle relaxants to relief painful muscular spasms and nonsteroidal anti-inflammatory drugs (NSAIDs) to address local pain and inflammation. Sometimes a cervical collar is also prescribed to reinforce the benefit of cervical traction.

When first-line treatment yields no benefit, steroid and anesthetic medication may be introduced into the site of pain in the form of a cervical epidural block or cervical facet joint block as the case deemed fit. When all else failed, surgery is the last available option but seldom recommended given the risk and consequence associated with its failure.

From a TCM perspective ...

Cervical spondylosis is categorically classified under occlusion or impediment conditions 痹证 whereby pathways to nutrition are obstructed 痹者闭也, meridians and collaterals are occluded 经络闭塞, numbness is present 麻痹不仁, or palpation causes aching 攻注作疼, or joints lack dexterity 凝结关节, or mobility is compromised to a point of paralysis 重着难移，手足偏废. Such conditions are also associated with blood stasis.[1]

As the proper function of the bones and sinews are intrinsically related to the kidney and liver respectively, the etiology of occlusion conditions, cervical spondylosis included, should logically be attributed to liver and kidney deficiencies. When kidney essence is lacking, bone marrows will be undernourished. When liver Yin and blood is insufficient, sinews shall be underdeveloped or ill-maintained leading to compromised mobility and impaired joint dexterity.

The invasion by exogenous pathogens of wind, cold and dampness are secondary factors to occlusion conditions. These three factors in concert engender phlegm, cause injury to bones and sinews and obstruction in meridians and collaterals with clinical manifestations of aversion to cold, aggravated aches/pains when exposed to wind and inclement weather. The condition is usually chronic.

Treatment is therefore directed at rectifying the underlying deficiencies of the liver, kidney and, if necessary, reinforce the spleen to boost Qi flow as well as providing symptomatic relief by dispelling blood stasis, evacuation of accumulated phlegm, improving blood circulation and alleviating local muscular spasm and edema. Expulsion of exogenous pernicious influence is also necessary if present.

Gua Sha Protocol for Adjuvant Therapy

a. Shoulder Sweep
b. Trapezius Sweep
c. Occipital-Cervical Sweep

d. Superior Bladder Meridian Dredge
e. Para-Vertebral Dredge T1-T12
f. Large Intestine Meridian Dredge (LI4-LI11) with emphasis on LI4 合谷 using acupoint 'press-and-hold' technique
g. Acupoint 'press-and-hold' for GB34 阳陵泉, GB39 悬钟, ST36 足三里, ST38 条口 for both legs
h. Acupoint 'press-and-hold' for LI11 曲池, LU7 列缺 for both hands
i. Acupoint 'press-and-hold' for BL23 肾俞 bilaterally on the torso

Execution — Unless TCM diagnosis suggests otherwise, moderation press-stroke recommended. Acupoints marked for application of 'press-and-hold' technique in each prescription form a set, each set to be repeated three times. 'Press-and-hold' maneuver should be attempted 10 times for each prescribed acupoint within each set. Use of skin lubricant that invigorates Qi and dispels blood stasis preferred. Observation of Sha appearance preferred.

Reference

1. Wang Qingren 王清任. *Correction of Errors in Medical Classics* 《医林改错·痹症有淤血说》1830.

Topic 58

Lateral Epicondylitis/Tennis Elbow

Lateral epicondylitis is an inflammation of the tendons that join the forearm muscles on the outside of the elbow. It is a painful condition caused by overuse or repetition of the same motions, commonly arising from playing tennis or other racquet sports. For the same reason, this condition, characterized by pain and tenderness on the outside of the elbow, is better known as Tennis elbow.

Aside from recreational activities, overuse of the elbow tendon may also be occupation-related; so long as the activity engaged involves repetitive lifting, gripping and grasping motions such as meat cutting, plumbing, painting or mechanical repair work that require straightening of the elbow and stabilizing the wrist. Trauma may also contribute to lateral epicondylitis as a direct blow to the elbow may result in swelling of the tendon leading to its degeneration as well as making the tendon more susceptible to an overuse injury.

The elbow joint is formed by three bones; humerus or the upper arm bone and the radius and ulna in the forearm. The epicondyles are protruding structures at the end of the humerus and the one facing outwards the elbow is the lateral epicondyle. In terms of musculature, the muscles on the forearm extend from wrist and fingers to elbow; and anchored down to the skeletal structure by tendons call extensors. At the elbow, the point of insertion or attachment for the tendon is at the lateral epicondyle.

The tendon usually associated with lateral epicondylitis is called the Extensor Carpi Radialis Brevis (ECRB). With lateral epicondylitis, there is degeneration of the tendon's attachment and weakening of the anchor site. The degeneration, caused by microscopic tears, in the tendon where it attaches to the lateral epicondyle leads to inflammation and therefore pain when the muscle is activated.

Like any degenerative condition, the symptoms develop progressively over time with increasing intensity. The pain usually starts at the outer part of the elbow and may travel down the forearm to the hand, weakening the grip strength.

Lateral epicondylitis, in many instances, is self-limiting and often time symptoms resolve within a year without treatment. In other more enduring situations, both non-surgical and surgical treatments are available, with the non-surgical option being the treatment of the first choice.

Non-surgical options include temporary abstinence from the offending activity, activity modification to reduce the incidence of further injury to the elbow, physical therapy, partial immobilization of injured tendon with counterforce braces, NSAIDs medication, steroid injections, acupuncture and possibly Autologous blood injections (ABI) or platelet-rich plasma (PRP) to accelerate tissue repair.

Surgery should only be considered when the pain is excruciating and did not respond to other forms of treatment for at least six months. Surgery involves removing the diseased, degenerated tendon tissue and reattaching healthy muscles to the lateral epicondyle. The surgery, in either open or arthroscopic format, would be performed in an outpatient setting. Rehabilitation typically follows surgery to restore normal strength, grip and mobility range.

From a TCM perspective ...

Lateral epicondylitis is a chronic degenerative disease, and in this regard, it shares very much the view of contemporary medicine. The etiology, however, is due to deficiencies in the liver and kidney in conjunction with invasion by external pathogens of wind, cold and dampness.

Energy expenditure, fatigue, and profuse perspiration 劳累汗出 can cause enervation or exhaustion of nutritive and defensive Qi in the body 营卫不固. When the meridians and collaterals coursing the elbow are being invaded by exogenous pathogens of cold and dampness nature during these moments, Qi stagnation and impediment in blood circulation arise. Impediment in blood circulation turns into blood stasis if this condition is allowed to perpetuate over time by engaging in the same strenuous activities, causing the nutrition-deprived tendon to become injured and inflamed. Pain arises when blood flow is impaired 不通则痛.

Although the etiology for lateral epicondylitis is one of combined deficiency-excess state syndrome, it manifests itself more as a musculoskeletal disorder. In this regard, the fundamental precept for its treatment is to focus on the coursing meridian for rapid relief 不盛不虚, 以经取之. The meridian of choice is, therefore, the Rising Yang Large Intestine Meridian of the Hand 手阳明大肠经 where Qi and blood are found in abundance. The Lesser Yang Triple Energizer Meridian of the Hand 手少阳三焦经 should also be employed for comprehensive treatment.

Gua Sha Protocol for Treatment and Symptomatic Relief

Gua Sha has a certain curative effect on the treatment of lateral epicondylitis as it can relieve the muscular spasm and pain, disperse Qi stagnation, stimulate blood circulation and dispel blood stasis in the collaterals. Execution of **item c** in this protocol is of particular importance.

a. Shoulder Sweep
b. Back Rejuvenation Dredge (T11-L4)
c. Large Intestine Meridian Dredge (LI4-LI14) for the affected arm with emphasis on LI4 合谷, LI10 手三里, LI11 曲池, LI12 肘髎, LI13 手五里, LI14 臂臑 using acupoint 'press-and-hold' technique
d. Acupoint 'press-and-hold' for ST36 足三里, SP6 三阴交
c. Acupoint 'press-and-hold' for affected arm on TE5 外关, TE10 天井, LU5 尺泽, HT3 少海, SI8 小海

Execution — Unless TCM diagnosis suggests otherwise, moderation press-stroke recommended. Acupoints marked for application of 'press-and-hold' technique in each prescription form a set, each set to be repeated three times. 'Press-and-hold' maneuver should be attempted 10 times for each prescribed acupoint within each set. Use of skin lubricant that invigorates Qi and dispels blood stasis preferred. Observation of Sha appearance preferred.

Topic 59

Lumbago/Lower Back Pain

Lumbago is a generic term that refers to lower back pain and in many instances, the two terms are used interchangeably. The lower back comprises of five vertebrae in the lumbar region (generally labeled as L1-L5). The lumbar structure is curved to support much of the weight of the upper body, but it also provides latitude for rotation, flexion, and extension so that the lumbar section may arguably be the next most flexibility structure in the spine aside from the cervical section or neck. The combined role of the lumbar in weight-bearing, as well as motion flexibility, makes it vulnerable to a wide range of back injury such that the lower back is where most back pain occurs.

Between each pair of vertebrae is a centimeter thick resilient intervertebral disk that prevents adjacent vertebrae from abrasion against each other when the body is subject to shock during motion. More importantly, the intervertebral disk provides healthy clearance or space between the vertebrae for spinal cord nerve roots to freely and laterally emerge from the foramen. Bands of tissue known as ligaments hold the vertebrae in place and provide cushioning against trauma from direct impact externally. Tendons attaching muscles to the spinal column yet form another added layer of robust protective structure for the delicate spinal cord.

Pain is a prominent feature of many musculoskeletal disorders, and its accurate and reliable determination is a prerequisite for its effective management. Lower back pain is no exception. Lower back pain can, however, be very elusive that makes accurate medical diagnosis difficult.

The lower back comprises of a composite mix of vertebrae with facet joints, intervertebral disk, nerve networks and surrounding soft tissues such as muscles, tendons, and ligaments; all intricately intermeshed. To coordinate this complex anatomical configuration with precision, a high level of overlapping nerve supply to these structures becomes necessary but the same arrangement also makes it confusing for the brain to pinpoint the exact source of pain signals when an injury occurs. As such, the intensity of pain often does not commensurate to the severity of the injury. In fact, a minor injury to an area where nerve supply is rich may elicit more pain than a serious one where nerve supply is less dense. Moreover, pain threshold is different among individuals, making an assessment of pain intensity a challenge.

Notwithstanding, diagnostic accuracy for lower back pain remains important as the pain may be indicative of some more serious underlying conditions especially if the pain is accompanied by weakness in the lower limbs, significant numbness, bowel and/or bladder dysfunction (voiding difficulty or incontinence), history of malignancy with significant unexplained weight loss, fever and chills or severe continuous abdominal pain and back pain. And when back pain is severe enough to wake one up from deep slumber, it is a sure tell-tale sign for medical attention.

Lower back pain that lasts for less than a month is deemed to be acute and is usually self-limiting with no residual loss of function after recovery. The pain is sub-acute when it extends between one and three months and pain that persists for any longer duration, despite treatment, is termed chronic.

By and large, there are three different types of lower back pain — axial, referred and radicular back pain.

Axial pain, which is self-limiting in nature, is the most common of lower back pain. Since the symptoms resolve with time, axial pain is deemed non-specific in that the anatomical structure responsible for the pain need not be identified for the purpose of treatment. Only in chronic and severe cases are further evaluation and diagnosis considered necessary.

Axial lower back pain can vary from severe sharp pain to a mild dull ache; continuous or intermittent. The pain is confined narrowly to the lower back area and does not radiate beyond the originating site to other parts of the body. The majority of axial lower back pain is mechanical in nature, i.e. causes functional disruption to the way the components of the back (spine, muscle, intervertebral discs, and nerves) fit together and move. As such it is characterized as a pain aggravated by the performance of specific motor functions or adoption of certain postures but rapidly relieved by rest.

Referred lower back pain is triggered by similar injuries that could have caused simple axial back pain and is often no more serious. Referred pain is usually felt in the low back area and tends to radiate into the groin, buttock and upper thighs. Less common than axial lower back pain or radicular lower back pain, the pain is often migratory but rarely extends below the knee. Seldom continuous, referred pain tends to be intermittent and varies in attribute and intensity but usually achy, dull, migratory and of lesser intensity.

Referred pain is pain perceived at a site other than where the stimulus is situated and results in the same pain signal being returned to the brain from the extensive network of interconnecting sensory nerves that supply many of the tissues of the low back, pelvis, and thigh. An injury to any of these structures causes pain to radiate — or be "referred" — to any of the other structures. It is important to understand that this type of pain is not associated with nerve compression or "pinched nerves".

Radicular lower back pain is often caused by compression or inflammation of a spinal nerve and the pain normally follows the involved dermatome in the leg — the area of distribution of the leg covered by the specific nerve. The most common symptom of radicular pain is sciatica when a nerve at L4-L5 or L5-S1 spinal segment is "pinched", involving the dermatome associated with the sciatic nerve that runs down the back of each leg to the foot. Similarly, compression of nerve roots at higher lumbar levels between L2 and L4 can cause radicular pain into the front of the thigh and the shin.

Radicular pain is often deep-seated and steady and could be faithfully reproduced with certain activities and positions, such as

Straight Leg Raise, also called Lasègue Test. Pain may also be accompanied by numbness and tingling, muscle weakness and loss of specific reflexes. When actual nerve dysfunction is noted, this is termed radiculopathy. With this condition, the leg pain is typically much worse than the low back pain.

All told, the vast majority of low back pain is mechanical in nature and associated with spondylosis or normal degeneration of the spine with aging. Such degeneration may be accelerated by physical abuse that causes overstretching or tearing of the supporting musculature, undue compression on the intervertebral disc as well as the loss of vertebral integrity. Herniated or ruptured discs occur when the intervertebral discs become over-compressed and can cause chronic pain. Even before degeneration sets in, extreme physical activities or accidents may result in traumatic injury that manifests as acute lower back pain. Severe traumatic injury may also cause an overly compressed intervertebral disc to rupture or herniate, exerting pressure on any of the nerves rooted to the spinal cord. When spinal nerves become compressed and irritated, back pain and sciatica result.

Radiculopathy is a condition caused by compression, inflammation and/or injury to a spinal nerve root. It can be caused by a herniated or ruptured disc pressing on the nerve root or by narrowing of vertebral foramen termed as spinal stenosis. Spinal stenosis puts pressure on the spinal cord and nerves causing pain or numbness and over time leads to weakness and sensory loss to the leg due to interruption of the nerve signal. A rare complication of a ruptured disc is Cauda Equina syndrome, where the disc material penetrated the spinal canal, damaging the lumbar and sacral nerve roots, and causing loss of bladder and bowel control.

Radiculopathy may also be caused by a tumor or cyst that impinges on the nerve or its roots or by spondylolisthesis. Spondylolisthesis is a condition in which a vertebra of the lower spine slips out of place, pinching the nerves exiting the spinal column. This is different from herniated, prolapsed or "slipped" disk where the intervertebral disk slipped out of place, compressing the spinal nerve.

Other less common conditions that predispose one to lower back pain include skeletal abnormality (scoliosis, lordosis), spinal infection(osteomyelitis), osteoporosis, endometriosis, abdominal aortic aneurysm, kidney stones, and even obesity and pregnancy.

Treatment of the first choice for lower back pain takes the form of conservative options such as physical therapy, NSAID medication, and topical analgesics, prescription spasmolytic/muscle relaxants and spine manipulation and traction.

Contrary to popular belief, complete bed rest following onset of lower back pain may actually aggravate the condition by reducing muscle tone and normal circulation essential for rapid recovery. Instead, strengthening of core muscle groups that support the lower back and cultivating proper posturing should be promoted and used in combinations with other interventions.

In the use of medication, there may a tendency for individuals to escalate from NSAIDs to opioids for chronic pain. Opioids should only be used under medical supervision and for a short duration as opioid tolerance can increase rapidly and develop into addiction and abuse.

Spinal manipulation may provide some small to moderate short-term benefit for chronic back pain but should not be deployed when the back pain is caused or accompanied by an underlying medical condition such as osteoporosis, spinal cord compression or arthritis. Similarly, traction that purports to improve skeletal alignment demonstrates no long-term benefit but may provide some transient relief when the traction is in force.

When necessary, more invasion options like selective spinal injections and even epidural nerve blocks therapy may be attempted.

If non-surgical interventions failed to reduce pain to a manageable level, surgical treatments may be considered on the basis of pain severity and/or in the presence of significant muscle weakness. Although there is a fairly large range of surgical options available for spinal nerve decompression, it is important to note that surgical procedures are not always successful. Anyone considering surgical approaches should be fully notified of all attendant risks before making an informed decision.

It is also instructional to note that unless definitive nerve compression or serious musculoskeletal anomalies can be unequivocally documented by imaging technology, the basis for surgery is likely to be ill-founded and the outcome likely to be unsuccessful.

From a TCM perspective ...

Lower back pain refers to a disorder caused by the invasion of exogenous pathogens of wind, cold and dampness genre at the lower back level or injury arising from physical labor or the impairment blood and Qi circulation due to kidney deficiency. Lower back pain is also closely associated with the dysfunction of the six principal meridians of the leg as well as disorder in the eight extraordinary meridians that course through the site of pain.

Performing heavy physical work in a state of Qi stagnation and blood stasis, adopting wrong postures for protracted durations, improper way of lifting heavy loads, traumatic accidents are risk factors to lower back pain.

There are five different sub-types of lower back pain namely, damp-heat type 湿热, blood stasis type 瘀血, phlegm accumulation type 痰积, kidney deficiency type 肾虚, and external injury type 挫闪.

Exogenous pathogens strike mostly those who reside or work in a damp environment or engage in heavy physical work under strong wind draft with perspiration-soaked clothes or frequently brave the inclement weather. Taking advantage of diminished immunity whilst the body is exhausted, the six exogenous pathogens invade the body causing an obstruction in the meridians coursing the waist region leading to Qi stagnation, blood stasis and lower back pain. When invaded by the cold pathogen, the kidney Yang is compromised; if invaded by the dampness pathogen which is heavy and thus gravitates to lower body, the Qi mechanism is impaired resulting in Qi and blood stagnation; if invaded by a damp-heat pathogen, heat injures Yin and dampness harms Yang. Thus, these pathogens singularly or in concert operate to impair the body's Yin, Yang, Qi and blood leading to lower back pain.

But the primary underlying cause for lower back pain remains with kidney deficiency, regardless of whether the insufficiency was congenital or otherwise. In fact, physicians in the past have attached such great significance to kidney deficiency and physical weakness as an important etiology of low back pain that Zhang Jiebin asserts that more than 80% of lower back pain may be attributed to kidney deficiency 腰痛之虚证十居八九.[1]

As the lower back is deemed the abode of the kidney 腰为肾之府, the choice of meridians for treatment would logically be the Kidney meridian 肾经 and those vessels that course through the lower back, namely Bladder Meridian, Governor Vessel 督脉, Penetration Vessel 冲脉, and Belt Vessel 带脉. The Kidney and Bladder systems, however, are intimately related as an exterior-interior dyad in TCM. In addition, the Bladder meridian serves the entire back region and is in closer proximity than the Kidney meridian. As such, the Bladder meridian becomes an excellent proxy for the Kidney meridian in this regard.

Gua Sha Protocol for Adjuvant Treatment and Symptomatic Relief

a. Sacral V Dredge
b. Iliac Contour Sweep
c. Back Rejuvenation Dredge
d. Spleen Meridian Dredge (SP1-5) with emphasis on SP1 隐白, SP2 大都, SP3 太白, SP4 公孙, SP5 商丘 using acupoint 'press-and-hold' technique
e. Acupoint 'press-and-hold' for GB34 阳陵泉, GB39 悬钟, BL60 昆仑, BL39 委阳, BL40 委中on both legs

Execution — Unless TCM diagnosis suggests otherwise, moderation press-stroke recommended. Acupoints marked for application of 'press-and-hold' technique in each prescription form a set, each set to be repeated three times. 'Press-and-hold' maneuver should be attempted 10 times for each prescribed acupoint within each set. Use of skin lubricant that invigorates Qi and dispels blood stasis preferred. Observation of Sha appearance preferred.

Other Considerations — So long as lower back pain is caused or accompanied by structural change or impairment, *Gua Sha* therapy may not improve the condition significantly unless the structural damage is rectified. Structural changes include herniated disk, displaced vertebra, ostcophytc, foraminal stenosis, osteoporosis, arthritis, etc. Like other physiotherapy modalities, *Gua Sha* can hardly rectify structural damage but will certainly improve functionality. Its therapeutic effect may be particularly appreciated when the patient makes compensatory adjustments by strengthening relevant core muscle groups and cultivate good posturing.

Supplementary Notes — Lumbar Herniated Disc/Sciatica

Intervertebral disks constitute one-third in length of the entire spinal column. A herniated disk is a condition that can occur anywhere along the spine, but most often in the lower back. Sometimes termed as a protruding or ruptured disk, it is one of the most common causes of lower back pain as well sciatica.

The intervertebral disk acts as a shock absorber for the spine when the body is in motion. The disk comprises of a soft, jelly-like center, the nucleus pulposus, surrounded by a tough flexible outer ring, the annulus fibrosus. Because of the high-water content in both components, the disk is capable of withstanding compression and the components work in concert to absorb shock to the spine with the nucleus pulposus providing the mobility and torsional flexibility.

Compression forces are mainly absorbed by the vertebral body's energy-dissipating mechanism. Conceptually, a disk herniates when its jelly-like nucleus pushes against the outer ring causing the disk to protrude posteriorly or posterolaterally into the spine. Mechanically-induced herniation experiments on healthy disk, however, demonstrate that during the application of maximal load it is more likely that the vertebral body fails rather than the disk.[2] It further appeared even in traumatic accidents, herniation occurs when there is loss in biochemical and hydrostatic behaviors in the disk due to degeneration.[3] This finding augurs well with the TCM theory that the majority of lower back pain is due to a deficiency state of the kidney system responsible for the well-being of the spine.

In degenerative disk, compression results in the nucleus pulposus pushing through the disk's outer ring, causing the ring to bulge and putting pressure on the spinal cord and the nearby nerve roots.

In addition, the disk when ruptured releases chemical irritants that contribute to nerve inflammation causing pain, numbness, and weakness in one or both legs, depending on whether the prolapse extends laterally or bilaterally.

The background of Sciatica has been duly covered under the main body of this topic and shall not be repeated.

Gua Sha Protocol for Adjuvant Treatment and Symptomatic Relief [Lumbar Herniated Disk]

a. Para-Vertebral Dredge
b. Sacral V Dredge
c. Iliac Contour Sweep
d. Back Rejuvenation Dredge
e. Spleen Meridian Dredge (SP1-5) with emphasis on SP1 隐白, SP2 大都, SP3 太白, SP4 公孙, SP5 商丘 using acupoint 'press-and-hold' technique
f. Acupoint 'press-and-hold' for GB34 阳陵泉, GB39 悬钟, BL60 昆仑, BL39 委阳, BL40 委中 on the affected limbs

Gua Sha Protocol for Adjuvant Treatment and Symptomatic Relief [Sciatica]

a. Para-Vertebral Dredge
b. Sacral V Dredge
c. Back Rejuvenation Dredge
d. Bladder Meridian Dredge (BL31-BL60) on the affected limb with emphasis on BL37 殷门, BL40 委中, BL54 秩边, BL57 承山, BL60 昆仑 using acupoint 'press-and-hold' technique
e. Acupoint 'press-and-hold' for GB30 环跳 on the affected limb

Execution — Unless TCM diagnosis suggests otherwise, moderation press-stroke recommended. Acupoints marked for application of 'press-and-hold' technique in each prescription form a set, each set to be repeated three times. 'Press-and-hold' maneuver should be attempted 10 times for each prescribed acupoint within each set. Use of skin lubricant that invigorates Qi and dispels blood stasis preferred. Observation of Sha appearance preferred.

References

1. Zhang Jiebin. *Complete Works of Jingyue* 《景岳全书·腰痛》 1640.
2. Roaf R. A study of the mechanics of spinal injury. *J. Bone Joint Surg.* **42B**(4): 810–823 (1960).
3. Virgin WJ. Experimental investigation into the physical properties of intervertebral disc. *J. Bone Joint Surg.* **33B**(4): 607–611 (1951).

Topic 60

Rotator Cuff Tendinitis

Rotator Cuff Tendinitis is a relatively common condition of the shoulders afflicting people of all ages. It is characterized by a pain in the shoulder that restricts the range of movement of the arm, that often worsen by resting or recumbency on the affected arm. The condition progresses with increasing pain at night as well as a loss of strength and restricted movement in the arm, especially when rotating the arm behind the back.

The shoulder comprises of three bones — humerus (upper arm bone), scapula (shoulder blade) and clavicle (collar bone). This skeletal structure is held together by a complex set of four muscle groups and tendons termed the rotator cuff that attaches the upper arm firmly to a shallow socket in the shoulder blade. Between the rotator cuff and the bone on top-end of the shoulder blade (acromion), there is a lubricating sac called a bursa that allows the rotator cuff tendons to glide freely when the arm moves.

This intricate musculoskeletal configuration that confers a wide latitude of motion for the arm is nevertheless susceptible to different mechanical issues of which rotator cuff is a frequent source of complaint. The rotator cuff tendons can be irritated, inflamed and damaged or even torn, giving rise to tendinitis. The bursa may also be inflamed with increased fluid accumulation causing painful subacromial bursitis. Pain is exacerbated by overhead movement of the arm and a painful arc may be present during the elevation of the arm from 60° to 120° when the acromion impinges upon the tendon and the bursa causing pain and irritation, manifesting shoulder impingement.

Individuals who repeatedly perform overhead or perhaps above-shoulder arm motion are vulnerable to developing rotator cuff injury. Engaging in such activities especially with load and over a protracted period of time invariably irritate or damage the tendons. The risk of rotator cuff injury increases with age resulting from progressive degeneration of tendon tissue. The condition could also develop as a consequence of a traumatic injury to the shoulder that did not receive timely and appropriate treatment.

Symptoms for rotator cuff tendinitis are usually minor at the onset with swelling and tenderness being localized at the anterolateral shoulder. Pain and stiffness may be experienced when the arm is abruptly lifted to or lowered from shoulder level. Occasionally, the pain may radiate from the front of the shoulder to the side of the arm. But the common complaint is always a mild but continuous (nagging) pain present both during activity and at rest.

Preliminary diagnosis for rotator cuff injury is usually a physical examination that involves motor and range extension tests. Because rotator cuff tendons are soft tissues, X-ray could reveal little but only associated structural anomalies like bone spurs. Magnetic resonance (MRI) and ultrasound imaging are more suited for examination of soft tissues for inflammation, fluid accumulation and perhaps tendon tears.

Minor rotator cuff injuries are usually self-limiting and will heal on its own especially with activity modification and rest. Symptomatic relief and function restoration are fundamental therapeutic objectives. The first treatment of choice is therefore conservative, starting with rest, NSAIDs medication, topical analgesics, and physical therapy. More persistent cases may be treated with steroid or combined steroid and anesthetic injection at the local site. Surgical treatment like subacromial decompression may be explored when non-invasive options failed.

Without treatment, rotator cuff injuries may develop into progressive degeneration of the shoulder joint when the individual adopts motion compensation to avoid pain. Keeping the shoulders immobilized for an extended period of time may also lead to adhesive capsulitis (frozen shoulder) when the connective tissue surrounding the glenohumeral joint of the shoulder, becomes inflamed, thickened and tight, greatly restricting motion and causing chronic pain.

From a TCM perspective ...

Rotator cuff tendinitis belongs to the category of "occlusion/impediment disorder 痹症" caused by the invasion of wind, cold and dampness-related exogenous pathogens when the arm and shoulder are subject to strain or trauma, leading to Qi stagnation and blood stasis 气血凝滞, obstruction in the attendant meridian and collateral 脉络痹阻 that manifest as pain and inflammation.

The pain is aggravated by either lifting or lowering the affected arm, often causing an abrupt and inhibiting pain when the adduction or abduction is between the range of 60° and 120°. This symptom differentiates rotator cuff tendinitis from adhesive capsulitis, better known as quinquagenarian shoulder 五十肩 in TCM, which presents a uniform restriction in all movement of the shoulder joint accompanied by severe pain.

During the acute phase, treatment of rotator cuff tendinitis is focused on warming and clearing the obstruction in the attendant meridian and collaterals to alleviate pain. In the chronic stage, therapy should aim to invigorate circulation, relax the spasmodic musculature and decongest the collaterals. For treatment, the meridians of choice are the three Yang meridians of the hand, namely the Large Intestine, Triple Energizer and the Small Intestine meridians.

Gua Sha Protocol for Treatment and Symptomatic Relief

a. Shoulder Sweep
b. Acupoint 'press-and-hold' for GB34 阳陵泉, GB39 悬钟 on both legs
c. Acupoint 'press-and-hold' for LI4 合谷, LI11 曲池, LI14 肩髃, TE3 中渚, TE5 外关, TE14 肩髎, SI9 肩贞, SI11 天宗 on the affected arm

Execution — Unless TCM diagnosis suggests otherwise, moderation press-stroke recommended. Acupoints marked for application of 'press-and-hold' technique in each prescription form a set, each set to be repeated three times. 'Press-and-hold' maneuver should be attempted 10 times for each prescribed acupoint within each set. Use of skin lubricant that invigorates Qi and dispels blood stasis preferred. Observation of Sha appearance preferred.

Glossary

Abduction and adduction are terms used to describe movements towards or away from the midline of the body. Adduction is the movement of a body part toward the body's midline, as in a person having his arm straight out at the shoulder level and bringing it down to his side in the path of an arc.

Abduction is a movement of a body part away from the body's midline, as in a person raising his arm out in an arc to the side of the body to shoulder level.

Neurological

TOPIC 61

Bell's Palsy/Idiopathic Facial Palsy

Bell's palsy is an unexplained episode of temporary facial muscle weakness or paralysis, resulting from damage or trauma to the facial nerves. This disorder, which is not related to stroke, starts abruptly but worsen progressively within days, usually affecting one of the paired facial nerves and therefore one side of the face only; though both sides may rarely be affected as an exception.

Bell's palsy afflicts both genders equally and usually between ages 15 and 60. Individuals who are immunocompromised, suffering from upper respiratory ailments, chronic inflammation (sarcoidosis, hypertension) or auto-immune diseases (Guillain-Barré syndrome, Myasthenia gravis, diabetes) are predisposed to the disorder. The condition often associated with pregnancy and recent infection, especially viral infection such as herpes simplex, meningitis or herpes zoster.

The facial nerve or 7th cranial nerve travels through the Fallopian canal (not Fallopian tube) to the muscles on each side of the face. Each facial nerve exerts full motor control on all muscles of facial expressions on one side of the face, including those that regulate eyelid motion. In addition, the facial nerve carries nerve impulses to the lacrimal or tear glands, the saliva glands and the muscles of the stapes, a small bone in the middle ear that conducts sound vibrations to the inner ear. The facial nerve also receives taste sensations from two-thirds of the tongue.

The complex function and pervasive reach of the facial nerve when disrupted by the onset of Bell's palsy prevents regular transmission of signals from the brain to the facial muscles and this interruption results in facial twitching, weakness or paralysis with a host of symptoms that may vary in severity and diversity with the individual.

These symptoms manifested on the affected side of the face include, but not limited to, loss of feeling and control of facial expressions, dizziness, difficulty in eating or drinking, drooping of the eyelid and corner of the mouth, drooling, dryness of the eye or mouth, taste impairment, impaired speech, ringing or hypersensitivity to sound in the affected ear and excessive tearing in one eye.

Treatment of Bell's palsy is made based on clinical presentations. Mild cases are usually deemed self-limiting and no treatment is required as symptoms usually disappear within a fortnight. In more severe cases, treatment is directed at reducing inflammation, relieving pain and, if necessary, containing viral proliferation. Medication like steroid prednisone for inflammation reduction, analgesics for pain relief and anti-viral acyclovir are often prescribed during the acute phase.

An almost mandatory treatment prescribed for Bell's palsy is eye protection. Bell's palsy can interrupt the eyelid's natural blinking ability during waking hours, exposing the eye to irritation and drying. Using lubricating eye drops, such as artificial tears, is an effective countermeasure until the function is restored. During slumber, the eyelid may not close completely leaving the cornea prone to drying and scratching. In this regard, patients are advised to tape down the affected eyelid with surgical tape as a form of nightly eye-care.

In recent years, complementary therapies such as vitamin therapy, facial massage, and acupuncture are also deployed which demonstrate potential in improving facial nerve function and pain relief, especially when administered early after onset.

The specific cause for Bell's palsy and attendant nerve damage is still unknown. Clinicians postulate that the disorder could be initiated by a viral infection causing the facial nerve to inflame in response to the infection. Now that the facial nerve is fitted snuggly within a rigid bony Fallopian canal, any inflammation will cause pressure to build up within the Fallopian canal causing ischemia that restricts blood and oxygen flow to the nerve cells. When ischemia is not severe and the damage is only limited to the myelin sheath of the nerve, recovery can be expected to be within a reasonable time; when the nerve itself is injured, recovery is, however, less predictable.

Bell's palsy is seldom a permanent disorder but the symptoms may remain, in part or in whole, for an extended period of time on exception. On rare occasions, the symptoms may never completely disappear. Affliction is not a proxy to immunity and the disorder may recur, either on the same or the opposite side of the face.

Notwithstanding, recovery would begin within a fortnight from the onset of symptom and, for most individuals, return to normal function may be expected within six months even without treatment. The extent of recovery and the rate of improvement is contingent on the extent of nerve damage.

Though there is no known cure for Bell's palsy currently, the prognosis for individuals with Bell's palsy remains very good.

From a TCM perspective...

This disorder is caused by the invasion of the wind and cold or heat-related exogenous pathogens whilst there is a weakness of or vacuity in the Yang meridians that converge at the head, leading to Qi stagnation and the fascia deprived of nutrients that in turn causes the musculature to lose tonus.

Palsy caused by exposure to windy draft during slumber is associated with invasion by cold wind pathogen and usually manifest no symptom of usual respiratory infection. On the contrary, palsy associated with invasion of a wind-heat pathogen is usually secondary to viral infection, otitis media or gingivitis and accompanied by pain in the inner ear and the mastoid on the affected side of the face.

The cheeks, being the largest exposed areas of the face and richly served by the Rising Yang and Lesser Yang meridians, receive the maximal effect of invading exogenous pathogens. Rapid onset of palsy and its involuntary movement are caused by wind pathogens that have attributes of being mobile and quick-acting. These symptoms are usually observed during the acute phase. In the sub-acute phase, endogenous heat is generated by the residing pathogens 邪郁化热 not evicted by the weak defensive Qi. The endogenous heat in turn consumed and deprived the body's vital essence and Yin 伤津灼阴, causing wind to be generated internally as a consequence of Yin-Yang imbalance 阴虚内风动. The internally generated wind further reinforces the perpetuation of the symptoms manifested during the acute phase, and may even aggravate them with muscular atrophy, making recovery less predictable.

In the treatment of Bell's palsy, the four major meridians to be acted upon are the Rising Yang Large Intestine Meridian of the Hand 手阳明大肠经, Rising Yang Stomach Meridian of the Foot 足阳明胃经, Lesser Yang Triple Energizer Meridian of the Hand 手少阳三焦经 and Lesser Yang Gall Bladder Meridian of the Foot 足少阳胆经. For these meridians, the therapeutic objectives should be to invigorate the blood 活血, decongest the meridians and collaterals 通络, and expel wind pathogens 祛风.

Gua Sha Protocol for Treatment and Symptomatic Relief

a. Occipital-Cervical Sweep
b. Shoulder Sweep
c. Lessor Yang Plough on the affected side
d. Acupoint 'press-and-hold' for ST36 足三里, ST40 丰隆, SP6 三阴交, LR2 行间 on both legs
e. Acupoint 'press-and-hold' for LI4 合谷 on both hands
f. Acupoint 'press-and-hold' for ST2 四白, ST4 地仓, ST6 颊车, TE17 翳风 on the affected side of the face

Additional Acupoints using 'press-and-hold' technique to be applied on the affected side
For Numbness — ST44 内庭, GB14 阳白,
For Spasm — TE23 丝竹空, BL2 攒竹,

Execution — Unless TCM diagnosis suggests otherwise, moderation press-stroke recommended. Acupoints marked for application of 'press-and-hold' technique in each prescription form a set, each set to be repeated three times. 'Press-and-hold' maneuver should be attempted 10 times for each prescribed acupoint within each set. Use of skin lubricant that invigorates Qi and dispels blood stasis preferred. Observation of Sha appearance not mandatory.

Glossary

Fallopian canal refers to a bony canal through which the facial nerve traverses the petrous temporal bone, from the internal acoustic meatus to the stylomastoid foramen. There are three segments of the canal, corresponding to the segments of the facial nerve they contain: labyrinthine, tympanic and mastoid. Discovered by the same anatomist who identified the Fallopian tube (gynecology), it is the longest bony canal through which a nerve passes in the human body.

Myelin sheath is an insulating layer that forms around nerves, including those in the brain and spinal cord. It is made up of protein and fatty substances. Like polymer covering on electric cables, the myelin sheath allows electrical impulses to transmit quickly and efficiently along the nerve cells. However, signal impulses slow down once the myelin sheath is damaged.

Topic 62

Headache — Migraine, Tension-Type Headache and Trigeminal Neuralgia

Headache, in general, is one of the most universal ailments that few have yet to experience. It is also one of the most complex disorders in neurology that require critical analysis before it may be accurately diagnosed. In this regard, The International Headache Society has compiled a 211-page comprehensive classification in 2018 to guide the medical community in the systematic evaluation of headache disorders. The International Classification of Headache Disorders — 3rd edition (ICHD-3) may be freely accessed from http://www.ihs-headache.org/ichd-guidelines/ihs-guidelines.

Headaches are broadly classified as primary, secondary, and painful cranial neuropathies & other facial pains.

Primary headache is any headache or headache disorder not caused by or attributed to another medical condition. Primary headache constitutes the vast majority of headache disorders, with migraine and tension-type headache (TTH) being the most prevalent. Cluster headache is the least common.

Secondary headache is any headache or headache disorder caused by another underlying condition. In ICHD-3, secondary headaches are attributed to the causative disorder. Headache arising from psychiatric disease is considered secondary but more common secondary headaches are those related to infection of CNS, vascular disease and trauma. Postural orthostatic tachycardia syndrome is an often-unrecognized cause of headache. The sudden and unprecedented onset of thunderclap headache may be a presenting feature of subarachnoid hemorrhage and other vascular accidents like arterial dissection, especially in the brain. Contrary to popular belief, brain tumors seldom cause alarming headaches, especially during the initial stages.

A secondary headache may share the characteristics of a primary headache but their timely recognition may prove to be an ominous symptom crucial for life-saving medical intervention. Of special mention is giant cell arteritis which is a matter of medical emergency.

Giant cell arteritis is an inflammation of the artery lining, usually the superficial temporal artery. The disorder affects older individuals, often women, with age above 70 years. The most prominent clinical feature is a persistent and severe headache, usually at the temporal area. Other symptoms include scalp tenderness, jaw claudication, visual loss and elevated inflammation markers (ESR and CRP).

Patients with a primary headache disorder are more susceptible to the development of headache when a secondary cause occurs. Their headaches may be phenotypically similar to their primary headache disorder. Therefore, a secondary cause should be considered in patients with pre-existing headache disorders who develop a significant increase in the number and severity of those attacks.[1]

Migraine is described as a recurrent headache disorder manifesting in attacks lasting between 4 and 72 hours. Typical characteristics of the headache are unilateral location, pulsating quality, moderate or severe intensity, aggravation by routine physical activity and association with nausea and/or photophobia and phonophobia.[2]

Diagnostic criteria for migraine stipulated in ICHD-3 documentation include a history of at least five repeated attacks, each lasting between 4 and 72 hours with attributes that substantially satisfy the typical characteristics.

The attacks are however episodic in nature with the patient preferring to remain motionless in a dark and quiet room during an attack but otherwise enjoys pain-free living.

For migraine with aura, the ICHD-3 guidelines describe the aura to be a progressive but transient visual, sensory, speech and/or language, motor, brainstem or retinal disturbance preceding the onset of pain. The aura may consist of seeing flashing lights or spreading scintillating scotoma (diminished sight), having numbness or tingling in the face or extremities, having a disturbed sense of smell, or having difficulty speaking. Each individual aura symptom may last between 5 and 60 minutes, with each aura typically occurring in succession to one another.

Migraine headaches are biased towards the female gender, could be genetically predisposed but not life-threatening. Its exact cause remains largely unclear. It is however postulated that genetically induced hypersensitivity of the brain to both internal and external homeostatic changes acts as headache triggers that influence the trigeminovascular pathway. The trigeminovascular system, consisting of neurons in the trigeminal nerve that innervate cerebral blood vessels, when stimulated releases neuropeptides and other substances that cause both local inflammation and distant amplification of neural circuitry in the brain, resulting in pain that often affects the periorbital area and the eye and intensifies when intracranial pressure increases.[3]

Tension-type headache (TTH) is another category of primary headache that is more common, less inhibiting and less dramatic than migraine. The pain is often described as a vice-like band around the forehead that often radiates to the posterior neck muscles. In its most extensive form, the pain distribution is almost "cape-like," radiating along the medial and lateral trapezius muscles covering the shoulders, scapular and interscapular areas.[4]

ICHD-3 documentation categorizes TTH into either episodic or chronic and further sub-classifies headache in these categories by whether they are associated with pericranial tenderness. Episodic is defined as recurring and remitting in a regular or irregular pattern of attacks of the headache of constant or variable duration whereas chronic refers to the high frequency of recurrence as opposed to persistence. By and large, episodic tension headache is usually of moderate intensity, self-limiting and associated with the occurrence of a stressful event. A chronic tension headache often recurs with high frequency and is associated with contracted muscles of the neck and scalp.

TTH is characterized by a headache disorder typically bilateral, pressing or tightening in quality and of mild to moderate intensity, lasting from 30 minutes to 7 days. The pain is not aggravated by routine physical activity and is not associated with nausea, although photophobia or phonophobia may be present. In some cases, patients may experience increased pericranial tenderness on manual palpation.[2]

Diagnostic criteria for TTH stipulated in ICHD-3 documentation include a history of at least 10 repeated episodes with attributes that substantially satisfy the typical characteristics and occurring <1 day/month on average (<12 days/year). Patients with attacks not exceeding 14 days in a month (<180 days/year) is deemed to be suffering from frequent episodic TTH and those suffering from more than 15 unremitting attacks per month would be considered as chronic TTH.

Circadian variation has also been observed in TTH pain pattern, with average intensity tending to be lower in the morning, building up in the afternoon and reducing again in the evening.[5]

Although tension-type headaches are common, the etiology and likely mechanism remain elusive. TTH was highly suspicious of muscular origin as the derivative pain exhibit characteristics typical of muscular or myofascial pain in that it is dull, radiating and poorly localized. However, as not all evidence seemed to support either ischemia or inflammation within the muscle structure, it is postulated that the disorder may be due to a combination of myofascial dysfunctions and a central nociceptive imbalance. TTH development from episodic to chronic TTH is thought to be accompanied by increasing central nociceptive dysfunction.[6]

According to ICHD-3 classification, Trigeminal Neuralgia is neither primary nor secondary headache but under the section of

"Painful Cranial Neuropathies, Other Facial Pains & Other Headaches".

In the same document, trigeminal neuralgia is described as a disorder characterized by recurrent unilateral brief electric shock-like pains, abrupt in onset and termination, limited to the distribution of one or more divisions of the trigeminal nerve and triggered by innocuous stimuli. It may develop without apparent cause or be a result of another diagnosed disorder. Additionally, there may be concomitant continuous pain of moderate intensity within the distribution(s) of the affected nerve division(s).[2]

Trigeminal neuralgia is sub-classified into classical, secondary and idiopathic types.

General diagnostic criteria for Trigeminal neuralgia stipulated in ICHD-3 documentation include recurrent paroxysms of unilateral facial pain in the distribution of one or more divisions of the trigeminal nerve with no radiation beyond the trigeminal dermatomes, pain that is electric shock-like, shooting, stabbing or sharp in quality with brief periods of intense pain that may increase in duration and intensity over time. This is further qualified by the pain located within the affected trigeminal distribution be precipitated by innocuous stimuli, ideally capable of being replicated in a clinical setting.

Other observations include contraction of facial muscles on the affected side when pain is extremely severe (tic douloureux), lacrimation (tearing) and/or redness of the ipsilateral eye, and there is usually a refractory period during which pain cannot be triggered following a painful episode.

Classical trigeminal neuralgia is a sub-form of the disorder provoked by neurovascular compression that fulfills all the general diagnostic criteria of unilateral facial pain mentioned above. Evidence of neurovascular compression should be beyond manual palpation but via definitive documentation by imaging (MRI) of anatomical changes reflecting nerve root atrophy and/or displacement due to neurovascular compression. Atrophic changes may include demyelination, neuronal loss, changes in the microvasculature and other morphological changes and such changes should relate to arterial compression as opposed to venous compression.

Pain in the classical sub-form usually appears in the second or third divisions of the trigeminal nerve. Presentation is mostly unilateral, perhaps appearing sequentially rather than concomitantly (bilateral). It may be preceded by a period of atypical continuous pain termed pre-trigeminal neuralgia but otherwise, most patients are asymptomatic between episodes. (except those suffering from concomitant continuous pain sub-form)

Secondary trigeminal neuralgia is caused by an underlying disease that is strongly correlated to the disorder and having general characteristics of trigeminal neuralgia referenced in the ICHD-3 guidelines. Lesion or tumor in the cerebellopontine angle, AV-malformation, and multiple sclerosis are known causes for secondary trigeminal neuralgia.

Idiopathic trigeminal neuralgia is a "catch-all" sub-form for the disorder when clinical presentations satisfy the diagnostic criteria for general trigeminal neuralgia but did not fulfill those of primary and secondary sub-forms for strict confirmation by electrophysiological and/or MRI investigations.

Except for idiopathic trigeminal neuralgia with concomitant continuous pain, individuals suffering from the pure paroxysmal sub-form are asymptomatic between episodes.

From a TCM perspective...

The head is regarded as the confluence of Yang Qi 诸阳之会 where all the six Yang meridians and the Governor Vessel that regulates the entire body's Qi meet. It is also the residence of the lucid Yang 清阳之府 by virtue that blood and essential fluids processed by the vital organs are infused into the head, nourishing the brain, the sea of marrow 髓之海, and the orifices that interface with the external environment. Given its close connection with the organ systems, the head would be hypersensitive towards internal and external homeostatic changes that impede the flow in meridians, disrupt nutrient supply to the head or occlude its orifices. This dysfunctional state is manifested symptomatically as headache.

There are two major categories of headaches in TCM, exogenous headache and endogenous headaches.

Exogenous headaches are caused by the invasion of external pathogens while body immunity is low. Exogenous pathogens usually attack the body in concert with and facilitated by wind-related pathogens. "Where an injury is caused by wind pathogen, the initial point of affliction is a superior location 伤于风者, 上先受之" and "injuries in superior locations can only be reached by wind pathogens 巅高之上, 唯风可到" are two observations in TCM that relate cerebral level disorders to assaults by wind-related pathogens. This occurs when exogenous pathogens enter the meridians of the head, interrupt the body's ascending Yang-Qi, causing flow of blood and Qi to stagnate in the head. When wind combined with cold pathogens, the cold Yin pathogen entraps the resident lucid Yang, causing sluggish blood circulation and musculature contraction resulting in pain; when wind combined with heat pathogens, heat irritates the head and its orifices, causing dysregulation in the flow of Qi and blood resulting in pain; when dampness pathogen with 'binding' characteristic 湿性粘滞 is facilitated by wind, pain is caused by occlusion of the lucid Yang 清阳不布 and obstruct the distribution of nutrient flow along with sluggish blood circulation. All told, the Yang energy is susceptible of being suppressed and stagnated by the invasion of wind, cold and dampness pathogens, the prime cause of headache. Notwithstanding, severe heat/toxin can also cause pain and distention of the feeding blood vessel via Qi stagnation and blood stasis 热极化瘀, 瘀郁化火.

Because exogenous headaches are induced by wind-led external pernicious factors, the onset is usually acute, severe in intensity, brief in duration, with the pain quality of scorching, distension, tightness, and pulsation.

Endogenous headaches, on the other hand, are associated with organ dysfunction and emotional issues. The brain, being the sea of marrow, draws much of its nutrients from essential fluids and blood processed by the spleen, stomach, liver and kidney systems. As the kidney is the guardian of bone and marrow, deficiency in kidney essence causes under-nourishment of the brain. A dysfunctional spleen that is ineffective in the transformation and transportation of nutrients to the head but produces dampness and phlegm instead, undermines the brain via under-nourishment as well as causing obstruction of the head orifices with generated phlegm.

Long term illness may cause generalized blood stasis similar to localized blood stasis experienced in traumatic head injuries. Though the underlying cause of headache in the two situations is the same, the nature of pain is different in that localized blood stasis produces intense stabbing pain while pain from generalized blood stasis would be less intense and throbbing. Blood stasis usually presents a headache that is persistent in which collaterals of the head may also affected.

Emotional disturbance and protracted stress cause liver Qi stagnation. Liver Qi stagnation prevents the liver in maintaining control over proper muscular function which is then interpreted by the brain as pain. With the passage of time, liver Qi stagnation transforms into internal heat 气郁化火 that consumes liver Yin, aggravating liver Yang, distending blood vessels including those in the head and induces a headache.

Endogenous headaches are slow in their onset, of longer duration with mild to moderate pain intensity, accompanied by lingering dull ache and dizziness. It is usually aggravated by physical exertion and may be relieved with rest.

Headaches may also be identified for treatment based on their proximity to the principal meridians.

Pains that are located at the forehead, vertex or *corona capitis*, occipital that extend to the neck, causing spasm to shoulders and back are associated with dysfunction of the Greater Yang Bladder Meridian. Occasionally, pain may also be found on the parietal bilaterally. Usually instigated by exogenous factors (exogenous headache), but could be endogenous with characteristics of the excess syndrome.

Pains located at the forehead, zygomatic region (cheek), and periorbital region especially eyebrows, that may extend to the mandible (lower jaw) region are associated with dysfunction of the Rising Yang meridians of the Stomach and a lesser extent the Large Intestines. Mainly of an excess-syndrome nature, the etiology is the invasion of wind-heat exogenous pathogens or, in the alternative, accumulation of damp-heat arising from indulgence in food and alcohol.

Temporal pains are closely associated with dysfunction of Lesser Yang Gall Bladder Meridian caused by an invasion of wind-heat pathogens or, in the alternative, internal heat by virtue of liver and gall bladder Qi stagnation.

Greater Yin Spleen headaches are characterized by either vague pain that permeates the entire head region not susceptible to palpation 按之不得 or a migratory pain 痛无定处 and accompanied by forgetfulness. The etiology is due to dysfunctional spleen not being efficacious in the transformation and transportation of essential nutrient to the brain; and in addition, generates phlegm that impairs the Lucid Yang 痰湿困清阳. Presence of phlegm, obesity and abdominal discomfort are the hallmarks of the disorder.

Lesser Yin headaches are associated with insufficiency of kidney essence failing to ascend the brain when this ascent was usurped by retrograde flow of Yang (Qi) of the Bladder meridian instead. Since the collateral of Bladder penetrates the brain, pain results. It is noteworthy that the Kidney and Bladder are organ dyads with the Kidney meridian being Yin and the Bladder meridian being Yang. The imbalance relating to the Yin deficiency and Yang excess within the two meridians created internal wind that rises upwards and in conjunction with an under-nourished brain causes headache.[7] Because the underlying cause of headache is related to deficiency syndrome, it manifests as a vague pain that permeates the entire head region.

> 张介宾注："头痛巅疾，实于上也。上实者因于下虚，其过在肾与膀胱二经。盖足太阳之脉从巅络脑，而肾与膀胱为表里，阴虚阳实，故为是病，甚则府病已而入于脏，则肾独受伤矣。"

Pain located primarily at the vertex of the head or *corona capitis* that permeates the entire head with extension to the periorbital region is associated with dysfunction of the Transiting Yin Liver meridian. The pain is due to retrograde flow of liver Qi arising from emotional disturbance. Blood propelled by the retrograde flow of Qi upwards causes pulsating blood vessels in the head and a feeling of distention. Distention also implies Qi stagnation and blood stasis that transform into internal heat in due course.

All told, the etiology of headache is due to the invasion of wind and cold exogenous pathogens 风寒外束, retrograde flow of liver Qi 肝阳上亢, obstruction of collaterals by blood stasis 瘀血阻络, occlusion of collaterals by wind-phlegm 风痰阻络, combined Qi and blood deficiency 气血两虚 and/or liver and kidney deficiency 肝肾亏虚.

Gua Sha Protocol for Treatment and Symptomatic Relief

Migraine

a. Trident Comb with emphasis on BL7 通天 using acupoint 'press-and-hold' technique on the affected side
b. Occipital-Cervical Sweep
c. Shoulder Sweep
d. Lessor Yang Plough on the affected side with an emphasis on TE17 翳风 using acupoint 'press-and-hold' technique
e. Acupoint 'press-and-hold' for LI4 合谷, LU7 列缺, on both hands
f. Acupoint 'press-and-hold' for ST36 足三里, ST40 丰隆, SP10 血海, GB34 阳陵泉, GB41 足临泣 on both legs

Tension-Type Headache

a. Four Spirit Extension or Trident Comb
b. Occipital-Cervical Sweep
c. Shoulder Sweep
d. Umbilicus-Pubic Sweep
e. Acupoint 'press-and-hold' for LI4 合谷, LI11 曲池, TE5 外关, LU7 列缺 on both hands
f. Acupoint 'press-and-hold' for SP6 三阴交, SP9 阴陵泉, SP10 血海, LR2 行间, LR3 太冲 on both legs

Trigeminal Neuralgia

a. Occipital-Cervical Sweep
b. Shoulder Sweep
c. Lessor Yang Plough on the affected side

d. Acupoint 'press-and-hold' for LI4 合谷 on hand of the affected side
e. Acupoint 'press-and-hold' for GB34 阳陵泉, ST41 解溪 on both legs

Distribution I — BL2 攒竹, ST6 颊车, LU7 列缺, EX HN5 太阳, GB14 阳白
Distribution II — ST2 四白, ST3 巨髎,
Distribution III — ST5 大迎, ST6 颊车, ST7 下关, CV24 承浆, GB43 侠溪
Execution — Unless TCM diagnosis suggests otherwise, moderation press-stroke recommended. Acupoints marked for application of 'press-and-hold' technique in each prescription form a set, each set to be repeated three times. 'Press-and-hold' maneuver should be attempted 10 times for each prescribed acupoint within each set. Use of skin lubricant that invigorates Qi and dispels blood stasis preferred. Observation of Sha appearance not mandatory.

Glossary

Remitting refers to periods of less severe symptoms that do not completely cease and is distinguished from relapsing that refers to a reappearance presentation of disease symptoms that become worse over time. Remission, which can be temporary or permanent, is the complete disappearance of symptoms of a disease.

Cerebellopontine angle is located between the cerebellum and the pons at the posteroinferior (back lower) part of the brain.

AV-malformation or arteriovenous malformation (AVM) is a tangle of abnormal blood vessels connecting arteries and veins in the brain. The cause of cerebral AVM is unknown and occurs when arteries in the brain connect directly to nearby veins without any intermediary (capillaries) between them.

References

1. Green MW. Secondary headache. *CONTINUUM: Lifelong Learning in Neurology* **18**(4): 783–795 (2012).
2. International Headache Society. The International Classification of Headache Disorders — 3rd Ed. *Cephalalgia* **38**(1): 1–211 (2018).
3. Burstein R, Noseda R, Borsook D. Migraine: multiple processes, complex pathophysiology. *J. Neurosci.* **35**(17): 6619–6629 (April 29, 2015).
4. Spira PJ. Tension headache. *Aust. Fam. Physician* **27**: 597–600 (1998).

5. Kikuchi H, Yoshiuchi Y, Komaki G, *et al.* Diurnal variation of tension-type headache intensity and exacerbation: an investigation using computerized ecological momentary assessment. *Biopsychosoc. Med.* **6**(1): 18 (2012).
6. Gold MS, Gebhart GF. Nociceptor sensitization in pain pathogenesis. *Nat. Med.* **16**(11): 1248–1257 (Nov 2010).
7. Unshuld P, Tessenow H. The generation and completion of the five depots. *Huang Di Nei Jing Su Wen*, Vol. 1《黄帝内经 素问·五脏生成》Berkeley & Los Angeles: University of California Press (2011), p. 196.

Annotation by Zhang Jiebin: "Headache and peak illness is repletion above. In the case of repletion above, there follows depletion below. The excess is located in the two conduits of the kidneys and bladder. The reason is, the major yang vessels of the foot move from the peak [of the skull] into the brain and the kidneys with the bladder represent outer and inner. Yin is depleted and yang is replete. Hence this disease." {literal translation}

Topic 63

Hyperhidrosis/Excessive Sweating

Humans have three different types of sweat glands: eccrine, apocrine and apoeccrine.

Eccrine sweat glands are abundantly distributed all over the skin, including the glans penis and prepuce, but not the clitoris, labia minora, oral lips and external auditory canals, and are the only true sweat glands in humans. Eccrine glands are of highest density on the armpits (axillae), palms (palmar), soles (plantar), and forehead. Eccrine sweat constitutes mainly water and electrolytes secreted through the surface of the skin where it cools the body by evaporation. Aside from being activated during thermoregulation, they are also triggered by emotional stimuli including anxiety and fear.

Apocrine glands are found only in hair-covered skin like the armpits, mammary, anal and genital areas. They secrete lipid-based substances containing proteins and steroids through hair canals. Apocrine glands are driven by adrenaline and hence, they increase in size during times of stress, sexual stimulation, anxiety, pain, and fright.

There is yet a third type of glands, the apoeccrine glands, that are found in the axillae and perianal regions. They can comprise up to 50% of all axillary glands and secrete watery fluids similar to eccrine glands. And because the apoeccrine glands have a capacity to produce much higher sweat output than the eccrine glands, they play a larger role in axillary sweating. Apoeccrine glands are stimulated by the cholinergic pathway but may also be activated via the adrenergic pathway.

Hyperhidrosis (HH) is a disorder of excessive perspiration under normal thermoregulatory requirements. HH is broadly classified into two categories: primary HH and secondary HH. Primary HH is, by definition, not associated with an underlying pathological condition. Genetic transmission is highly suspected as family history is often indicated by more than two-thirds of patients affected by HH. Male and female genders appear to be equally affected.

Secondary HH, in contrast, may be attributed to a number of other conditions, including endocrine disturbances, drugs, certain malignancies, infections, and central nervous system abnormalities. Menopausal women often experience vasomotor symptoms of menopause which cause excessive sweating; frequently nocturnal sweats. Lymphoma, cancer and even tuberculosis can cause excessive sweating, especially of the nocturnal type. Parkinson's disease, multiple sclerosis, and other neurological diseases may cause hyperhidrosis. Hyperhidrosis can also occur in patients of cerebrovascular accidents with excessive sweating localized on the paralyzed side.

HH can be further distinguished by anatomic distribution of affected regions and by laterality: unilateral versus bilateral and symmetrical. HH that affects numerous parts of the body is termed "generalized", whereas "focal hyperhidrosis" refers to excessive sweating in a local, bilateral, and symmetrical distribution.

Notwithstanding the above, HH is usually presented in two combinations, primary focal HH and secondary generalized HH. It is further observed in a clinical setting that focal HH is in most cases a primary condition, regional HH is usually a neurological cause and generalized HH is often time organic in nature.

Primary focal HH refers to excessive sweating not caused by another medical condition, nor is an adverse effect of medication. Sweating is "focus", occurring in very specific areas of the body and is usually relatively "symmetric" affecting both sides of the body similarly. The most common focal areas are the palmar, plantar, axillae regions and face or head. And often time in one or more areas concurrently, e.g. those with sweaty palms almost always have sweaty feet. The onset of primary focal HH is typical during childhood or adolescence with weekly or more frequent sweating episodes. Primary HH, however, does not occur during sleep.

Secondary generalized HH is caused by an underlying medical condition or is a side effect of some medication. As such, the disorder may be resolved once the underlying medical condition or medication causing it is identified. It should also come as no surprise that the onset of this disorder is biased towards adulthood. Sweating is "generalized" as sweating affects larger or other areas of the body and may often be experienced while sleeping.

Between normal individuals and those suffering from hyperhidrosis, there is no difference in the structure nor size or increase in the count of sweat glands. This led clinicians to believe that the condition is caused not by hypertrophy but rather hyperfunction of the sweat glands. Recent research also demonstrates that sympathetic ganglia of HH patients have significantly higher expression of acetylcholine receptors and significantly larger sympathetic chain ganglia. Given the normal thermoregulatory mechanisms are centrally controlled through the anterior hypothalamus, sweating associated with primary HH may, therefore, be related to a dysfunction of the sympathetic nervous system and hypothalamus.

Treatment for hyperhidrosis ranges from topical applications, oral medication, botulinum toxin A injections to surgery.

From a TCM perspective ...

Perspiration becomes pathological when it is not a physiological response of thermoregulation. This is synonymous to hyperhidrosis. TCM further differentiates abnormal sweating in a conscious state as spontaneous sweating 自汗 and excessive sweating during slumber as nocturnal sweating 盗汗.

Spontaneous sweating is mostly caused by Qi or Yang deficiency resulting in a failure to regulate the skin pores from closing that permits the untoward outflow of perspiration. On the contrary, nocturnal sweating is the outcome of yin deficiency causing a build-up of internal heat 阴虚内热 such that perspiration becomes necessary to maintain the appropriate core temperature.

The attributes of perspiration may also assist in the diagnosis of sweating. Perspiration that leaves yellow stains is associated with damp-heat trapped in the spleen and stomach. Perspiration with a tinge of red is a reflection of deficiency-induced extreme heat 阴虚化火. Lipid-like perspiration is secreted by patients with life-threatening ailments when the Yang and Qi are severely deficient to a point that the separation of Yin and Yang becomes imminent.

The anatomic region where perspiration is distributed is indicative of the cause of pathological sweating.

When perspiration is restricted to the head region only, the cause is usually Yang in nature since the head is the confluence of Yang meridians. The usual indications are the ascent of heat 火热上攻, the uprising of damp-heat to head 湿热熏蒸, gynecological-related bacteremia or sepsis 热入血室, biliary heat leading to Qi stagnation 胆热气郁, alcohol toxemia 饮热相结, postpartum blood deficiency 产后血虚, and blood stasis 瘀血阻滞.

When perspiration is restricted to the chest area, the cause is due to an over-labored heart, possibly associated with respiratory issues.

When perspiration is restricted to the four extremities accompanied by constipation, the cause is due to heat in the stomach meridian since the stomach dominates the extremities 胃主四肢. When perspiration is consistently present at the four extremities, dampness in the spleen and stomach is generally the cause. Above all, when the center of the palms and feet are cold to touch, a general state of Yang deficiency must be considered during treatment. Similarly, when the center of the palms and feet are warm to feel, it is indicative of a deficiency in Yin and blood.

Perspiration at the inguinal and genital regions are indicative of dampness, the latter may combine with heat or cold in its presentation.

When perspiration is unilateral, the cause is usually due to occlusion of meridians and collaterals by phlegm, dampness or embolism as observed in post-stroke individuals.

In fact, the anatomic distribution of perspiration in relation to organ system dysfunction was succinctly expressed in "Wang's Medical Preservation 王氏医存" of the Qing Dynasty as "Any of the five organ systems may cause perspiration; not just the heart alone.

These presentations are related to deficiency syndromes; with heart deficiency, the perspiration shall be located at the head; with liver deficiency, perspiration will manifest at the spinal region; perspiration at the groin reflects kidney deficiency; perspiration at the chest reflects lung deficiency; and perspiration at the hands and feet reflects spleen deficiency. Indeed sweating at a single location with chronic clinical presentation reflects deficiency at the meridian level pertaining to the organ system.

> 《王氏医存》:"五脏皆有汗，不独心也：汗皆为虚，心虚则头汗，肝虚则脊汗，肾虚则囊汗，肺虚则胸汗，脾虚则手足汗，人弱而专一处之汗，久而不愈，即此经虚也"

In summary, the etiology of abnormal sweating (hyperhidrosis) may be categorized under two major branches — Yin and Yang deficiency syndromes.

In the Yang deficiency syndrome sub-form, the causes are Lung Qi deficiency, Heart Yang deficiency, Spleen Yang deficiency, and Kidney Yang deficiency. Yang deficiencies could lead to the coalesce of dampness into phlegm that obstructs meridians and collaterals or forms a complex with heat; in both cases cause abnormal sweating.

In the Yin deficiency syndrome sub-form, the causes are Heart Yin deficiency and Kidney Yin deficiency. Yin deficiency implies a lack of vital essence and presence of internal heat, of which two organs are frequently involved — the heart 心火旺 and liver 肝火旺.

But in a clinical setting, complex or hybrid sub-forms exist and these are combined deficiency in Qi and Yin 气阴两虚 and combined deficiency in heart and spleen 心脾两虚. There is however yet another cause — blood stasis with latent heat pathogen 瘀血阻滞，热邪内伏. As recorded in the Correction of Errors in Medical Classics 医林改错 "when Qi tonification, immunity reinforcement, Yin nourishing or heat lowering therapeutic methods bore no results but instead caused a deterioration in the condition, this is because there was a lack of knowledge that blood stasis can cause spontaneous sweating and nocturnal sweating. The condition would certainly improve after the patient imbibed one or two prescriptions of Blood Stasis Dispelling Concoction 血府逐瘀汤".[1]

《医林改错》: "竟有用补气、固表、滋阴、降火之不效而反加重者, 不知血瘀亦能令人自汗、盗汗, 用血府逐瘀汤, 一两付而汗止".

Gua Sha Protocol for Treatment and Symptomatic Relief

a. Occipital-Cervical Sweep
b. Trapezius Sweep
c. Governor Vessel Dredge
d. Superior Bladder Meridian Dredge (T1-T9)
e. Sternal Sweep
f. Acupoint 'press-and-hold' for ST36 足三里, KI7 复溜, on both legs
g. Acupoint 'press-and-hold' for LI4 合谷, PC6 内关, HT6 阴郄, HT7 神门, LI11 曲池, SI3 后溪, on both hands

Execution — Unless TCM diagnosis suggests otherwise, moderation press-stroke recommended. Acupoints marked for application of 'press-and-hold' technique in each prescription form a set, each set to be repeated three times. 'Press-and-hold' maneuver should be attempted 10 times for each prescribed acupoint within each set. Use of skin lubricant that invigorates Qi and dispels blood stasis preferred. Observation of Sha appearance not mandatory.

Glossary

The adrenergic pathway is better known as the sympathetic nervous system (SNS) while the cholinergic pathway is the parasympathetic nervous system (PNS). Generally, the SNS or adrenergic pathway induces 'fight or flight' responses while the PNS or cholinergic pathway induces 'rest and digest' effects. These effects are triggered by different neurotransmitters sensitive to the pathways, being norepinephrine or epinephrine for SNS and acetylcholine (ACh) for PNS.

Reference

1. Wang Qingren 王清任. *Correction of Errors in Medical Classics*《医林改错•血府逐瘀汤所治之证目》1830.

Topic 64

Insomnia

Sleep is essential to the human body as sleep is profoundly involved in the maintenance of many vital physiologic functions including brain development, energy conservation, neural housekeeping/waste clearance, memory consolidation, modulation of immune responses, hormonal regulation, cognition, and performance conditions.

Human sleep typically cycles between non-rapid eye movement sleep (NREMS) and rapid eye movement sleep (REMS) for about four to five times during the night in an ultradian manner. Sleep architecture consists of three stages of NREMS and a single REMS phase that progress from Stage 1 to Stage 3 NREMS and REMS within each recurring cycle. About half of total sleep time is spent in Stage 2 NREMS and only 20 percent in REMS.

Stage 1 NREMS, the transition from wakefulness to sleep, is relatively light sleep characterized by slowing down of brain waves, heart rate, respiration, eye movements, and muscle motor activity. It is an easily awaken state.

Stage 2 NREMS witnesses further relaxation in heart rate, breathing, and muscle motor activity. Body temperature drops and eye movements stop as sleep becomes deeper. Brain wave activity slows but is marked by occasional bursts of rapid waves called sleep spindles.

Stage 3 NREMS is the period of deep restorative sleep that occurs in longer durations during the first half of the night. Heart rate, respiration, and brain waves slow to their lowest levels during sleep. Extremely slow brain waves, the *delta* rhythm, begin to appear and populate the entire session before the REMS phase.[1] There is no eye movement or muscle activity such that it may be difficult to awaken the person. People awakened during this stage do not adjust immediately and often feel disoriented momentarily after being awakened. Protein synthesis leading to physiological body repair, tissue regrowth, and immunity reinforcement are performed during this stage. *Delta* rhythmic activity during sleep is associated with enhanced cognitive performance and attentive focus during wakefulness.

REM sleep first occurs about 90 minutes after falling asleep. The eyes jerk rapidly in various directions behind closed eyelids. Respiration becomes more rapid, shallow and irregular, and heart rate and blood pressure increase to near wakeful levels. Males develop penile erections. *Theta* rhythm, which is of shorter frequency than *delta* rhythm, dominates this stage as the brain is reactivated with mixed frequency brain wave activity more akin to that during wakefulness. Most dreams occur during REMS, but dreams are prevented from being acted out by temporary paralysis of skeletal muscles.

A complete sleep cycle takes 90 to 110 minutes on average. Initial sleep cycles each night contain short REMS relative to Stage 3 NREMS (deep sleep). The length of time for Stage 3 NREMS, however, decreases in favor of REMS as the night progresses such that restorative sleep almost always disappears before dawn. REMS duration, however, declines with aging.

Physiologically, sleep is induced by the anterior hypothalamus while wakefulness is promoted by the posterior hypothalamus. Within the hypothalamus, the suprachiasmatic nucleus (SCN) synchronizes sleep with light exposure to match circadian rhythms. It transmits signals to the pineal gland to upregulate hormone melatonin production during darkness to induce sleep. As such, it is postulated that fluctuation in melatonin against time matches the body's circadian rhythm to the external light-dark cycle.

To induce sleep, the hypothalamus and the brain stem produce neurotransmitter GABA that reduces activity level in their respective arousal centers. During REMS, the brain stem ensures that skeletal muscles are "disengaged" so that dreams are not acted out. The thalamus, the bridge between external signals and the cerebral cortex during wakefulness or arousal, is also inactivated during most sleep stages except REMS where it serves to construct dreams by hashing stored images, sounds and other sensations from the cortex.

Insomnia, a symptom as well as a complex disorder, is defined by at least three different medical affiliations with slightly different connotations and therefore diagnostic criteria (refer to Topic 64 Glossary).[2] Notwithstanding, the disorder may be succinctly defined as repeated difficulty in sleep initiation, maintenance or consolidation or sleep that is chronically nonrestorative in quality, despite being accorded adequate opportunity and conditions; that result in clinically significant distress or functional impairment and these symptoms occur in absence of any known causative organic factor.

Insomnia is generally transient and lasts less than a month but, when left untreated, may deteriorate into a chronic condition. Acute insomnia or sometimes known as adjustment insomnia is usually associated with a precipitating factor or specific stressor. The stressor can be psychological, physiologic, environmental, or physical. This disorder usually resolves when the stressor is removed.

Psychophysiological insomnia is a form of chronic insomnia that is present for at least one month and is characterized by muscle tension, a pre-occupation with an inability to sleep, a raised level of anxiety that often intensifies when lying awake in bed and absence of deep sleep caused by a heightened sense of situational awareness. Patients suffering from this form of 'learned' insomnia should attempt to distance themselves from 'learned' sleep-preventing agents, with some reporting that they sleep better away from home.

Paradoxical insomnia is a relatively rare form of severe insomnia that occurs without evidence of objective sleep deprivation and without appreciable daytime impairment. The patient often reports little or no sleep on most nights over long periods of time. Sleep study reveals normal sleep architecture with normal sleep onset latency and sleep efficiency, but with subjective patient reports indicating prolonged sleep onset latency and poor sleep efficiency.

Idiopathic insomnia is a long-standing form of insomnia that has an insidious onset mostly early in life or even in childhood. Usually persistent and without periods of remission, it is characterized by short sleeping times, numerous nocturnal awakenings that are without cause, and difficulty falling asleep even when fatigue is present. There are often no precipitating factors associated with the onset of this insomnia.

Another sleep disorder that is often reckoned as insomnia by individuals is Circadian Rhythm Sleep Disorder. The underlying issue is a persistent or recurrent misalignment between the patient's sleep pattern and a pattern that is desired or dictated by societal norms, leading to the patient not being able to sleep when sleep is desired, needed or expected and thus a complaint of insomnia. However, in most instances, it was observed that the duration of major sleep episodes is normal with typical REM and NREM cycling once sleep is initiated.

More commonly observed sleep pattern misalignments are delayed sleep phase type or advanced sleep phase type depending if the misalignment was a delay or advance in the phase of the major sleep period in relation to the desired sleep time and wake time. This may be associated with an individual's choice guided by behavioral, social, or professional demands. When no clearly defined circadian rhythm of sleep and wakefulness can be detected in the misalignment, the disorder is termed irregular sleep-wake type, often seen in institutionalized older adults and is associated with a lack of synchronizing agents, such as light, activity, and social activities. Jet lag and shift work that temporarily disrupt the operation of the endogenous circadian clock can also cause a temporal mismatch between the timing of the sleep-wake cycle.

The etiology and pathophysiology of insomnia are largely unclear though much work has been performed across multiple levels of analysis to develop a compelling model. However, converging lines of evidence from psychological and physiological studies suggest an overarching role of hyperarousal as a causative factor of insomnia.[3]

Cognitive (thought) and affective (emotional/feeling) hyperarousal in insomnia due to physiologic or neurophysiologic factors have been demonstrated in both clinical reports and experimental results. As markers of increased arousal, physiological indicators include elevated plasma and urinary cortisol/ACTH during evening hours that suggests a hypothalamic-pituitary-adrenal axis involvement in the pathology, increased heart rate and decreased heart rate variability in all sleep stages of insomniacs, and increased whole-body metabolic rate.[4]

PET imaging also supports the hypothesis of hyperarousal in that insomniacs exhibited greater cerebral glucose metabolism during wakefulness and REMS states; with cerebral glucose metabolism being an indirect measure of whole-brain metabolism. EEG markers of increased arousal include increased activity was also observed.

Treatment for insomnia include pharmacological prescriptions, psychological and behavioral therapies.

Secondary forms of insomnia that occur when sleep deprivation is a symptom of a medical or psychiatric illness, another sleep disorder, or substance abuse, shall not be a subject of this topic.

From a TCM perspective ...

The earliest explanation for the cause of insomnia is found in the book of 'HuangDi's Internal Classics — Miraculous Pivot' 黄帝内经·灵枢·大惑论 in the form of a dialogue between Huangdi and his advisor:

> "The Defensive Qi that permeates the body surface (Yang) during wakefulness failed to re-enter the internal organs (Yin) when it is time to sleep and instead remains at the body surface. When this happened, Yang and Qi will be in excess and overflowing, causing the Yang Heel Vessel 阳蹻脉 to be highly excitable. The Defensive Qi failing to reunite with Yin essence also causes a deficiency in Yin, thus maintaining wakefulness."
>
> 黄帝曰：病而不得卧者，何气使然？
>
> 岐伯曰：卫气不得入于阴，常留于阳。留于阳则阳气满，阳气满则阳蹻盛，不得入于阴则阴气虚，故目不瞑矣。

The Yang Heel Vessel, one of the eight Exceptional Vessels, is an offshoot from the Bladder meridian that ascends from the lateral heel towards the brain. The Yin Heel and Yang Heel Vessels converge at the *medial canthus* (inner corner of the eye) before entering the brain. Another section from the same text further qualified that excess Yang is associated with wakefulness while excess Ying will cause somnolence 阳气盛则目，阴气盛则瞑目《灵枢·寒热病》, which implies that insomnia shall result when the Yang Heel Vessel is in a highly excitable state.

The Complete Works of Jingyue[5] 景岳全书·不寐 is perhaps more explicit in stating that sleep, being fundamentally a Yin element and dominated by the spirit/mind, will only avail when the spirit/mind is composed and vice versa (refer hyperarousal theory above); and the cause for agitated spirit /mind is two-fold, invasion by exogenous pathogens and/or deficiency in nutritive Qi.

> 《景岳全书·不寐》: 盖寐本乎阴，神其主也，神安则寐，神不安则不寐。其所以不安者，一由邪气之扰，一由营气之不足耳

The heart is the abode of the spirit/mind 心藏神 and the spirit/mind is associated with Yang. However, the spirit/mind requires nourishment from blood and Yin essence in order to remain composed, of which sleep is predicated.

From the foregoing, the etiology of insomnia that closely associates vital essence, spirit/mind, and Qi or the three treasures of life 生命三宝 精、气、神, is therefore in alignment with the "hyperarousal" hypothesis postulated by contemporary medicine.

Although TCM did not analyze sleep architecture at a micro level, it observed insomniacs encounter two issues: failing to sleep 不眠 and easily awaken 易醒.

There are 10 syndromes (clinical presentations) for insomnia that may be classified under three categories — agitation by heat, deficiency syndrome and other complexities.

In the agitation by heat category, there are three subtypes related to invasion by exogenous pathogens or excessive emotions — constipation-induced heat disturbance of the mind 热扰神明, heat transformed from liver repression 肝郁化火 and agitation by phlegm-heat 痰热内扰.

There are however four subtypes in the deficiency syndrome category, namely heart-spleen weakness 心脾两虚, Qi deficiency of heart and gall bladder 心胆气虚, blood deficiency arising from liver repression 肝郁血虚 and internal heat arising from Yin deficiency 阴虚火旺.

In the other complexities category, the three subtypes are retrograde of stomach Qi or GERD 胃气失和, blood stasis 瘀血内阻 and disharmony of heart and kidney 心肾不交. These subtypes are more akin to secondary insomnia as these clinical presentations arise from other medical conditions.

In the treatment of insomnia, the therapeutic objectives are to rectify the deficiency, address the dysfunctional organ system(s) and compose the spirit/mind. Dissipation and clearing of heat, both exogenous and endogenous, may be necessary as a means to achieve spirit/mind tranquility.

Gua Sha Protocol for Treatment and Symptomatic Relief

a. Four Spirit Extension
b. Occipital-Cervical Sweep
c. Trapezius Sweep
d. Superior Bladder Meridian Dredge (T1-T12)
e. Para-Vertebral Dredge (T1-T12)
f. Epigastric-Umbilicus Sweep
g. Sacral V Dredge
h. Acupoint 'press-and-hold' for ST36 足三里, ST40 丰隆, SP6 三阴交, KI1 涌泉, KI3 太溪, LR2 行间, LR3 太冲 on both legs
i. Acupoint 'press-and-hold' for PC6 内关, HT7 神门, TE2 液门, TE3 中渚, TE5 外关 on both hands

Execution — Unless TCM diagnosis suggests otherwise, moderation press-stroke recommended. Acupoints marked for application of 'press-and-hold' technique in each prescription form a set, each set to be repeated three times. 'Press-and-hold' maneuver should be attempted 10 times for each prescribed acupoint within each set.

Use of skin lubricant that invigorates Qi and dispels blood stasis preferred. Observation of Sha appearance not mandatory.

Glossary

Ultradian rhythm is a biological cycle that recurs more than once within a 24-hour day.

Circadian rhythm is a biological cycle that completes itself once within a 24-hour day, e.g. body temperature cycle.

Diurnal rhythm is a biological rhythm that is synchronized with the day/night cycle and may or may not be a circadian rhythm.

Infradian rhythm is a biological cycle that spans longer than a day, e.g. human menstrual cycle.

ACTH (adrenocorticotropic hormone) is produced by the anterior pituitary gland. ACTH levels are generally high in the morning and fall throughout the day (reaching the lowest level during sleep), following a diurnal (circadian) rhythm. When ACTH reaches the adrenal glands, it binds to receptors causing the adrenal glands to secrete cortisol, resulting in higher levels of plasma cortisol.

Cortisol is a steroid hormone that regulates a wide range of processes in the body, including metabolism and the immune response. Almost every cell contains cortisol receptors for cortisol to act on. Like ACTH, levels of cortisol are generally high in the morning and fall throughout the day. It plays a very important role in helping the body respond to stress.

World Health Organization: International Statistical Classification of Diseases and Related Health Problems, 10th Revision (ICD-10)

A. A complaint of difficulty falling asleep, maintaining sleep or non-refreshing sleep.
B. The sleep disturbance occurs at least three times per week for at least one month.
C. The sleep disturbance results in marked personal distress or interference with personal functioning in daily living.
D. Absence of any known causative organic factor, such as a neurological or other medical condition, psychoactive substance use disorder or a medication.

American Psychiatric Association: Diagnostic and Statistical Manual of Mental Disorders, 5th ed (DSM V)

A. A predominant complaint of dissatisfaction with sleep quantity or quality, associated with one or more of the following symptoms:

   1. Difficulty initiating sleep (in children, this may manifest as difficulty initiating sleep without a caregiver intervention).
   2. Difficulty maintaining sleep, characterized by frequent awakenings or problems returning to sleep after awakenings (in children, this may manifest as difficulty returning to sleep without a caregiver intervention).
   3. Early morning awakening with inability to return to sleep.

B. The sleep disturbance causes clinically significant distress or impairment in social, occupational, educational, academic, behavioral or other important areas of functioning.
C. The sleep difficulty occurs at least three nights per week.
D. The sleep difficulty is present for at least three months.
E. The sleep difficulty occurs despite adequate opportunity for sleep.
F. The insomnia is not better explained by and does not occur exclusively during the course of another sleep disorder (e.g., narcolepsy, a breathing-related sleep disorder, a circadian rhythm sleep-wake disorder, parasomnias).
G. The insomnia is not attributable to the psychological effects of a substance (e.g., drug abuse or medication).
H. Coexisting mental disorders and medical conditions do not adequately explain the predominant complaint of insomnia.

American Academy of Sleep Medicine: International Classification of Sleep Disorders (ICSD) 3rd ed (ICSD-3)

A. The patient reports, or the patient's parent or caregiver observes, one or more of the following:

   1. Difficulty initiating sleep.
   2. Difficulty maintaining sleep.
   3. Waking up earlier than desired.

4. Resistance to going to bed on an appropriate schedule.
5. Difficulty sleeping without parent or caregiver intervention.

B. The patient reports, or the patient's parent or caregiver observes, one or more of the following related to the night-time sleep difficulty:

1. Fatigue/malaise.
2. Attention, concentration or memory impairment.
3. Impaired social, family, occupational or academic performance.
4. Mood disturbance/irritability.
5. Daytime sleepiness.
6. Behavioral problems (e.g., hyperactivity, impulsivity, aggression).
7. Reduced motivation/energy/initiative.
8. Proneness for errors/accidents.
9. Concerns about or dissatisfaction with sleep.

C. The reported sleep/wake complaints cannot be explained purely by inadequate opportunity (i.e., enough time is allotted for sleep) or inadequate circumstances (i.e., the environment is safe, dark, quiet and comfortable) for sleep.
D. The sleep disturbance and associated daytime symptoms occur at least three times per week.
E. The sleep disturbance and associated daytime symptoms have been present for at least three months.
F. The sleep/wake difficulty is not better explained by another sleep disorder.

References

1. Zielinski MR, McKenna JT, McCarley RW. Functions and mechanisms of sleep. *AIMS Neurosci.* **3**(1): 67–104 (2016).
2. Thorpy MJ. Classification of sleep disorders. *Neurotherapeutics* **9**: 687–701 (2012).
3. Levenson JC, Kay DB, Buysse DJ. The pathophysiology of insomnia. *Chest* **147**(4): 1179–1192 (Apr 2015).
4. Roth T. Insomnia: definition, prevalence, etiology, and consequences. *J. Clin. Sleep Med.* **3**(5 Suppl): S7–S10 (Aug 15, 2007).
5. Zhang Jiebin 張介賓. *Complete Works of Jingyue*《景岳全書》1640.

Topic 65

Post Cerebrovascular Accident Syndrome

A cerebrovascular accident (CVA) or generally termed as a stroke, can be broadly classified as either ischemic or hemorrhagic. In either category, the end result is an interruption of blood flow, nutrients, and oxygen to a region of the brain, resulting in brain tissue damage and subsequent neurological deficits. In an infarcted brain, some brain tissues are destroyed and the effects of stroke shall be permanent. If the brain is ischemic, the brain tissue in the area is injured only and recovery of function is more hopeful.

Common causes of stroke are chronic hypertension, arteriosclerosis, and embolism resulting from atrial fibrillation or rheumatic fever. In younger patients, possible causes include clotting disorders and various forms of vasculitis.

The effects of a stroke depend largely on the part of the brain that is injured and the severity of the injury assessed after the stroke is stabilized. A very severe stroke can cause protracted comatose, permanent loss of faculties and even death. The road to recovery from a cerebrovascular accident can be long and tortuous that demands patience and perseverance from the stroke survivor who has to overcome many of the post-stroke conditions enumerated hereinunder.

Dysphagia is a condition that the individual finds difficulty in swallowing, partially caused by poor tongue control and loss of gag reflex. This is often manifested as coughing/gagging while swallowing, choking when food gets stuck, with food backing up through the nose. In serious cases, instead of being swallowed into the esophagus and stomach, food, saliva, or liquids, might get caught in the lungs or airways leading to aspiration pneumonia. Drooling is a common sight.

Post-stroke fatigue is a significant problem encountered by more than half of stroke patients and is a major deterrent against rehabilitation and thus therapeutic progress. Post-stroke fatigue can range from relatively mild to severe with the intensity of the listlessness appearing independent of the severity or type of CVA. It is also non-bias towards CVA type with both ischemic and hemorrhagic stroke having an equal share. Because rest does not always alleviate post-stroke fatigue, clinicians postulated that the cause involves a mixture of physical and emotional factors. Other contributory factors include sleep adequacy, side effects of medication and pain. There is no specific treatment or medication to treat post-stroke fatigue.

Hemiparesis is contralateral weakness or loss of functional power on one side of the body occurring on the side opposite to the brain that sustained the CVA; a left-sided CVA results in right-sided hemiparesis and vice versa. When hemiparesis is so severe that it turns into paralysis or inability to move one side of the body, the condition is termed hemiplegia. Hemiparesis hampers the performance of normal daily activities due to patient's impaired sense of balance, lack of coordination, impaired motor precision and range, muscular fatigue, and reduced mobility. **Foot drop** is a common observation in stroke patients where weakness or paralysis limits the ability to raise the front part of the foot. The cause is generally due to nerve damage. Rehabilitation treatments, electric nerve stimulation, home-based exercises, acupuncture, and assistive devices can help improve mobility and hasten recovery of hemiparesis.

Hemiparesis is a common presentation. A stroke occurring in the brain stem can affect both sides of the body, leaving the patient in a 'locked-in' state that deprives the victim speech and/or motor capabilities.

Incontinence can come in the form of urinary incontinence (loss of bladder control) and/or fecal incontinence (loss of bowel control). Urinary incontinence is more common among stroke survivors. Early treatment is important to prevent possible complications such as urinary tract infections or skin breakdown. Treatment options that offer differing effectiveness include behavioral and physical therapies, medication, bladder and bowel training, use of bladder bag and surgery. Making modifications to bowel habit, diet and fluid intake could also be helpful for fecal incontinence.

Post-stroke pain is generally categorized into two types: local and central. Local pain is usually felt in the joints, with the shoulder being a common location. Central post-stroke pain (CPSP) is a neuropathic pain condition characterized by pain and sensory abnormalities that manifest in the body parts that correspond to the area of the brain that has been injured by the cerebrovascular lesion. Any slight sensation on the skin, as in physical stimulus of touch, warmth or cold, is registered by the brain as a moderate to severe pain. The pain could be constant, with attributes of aching, burning, sharp, stabbing or itching.

Seizures, characterized by spasms or convulsions, are caused by sudden disorganized electrical activity in the brain as a result of a CVA. Seizures are more closely associated with hemorrhagic stroke or a CVA involving the cerebral cortex and the onset normally happens within 24 hours of the stroke. Though stroke is the most common cause of seizures especially in elderly people, the risk of stroke-induced seizure is relatively low (5%) and decreases over time. Those who suffered frequent recurring seizures may progress to develop epilepsy. Epilepsy is a neurological disorder in which recurrent seizures that occur cannot be associated with other specific causes. Stroke-related epilepsy may be controlled with anticonvulsant medications or the installation of a vagus nerve stimulator (VNS) — 'the pacemaker for the brain'.

Insomnia in the generalized form has been deliberated in the previous topic and shall therefore not be repeated here. Notwithstanding, insomnia secondary to CVA is complex but usually alleviates when the primary cause is addressed.

Spasticity is characterized by a spasm that is unidirectional and exhibited in rapid joint movements. After a stroke, damage to the brain can block messages between muscles and the brain causing arm and leg muscles to cramp or go into spasm (spasticity) that limits coordination and muscle movement. Commonly observed presentations of spasticity are clenched fist, bent elbow, stiff knees and stiffness in other joints. Protracted spasticity in major muscle groups can cause strong contractions and painful muscle spasms. Treatment options include the use of braces, physiotherapy, medication, injection, and surgery.

Visual impairment for stroke survivors can be classified under two broad categories, visual field loss and perception issues.

Visual field loss appears as blind spots in the field of vision. Loss of visual field should be differentiated from blindness in an affected eye, the latter due to impairment of the visual pathway on the same side before the optic chiasm. Normally, the right side of each eye sees the left part of the visual field, while on the left side of each eye see the right part of the visual field. Anatomically, this is achieved by a crossing of optic nerves at the optic chiasm in the brain that redirects optic signals towards the occipital lobe of the brain. The optic nerves (CN II) in each eye, however, is exposed to the full visual field on its side before the optic chiasm.

Hemianopia is the loss of half normal visual field due to a stroke-related impairment while quadrantanopia means loss of a quarter of the normal visual field. The most common form is homonymous hemianopia, the loss of vision is on the same side of each eye, due to impairment of the visual pathway after the optic chiasm. This cause a loss of half normal visual field contralateral to the stroke injury. Loss of peripheral (temporal) vision is caused by injury at the optic chiasm. Medically known as bitemporal hemianopia, the stroke survivor loses the outside half of the visual field giving rise to a tunnel vision and occasionally 'depth of view' impairment. Scotoma refers to an island-like area of blindness, typically smaller than hemianopia or quadrantanopia.

Vision Perception issues are ocular motility impairment created when the stroke lesion damages the brainstem and/or cerebellum causing difficulties in processing what the eye sees. The brain stem and cerebellum play an important role in sensation. The brain stem houses three pairs of nerves, Oculomotor (CN III), Trochlear (CN IV), and Abducent (CN VI), that control eye movement. When damaged or compressed, these nerves may not allow one or both eyes to blink, stay aligned or coordinated, resulting in dry eyes and blurred vision, double vision or visual midline shift. Visual midline shift may further induce dizziness or cause unnecessary body tilt to compensate for the perceived shift.

Visual neglect or visual inattention is a reflection of the brain stem or cerebellum injury. It causes the stroke survivor to be oblivious to objects in the vicinity. Fortunately, recovery from visual neglect is often possible and complete.

In the long term, stroke-related visual field impairment may improve in part or in whole, although these are often permanent deficits.

Communication impairment or aphasia is difficulty in expressing oneself *when speaking*, trouble understanding speech, and difficulty with reading and writing. Aphasia is not a disease, but a symptom of brain damage commonly observed in adult stroke survivors immediately after the ordeal. Clinical presentation for aphasia is unique to each survivor in that the effect is dependent on the location of stroke lesion in the brain.

Generally, aphasia can be divided into four broad categories: Broca's or expressive aphasia when the survivor failed to construct a sentence even though thought remains lucid; Wernicke's or receptive aphasia when the survivor failed to comprehend or interpret presented communication, be it verbal or written; anomic or amnesia aphasia when the survivor failed to use appropriate names for objects, people, places, or events; and global aphasia which is a combination of expressive and receptive aphasia caused by significant damage to the left side (language area) of the brain.

Vascular dementia is an impairment of cognitive/thinking function or information process abilities caused by brain damage from impaired blood circulation to the brain, depriving the brain of vital oxygen and nutrients, and leading to memory loss, confusion, decreased attention span, aphasia, impaired problem-solving ability, impaired visual orientation and possible impaired motor skills. Not all CVAs will develop into vascular dementia, but left-hemisphere strokes are commonly associated with vascular dementia. The risk of vascular dementia increases in recurring stroke.

From a TCM perspective ...

The basic pathogenesis of stroke is due to qi deficiency, improper diet, emotional stress, physical fatigue and organ dysfunction that induce blood and Qi to circulate in a discordant and irregular manner, resulting in the production of internal wind, internal heat, phlegm, and embolism. These pathological by-products, in turn, cause an obstruction in the cerebral blood vessels (ischemia) 脑脉痹阻 or escape of blood from ruptured blood vessels (hemorrhage) 血溢脑脉之外. The Book of Plain Questions in the Internal Classics recorded that when both blood and Qi ascend upwards in unison, there will be stupor, unconsciousness and sudden death.

《素问·调经论》：“血之与气，并走于上，则为大厥，厥则暴死”

In the second volume of 'Internal Classics — Miraculous Pivot', post-stroke symptoms are described on a broad front as "pathogenic factors having a propensity to reside in half the body and work insidiously into the nutritive and defensive Qi layer; and when this layer is consumed and the constitution spent, only pathogenic factors remain to further cause unilateral wasting (hemiplegia) to the body"

《灵枢·刺节真邪》：“虚邪偏客于身半，其人深，内居营卫，营卫稍衰，则真气去，邪气独留，发为偏枯。”

Synopsis of Prescriptions of the Golden Chamber 金匮要略 further explains the development and progressive staging of post-cerebrovascular events in that “pathogenic factors at the collateral level cause numbness to the flesh; pathogenic factors at the meridian level cause severe weakness in skeletal muscles; pathogenic factors at the visceral level brings stupor and mental confusion; pathogenic factors at the organ level induces loss of speech and foaming at the mouth (seizure)”

《金匮要略·中风历节病脉证并治》：“邪在于络，肌肤不仁；邪在于经，即重不胜；邪入于腑，即不识人；邪入于脏，舌即难言，口吐涎。”

Clinical presentations of post-stroke sequelae are therefore reflective of the degree of cerebral damage corresponding to whether the injury or lesion is at the meridian-collateral level 中经络 and/or organ-viscera level 中脏腑 as indicated by the state of consciousness or neurological lucidity.

In TCM, stroke is an outcome of mounting pathological afflictions and physiological dysfunction in the light of general deficiency 积损正衰 culminating in an impairment to the brain; and is closely associated with Yin deficiency of the liver and kidney and Qi deficiency in the heart and spleen systems but marked by internal wind and heat, accumulation of phlegm and blood stasis.

Post-stroke sequelae are natural progressions of undertreated or unaddressed stroke conditions that generally classified as Qi deficiency-Blood stasis syndrome 气虚血瘀证, Yin deficiency-Internal heat syndrome 阴虚内热证, Liver and Kidney deficiency syndrome 肝肾不足证, Heart-Spleen Yang deficiency syndrome 心脾阳虚证, Obstruction of collaterals by Wind and Phlegm syndrome 风痰阻络证 and Phlegm-Blood coagulation syndrome 痰瘀互结证.

Treatment is often complex and therapeutic strategies employed include dispersion of blood stasis by promoting blood circulation

活血化瘀, unblocking collaterals through dissipation of phlegm 化痰通络, suppression of internal wind by sedating the liver 平肝熄风, dissipation of phlegm-heat through bowel evacuation 通腑化痰清化痰热, promotion of blood circulation by invigorating Qi 益气活血, suppression of internal wind by nourishing Yin 育阴熄风 and, when necessary, restoration of consciousness by unblocking the orifices 醒神开窍.

Gua Sha Protocol for Adjuvant Treatment and Symptomatic Relief

Gua Sha is more relevant in the restoration of post-CVA motor dysfunction and improvement of patient's general well-being.

a. Four Spirit Extension or Trident Comb
b. Occipital-Cervical Sweep
c. Shoulder Sweep
d. Governor Vessel Dredge
e. Superior Bladder Meridian Dredge (T1-S4),
f. Large Intestine Meridian Dredge (LI4-LI15) with emphasis on LI4 合谷, LI10 手三里, LI11 曲池, LI15 肩髃 using acupoint 'press-and-hold' technique
g. Stomach Meridian Dredge (ST31-ST41) with emphasis on ST31 髀关, ST32 伏兔, ST36 足三里, ST41 解溪 using acupoint 'press-and-hold technique
h. Gall Bladder Meridian Dredge (GB30-GB39) with emphasis on GB30 环跳, GB34 阳陵泉, GB39 悬钟 using acupoint 'press-and-hold' technique
i. Acupoint 'press-and-hold' for TE4 阳池 for hand on the affected side

Execution — Unless TCM diagnosis suggests otherwise, moderation press-stroke recommended. Acupoints marked for application of 'press-and-hold' technique in each prescription form a set, each set to be repeated three times. 'Press-and-hold' maneuver should be attempted 10 times for each prescribed acupoint within each set. Use of skin lubricant that invigorates Qi and dispels blood stasis preferred. Observation of Sha appearance not mandatory.

Glossary

Spasticity is characterized by abnormally high muscle tone (spasm) that often asymmetrically affects antagonistic muscle groups (unidirectional). It is both amplitude and velocity-dependent which is clearly observed in rapid joint movements. Rigidity differs from spasticity in that the increased tone remains constant throughout the range of movement of the joint, is independent of velocity and therefore detectable with very slow movements. It is present in flexors and extensor muscle groups equally, giving rise to a uniform quality in all directions (bidirectional) often described as "lead pipe" rigidity.

Optic chiasm is an X-shaped space, located in the forebrain and directly in front of the hypothalamus. Crucial to vision, the left and right optic nerves intersect at the chiasm, thus creating the hallmark X-shape. Half of each nerve's axons (nasal half but not the temporal half) enters the opposite tract at this location, making it a partial crossing. The partial crossing of optic nerve fibers allows the depth of view or binocular vision (3-dimensional view).

Broca's or Expressive aphasia results from damage to a part of the brain called Broca's area. Broca's area is a functionally defined structure in the left frontal lobe of the brain involved mainly in producing speech, writing, and also language processing and comprehension.

Wernicke's or Receptive aphasia results from damage to a part of the brain called Wernicke's area located in the temporal lobe on the left side of the brain responsible for the comprehension of speech.

Topic 66

Vertigo/Meniere's Disease

Vertigo is a multisensory and sensorimotor syndrome involving a perceived self-movement or object-movement or both when in reality the individual and the environment are stationary. Subjective vertigo refers to an episode when the person feels self-motion with respect to a stationary surrounding whereas objective vertigo refers to an episode when the person has the sensation that only stationary objects in the environment are moving. There is yet a third type known as pseudo vertigo which an intensive sensation of rotation is felt inside the person's head.

Vertigo is caused by a mismatch between the vestibular, visual, and somatosensory systems, due to a pathological dysfunction of any of the stabilizing sensory systems resulting in asymmetric input into the vestibular nuclei. Typically aggravated by head movement, the usual sensations of swaying, spinning or rotation are commonly associated with nausea, vomiting, postural instability and possibly falls.

Vertigo is classified according to the location of the dysfunction within the vestibular pathway. The inner ear or vestibular system is broadly categorized into both peripheral and central components. The peripheral system is bilaterally composed of 5 vestibular end organs — three semi-circular canals (posterior, superior, lateral) and two otolithic organs (saccule and utricle). The semi-circular canals, structured at a vertical plane to each other, are sensitive to angular acceleration (direction and amplitude of head rotation in 3 dimensions) while the utricle and saccule respond to horizontal linear acceleration and gravity respectively. These vestibular organs when excited stimulate the central vestibular system.[1]

The vestibular end organs communicate via the vestibular branch of the vestibulocochlear nerve (CN VIII) with vestibular nuclei in the brainstem and the cerebellum that perform much of the processing necessary to compute head position and motion. The vestibular nuclei are important centers of integration, receiving input from the vestibular nuclei of the opposite side, as well as from the cerebellum and the visual and somatic sensory systems to maintain the sense of balance and position.[1]

Peripheral vestibular disorders are limited to the vestibulocochlear nerve (CN VIII) and all distal structures. Individuals with a peripheral disorder demonstrate nystagmus to the contralateral side which suppresses with visual fixation. Nystagmus improves with a gaze towards the lesion and worsens with gaze opposite the lesion. Patients may also report a falling sensation. Loss of appetite and weight, nausea, vomiting, and possibly sweating and bradycardia are common symptoms. Age and severity operate against recovery.

Vertigo caused by a disorder of the vestibular system and the vestibular nerve is termed as peripheral, otologic or vestibular vertigo. The most common cause is benign paroxysmal positional vertigo (BPPV), which accounts for a third of all peripheral vertigo. Another usual cause is Ménière's disease. Labyrinthitis (inner ear inflammation) resulting from viral and bacterial infections may also lead to transient vertigo. Motion sickness causes physiologic vertigo.

Some medication, including gram-negative antibiotic aminoglycoside (-micins and -mycins), loop diuretics (furosemide), platinum-based chemotherapy agents (cisplatin, carboplatin, vincristine), and some NSAIDS, have been shown to be ototoxic and can induce sensorineural hearing loss, oscillopsia (gaze instability) and balance impairments and thus vertigo.

Peripheral vertigo is typically presented with mild to moderate imbalance, nausea, vomiting, hearing loss, tinnitus, fullness and pain in the ear. Due to rapid compensation, acute vertigo as a result of a peripheral lesion tends to improve in a short period of time.

Vertigo arising from injury to the balance centers of the central nervous system (CNS), usually from a lesion in the brainstem or cerebellum, is called central vertigo. Conditions involving the CNS that might lead to vertigo include lesions caused by infarction, hemorrhage or tumors in the cerebellopontine angle, epilepsy, cervical spondylosis, transient ischemic attack (TIA), degenerative ataxia disorders, migraine, Chiari malformation, multiple sclerosis, and parkinsonism. Depending on the severity of traumatic brain injury (skull fractures), vertigo could be either peripheral or central.

Clinical presentations of central vertigo with nausea, vomiting, and auditory symptoms (tinnitus, hearing loss) may be similar to but are generally less pronounced than those of peripheral vertigo. The onset of central vertigo is often more gradual in comparison to vertigo of peripheral origin and accompanied by neurologic deficits (e.g. slurred speech, double vision).

Central pathology can cause disequilibrium, a sensation of being off-balance. The balance disorder associated with central lesions causing vertigo is often so severe that many people are unable to stand or walk. Central vertigo may not improve or may do so more slowly than vertigo caused by a disturbance to peripheral structures.

Recurrent episodes of vertigo are common and vertigo episodes may also be classified by duration as either a persistent (insidious) onset or an episodic (sudden) onset. Persistent onset vertigo is characterized by symptoms lasting for longer than a day and is caused by degenerative changes that affect balance as people age. Age-related degeneration of different neural structures affects balance, including vestibular receptors, central vestibular neurons, cerebellum, and the visual and proprioceptive pathways. Persistent onset is commonly paired with central vertigo signs and symptoms.

Episodic onset vertigo is indicated by symptoms lasting for a shorter, more memorable amount of time, typically lasting for only seconds to minutes. Typically, episodic vertigo is correlated with peripheral symptoms.

Benign paroxysmal positional vertigo (BPPV) is the most common vestibular disorder that occurs when free particles, suspended in the fluid (endolymph) of a patient's vestibular labyrinth, find their way into one of the semi-circular canals. Normally, the canals are excited only by head rotation; when particles denser than endolymph are present in the lumen, however, canals become gravity sensitive, pathologically responding to changes in head position. People with BPPV may experience brief periods of vertigo, usually under a minute, which occur with postural change. It is, therefore, more likely to be recurring with movement but otherwise normal between episodes. BPPV may be diagnosed with the Dix-Hallpike test that typically produces a period of rapid eye movements known as nystagmus in this condition, and could possibly be treated with repositioning movements such as the Epley maneuver.[2]

Ménière's disease (MD) is a vestibular dysfunction characterized by the clinical triad of recurrent rotatory vertigo, sensorineural hearing loss and tinnitus (ringing in the ears); often accompanied by a sensation of aural pressure and fullness that precedes an onset. Hearing loss usually involves low-frequency spectrum, especially in the early stages of the disorder, and may not be noticeable in the light of more perturbing tinnitus. Initially, only one ear may be affected but over time both ears may be involved with the mean conversion time of 7 years. The hearing loss and tinnitus may turn from episodic to persistent and with greater severity as the dysfunction progresses. Episodes generally last from 20 minutes to a few hours.

The most common age for the onset of MD is in the forties and the disorder is unbiased in its affliction towards both genders. The cause of MD remains elusive but is thought to be caused by endolymphatic hydrops, an excessive build-up of endolymphatic fluid present in the labyrinth of the inner ear.

From a TCM perspective ...

The basic etiology of vertigo is the functional disruption in the superior orifices 上扰清窍, especially the vestibular and ocular components, by internal wind, endogenous fire, phlegm, blood stasis or, in the alternative, deficiencies in vital essence and blood failing to nourish these superior orifices causing dysfunction. The resulting dysfunction could originate from emotional distress, eating disorders, general debility, blood loss, chronic physical exhaustion, trauma or even surgery.

The relationships between vertigo and various organ-systems have been duly documented in the ancient Internal Classics. In the book of Plain Questions, it categorically states that dizziness and vertigo intrinsically resulted from a disorder of the liver system. It further qualified that the clinical presentation of vertigo with tinnitus and perceptual distortion is due to neurologic deprivation arising from Qi deficiency in the superior (head) region.

> 《素问·至真要大论》:"诸风掉眩，皆属于肝"
> 《灵枢·口问》：“上气不足，脑为之不满，耳为之苦鸣，头为之苦倾，目为之眩”

The notion of "no vertigo is without phlegm 无痰不作眩 was first mooted by Zhang Zhongjing 張仲景 of the Han dynasty and later elaborated by Zhu Zhenheng 朱震亨 during the Yuan dynasty. Zhu surmised that vertigo is caused by a combination of phlegm, Qi deficiency, and endogenous heat. Treatment should, therefore, be prioritized with the expulsion of phlegm in the first instance, then the promotion of Qi and followed by reducing heat. There is no vertigo without phlegm, of which the phlegm is propelled by endogenous heat; which therefore necessitates differentiation between damp-phlegm and heat-phlegm.

> 《丹溪心法·头眩》：“头眩，痰挟气虚并火，治痰为主，挟补气药及降火药。无痰不作眩，痰因火动，又有湿痰者，有火痰者”

Vertigo etiologies were further expanded upon during the Ming dynasty by Zhang Jiebin 张介宾 in his work 'The Complete Works of Jingyue 景岳全书'. He postulated vertigo is fundamentally a deficiency syndrome 虚者居其八九 and elaborated that though vertigo is due to a deficiency in the superior region, the inferior region would certainly be involved; a fundamental TCM concept of Yin-Yang mutual dependency 阴阳互根. This is because a deficiency in the superior region is considered as a Yang within Yang deficit whereas a deficiency in the inferior region is a Yin within Yang deficit. Yang within Yang deficit should be addressed by rectification of Qi whereas for a Yin within Yang deficit the prescribed therapy should be nourishing the vital essence. As in cultivating a plant, curtailment at the roots (inferior region) sees wilting at the leaves (superior region) whilst nurturing a sapling requires nourishing the roots. For the same reason, treatment of deficiency in the superior region (head) requires mandatory tonification of both blood/vital essence and Qi to achieve nourishing the mutually rooted Yin and Yang.

《景岳全书·眩晕》中说："头眩虽属上虚，然不能无涉于下。盖上虚者，阳中之阳虚也；下虚者，阴中之阳虚也。阳中之阳虚者，宜治其气……。阴中之阳虚者，宜补其精……。然伐下者必枯其上，滋苗者必灌其根。所以凡治上虚者，犹当以兼补气血为最，…补阴补阳…。"

Prior to the above, Xu Chunxi 徐春甫 in his work 'Ancient and Contemporary Medical System 古今医统' observed that vertigo in the obese is caused by phlegm in the presence of Qi deficiency whereas vertigo in the scrawny is caused by blood deficiency in combination with endogenous heat. Emesis arising from invasion of exogenous pathogens invariably results in Yang deficiency.

《古今医统·眩晕宜审三虚》："肥人眩运，气虚有痰；瘦人眩运，血虚有火；伤寒吐下后，必是阳虚。"

Empirical observations provided TCM with guidelines for diagnosis and treatment of vertigo and may be summarised as follows:

a. No vertigo is without wind 无风不作眩 — implies that one of the root causes of vertigo is wind resulting from the dysregulation of/maladjustment in liver Qi. In TCM, the Liver is associated with wind and wood elements and is characterized by mobility and ascent. Emotional distress can result in liver dysfunction, Qi stagnation, endogenous heat, the excessive ascent of liver Yang and internal wind in the liver. The outcome would be a disruption of functions of the superior orifices leading to vertigo. The appropriate treatment strategy would be to placate the liver and settle the internal wind 平肝熄风.

b. No vertigo is without phlegm 无痰不作眩 — implies that obstruction by accumulated phlegm is another root cause. Excessive eating and a poor imbalanced diet can cause nutritive transformation and transportation dysfunctions associated with the spleen and stomach that result in the accumulation of dampness and phlegm at inappropriate locations, obstructing the ascent of the nutritive Yang to the superior orifices. Treatment methods should be based on dispelling dampness and expelling phlegm 化湿祛痰.

   The phlegm theory of vertigo in TCM appears to be in congruence with the association between elevated plasma anti-diuretic hormone (p-ADH) and endolymphatic hydrops in contemporary medicine.

   Phlegm, in the earlier discussions, was defined as misplaced vital essence and excess fluids accumulated at inappropriate locations in the body. ADH is a hormone produced by the hypothalamus, stored in the posterior pituitary gland and released on demand to maintain the fluid balance in the body by regulating and balancing the amount of water in the blood. When the p-ADH level is elevated, there is a tendency for water retention. A significant elevation of plasma anti-diuretic hormone (p-ADH) level has frequently been observed in patients with Meniere's disease and others with endolymphatic hydrops. This elevated ADH level is especially pronounced during the acute phase of the disorder in comparison to that in the remission phase. Individuals with persistently high p-ADH levels tended to have frequent vertigo attacks and these observations led to the assumption that disorders of ADH-dependent hormonal control in the inner ear may constitute the possible mechanism underlying vertigo attacks and deafness in patients with endolymphatic hydrops.[3,4]

c. No vertigo is without deficits 无虚不作眩 — implies that deficiencies in Qi and blood are also causes of vertigo. The constitutional foundation of an individual is generally determined by both nature and nurture. Nature implies congenital endowment 先天之本 bestowed by the parents and this vital essence is stored in the kidneys whereas nurture refers to post-natal development from nutritive absorption. The spleen dominates the transformation and transportation of nutrients in the body as well as generates Qi and blood. Emotional burdens and physical stress and/or eating disorders can the injure the spleen and stomach such that the production of nutritive essence, Qi and blood is compromised. Vertigo, therefore, occurs when nutrients and blood reaching the superior region is not adequate to nourish the brain and the superior orifices.

On the other hand, excessive coitus, disease of nocturnal emission or simply aging can cause a decline the stored genetic essence in the kidneys and therefore the functional level. The brain is the 'sea of marrow' and the kidney governs the marrow producing function. Any decline in kidney function correspondingly affects the integrity of the brain and thus induces vertigo. Treatment should focus on nourishing and invigorating the heart, spleen, and kidney as well as in cultivating Qi and blood 补益心脾肾，培补气血.

Within the clinical setting, TCM identifies six different sub-forms of vertigo, namely Excessive Liver Yang (Yin Deficiency) 肝阳上亢, Ascending Endogenous Liver Heat 肝火上炎, Obstruction of Superior Orifices by Ascending Phlegm 痰浊上蒙, Obstruction of Superior Orifices by Blood Stasis 瘀血阻窍, Deficiency of Qi and Blood 气血亏虚 and Yin Deficiency in Liver and Kidney 肝肾阴虚.

Gua Sha Protocol for Adjuvant Treatment and Symptomatic Relief

a. Occipital-Cervical Sweep
b. Four Spirit Extension or Trident Comb
c. Lesser Yang Plough
d. Epigastric-Umbilical Sweep

e. Trapezius Sweep
f. Acupoint 'press-and-hold' for ST36 足三里, ST40 丰隆, SP6 三阴交, KI3 太溪, LR3 太冲 on both legs
g. Acupoint 'press-and-hold' for LI4 合谷, PC6 内关, HT7 神门 on both hands

Execution — Unless TCM diagnosis suggests otherwise, moderation press-stroke recommended. Acupoints marked for application of 'press-and-hold' technique in each prescription form a set, each set to be repeated three times. 'Press-and-hold' maneuver should be attempted 10 times for each prescribed acupoint within each set. Use of skin lubricant that invigorates Qi and dispels blood stasis preferred. Observation of Sha appearance not mandatory.

Glossary

In TCM, there are nine openings or orifices, including seven orifices of the head (2 for eyes, 2 for nostrils, 2 for ears and 1 for mouth) plus one for the genitals and another for the anus; a total of nine orifices. The seven orifices of the head are also known as the "superior orifices 上窍 or clear orifices 清窍" while the genital and anus are termed as "inferior orifices 下窍 or turbid orifices 浊窍"

References

1. Purves D, Augustine GJ, Fitzpatrick D, *et al.* (eds.). *Neuroscience, 2nd edition.* Sunderland (MA): Sinauer Associates (2001), Chap. 14: Central vestibular pathways: eye, head, and body reflexes.
2. Zatonski T, Temporale H, Holanowska J, *et al.* Current views on treatment of vertigo and dizziness. *J. Med. Diagn. Meth.* **3**: 1 (2014).
3. Takeda T, Kakigi A, Saito H. Antidiuretic hormone (ADH) and endolymphatic hydrops. *Acta Otolaryngol. Suppl.* **519**: 219–222 (1995).
4. Aoki M, Ando K, Kuze B, *et al.* The association of antidiuretic hormone levels with an attack of Meniere's disease. *Clin. Otolaryngol.* **30**(6): 521–525 (Dec 2005).

Respiratory

Topic 67

Asthma

Asthma is a heterogeneous, multifactorial disease affecting the lower respiratory tract with variable and mostly reversible respiratory pathway obstruction caused by a chronic bronchial inflammatory reaction. It is characterized by episodic or persistent symptoms of cough, rhonchus, wheezing, chest tightness or shortness of breath that are variable and correlated with expiratory flow limitation. Symptoms are usually worse at night or in the early morning.

The above highlighted three important characteristics of the disease — expiratory airway limitation that is reversible spontaneously or with treatment, inflammation of the bronchi and hyper-responsiveness of the airway as an inflammation response. The interaction of these pathophysiological changes, operating in an extremely complex manner, determines the clinical manifestations and severity of asthma. As the pathophysiology of asthma is still not completely understood, many a clinician choose to diagnose and treat patients based on clinical presentations for asthma.

Due to the heterogeneity of the disease, asthma can manifest itself in a number of different phenotypes. These are Allergic asthma, Non-allergic asthma, Pediatric asthma/recurrent obstructive bronchitis, Late-onset asthma, Asthma with fixed airflow obstruction, Obesity asthma, Occupational asthma, Exercise-induced asthma, Asthma in the elderly and Severe asthma. Understanding and being able to distinguish between the phenotypes would be relevant to and advantageous for disease management.[1]

Central to the various asthma phenotypes is the presence of underlying airway inflammation, which is variable and has distinct but overlapping patterns that reflect different aspects of the disease, such as intermittent versus persistent or acute versus chronic manifestations. Acute symptoms of asthma usually arise from bronchospasm. Acute and chronic inflammation can affect not only the airway caliber and airflow but also the underlying bronchial hyper-responsiveness that enhances susceptibility to bronchospasm.[2]

As a chronic inflammatory disorder of the airways, many cellular elements, particularly mast cells, eosinophils, T lymphocytes, macrophages, neutrophils, and epithelial cells, interact and result in the pathophysiological feature of the disease: bronchial inflammation leading to airflow limitation and the subsequent cascade of events. The pattern of airway inflammation in asthma, however, does not necessarily vary with severity, persistence, and duration of disease.

Airflow limitation is a dominant physiological event leading to clinical symptoms in asthma and is caused by the narrowing of airways where the change can come in a variety of ways including bronchoconstriction, airway edema, airway hyper-responsiveness, and airway remodeling.

In acute asthma, bronchoconstriction or bronchial smooth muscle contraction rapidly narrows the airways in response to exposure to a variety of stimuli including allergens or irritants. The bronchoconstriction could be Immunoglobulin E (IgE) mediated or pro-inflammatory cytokine-mediated. In asthmatics who are atopic (i.e. those who generate allergen-specific IgE that binds to mast cells in the airways), the inhalation of an allergen triggers the mast cells to release histamine and leukotriene B4, which are powerful broncho-constrictors.

As the disease develops persistence and chronic inflammation progresses, the airway becomes hyper-reactive, causing structural changes to the airway that lead to occlusion of the airway lumen. These changes include edema, increased mucous secretion leading to the formation of inspissated mucus plugs, loss of surface epithelial cells, thickening of the basement membrane and hypertrophy and hyperplasia of the bronchial smooth muscle. The mucous plugs are composed of mucus and secretory immune cells eosinophils and lymphocytes. Histologic examination of airway lumen in fatal asthma attack victims supported these observations and when the grossly overdistended lungs of the dead are dissected, gelatinous mucous plugs are found in most of the bronchial branches down to the terminal bronchioles.

Airway hyper-responsiveness or bronchial hyperreactivity in asthma is an exaggerated response to exogenous and endogenous stimuli. The mechanisms involve direct stimulation of airway smooth muscle or indirect stimulation by pharmacologically active substances. The degree of airway hyper-responsiveness generally correlates with the clinical severity of asthma. Inflammation appears to be a major determinant of airway hyper-responsiveness and treatment directed toward reducing inflammation, such as steroid administration, can ameliorate airway hyper-responsiveness.

Airway remodeling involves permanent, non-reversible structural changes in the airway that increase airflow obstruction associated with progressive loss of lung function and decreased response to therapy. These structural changes include thickening of the subbasement membrane, subepithelial fibrosis, airway smooth muscle hypertrophy and hyperplasia, blood vessel proliferation and dilation, and mucous gland hyperplasia and hypersecretion earlier mentioned.

Management of asthma requires avoidance of aggravating environmental factors, use of inhaled short-acting β_2-adrenergic agonists (salbutamol, terbutaline sulfate) for rapid relief of acute symptoms and daily maintenance use of inhaled corticosteroids for persistent asthma. Combination therapy, including inhaled corticosteroids and long-acting β_2-adrenergic agonists, should be attempted for patients who inhaled corticosteroids alone lack effectiveness. Long-acting β_2 agonists are not recommended for the treatment of acute asthma due to a slower onset of action.

From a TCM perspective …

The modern-day description of asthma was articulated during the Qing dynasty by Li Yongcui 李用粹 in his work 'Supplemental Compilation for Therapy 证治汇补' as a disorder of which the interior (chest) is congested with by air or gaseous substance, the exterior (environment) is presented with aggravating stimuli and the thoracic region (lungs) is filled with gelatinous inspissated phlegm.

《证治汇补》：内有壅塞之气，外有非时之感，隔有胶固之痰

Asthma is due to constitution weakness arising from congenital deficiency, organ-visceral dysfunction and aggravated by the invasion of exogenous pathogenic factors, eating disorders, emotional distress or neglect in maintaining warmth; thus causing phlegm to accumulate in the lungs. Dwelling in chilly humid or hot arid environment on a protracted basis, that promotes the production of cold or heaty phlegm, could also be a causative factor.

Acute exacerbation of asthma is usually manifested as an excess syndrome, while asthma during the remission period is reflective of a deficiency syndrome. Recurring episodes of this chronic illness can, however, lead to the deficiency of the lungs, kidneys, and spleen, which characterized the disorder at this stage by underlying symptoms of deficiency with superficial excess-related clinical presentations; the hallmark of a combined excess-deficiency syndrome. It is very common for patients who have recurrent asthma attacks to have Kidney Deficiency. When under attack, such patients are said to have upper excess with lower deficiency 上实下虚. Upper excess refers to phlegm stagnation in the lung whereas lower deficiency refers to a deficiency of Kidney Qi.

According to TCM, the pathogenesis of asthma is due to congenital deficiency or organ-visceral dysfunction leading to phlegm being collected at the lungs and developing into phlegm-heat that damages the delicate lung. This increases the individual's susceptibility to exogenous pathogens. During the acute phase, asthma is represented by a strong presence of pathogenic factors at the lungs but the root cause of the disorder is closely associated with kidney and spleen. In the 'Classification & Treatment of Syndromes 类证治裁', Lin Peiqin 林佩琴 postulated that though the lung governs breathing, the roots of respiration lies with the kidney; while the lung determines expiration, the kidney determines inspiration; ventilation is harmonious when the two organs work in tandem and breathlessness arises when the organs did not function in synchrony.

《类证治裁》: "肺为气之主, 肾为气之根, 肺主出气, 肾主纳气, 阴阳相交, 呼吸乃和, 若出纳升降失常, 斯喘作焉"

In TCM, the lung is the storage device for phlegm 肺为贮痰之器 and the spleen is the source of phlegm production 脾为生痰之源. Phlegm would, in this instance, be produced from stagnated nutrients in the spleen, ascend and be accumulated in the lungs as well as obstruct the airways if the spleen is dysfunctional in the transformation and transportation of fluids. In addition, by virtue of the Five Elements 五行 Theory, the Spleen (Earth) is the mother of Lung (Metal) which implies that weakness in spleen shall impinge upon the lung causing inadequate Qi metabolism/transformation, leading to breathlessness.

As a causative factor in the onset of and recurrence in asthma, phlegm can be generated under three situations: spleen deficiency, kidney Yang deficiency and Qi deficiency of the Lung. This is because phlegm is a pathological by-product from coalesced dampness and body fluids. Spleen deficiency causes stagnation in fluid transport; kidney Yang deficiency leads to excessive fluid retention in the body, and Qi deficiency of the lung means loss of 'ascending and descending' action that mandates the proper distribution of fluids in the body. This is succinctly stated by Wang An 汪昂 in his work 'Medical Prescription 医方集解' that the lung is the superior source of fluids and the kidney is the inferior source of fluids, which explains that body fluids are produced at the spleen, distributed by the lungs and excreted by the kidney. Dysfunction in any of these organs will, therefore, give rise to excess fluid retention and thus phlegm formation.

《医方集解》: "肺为水之上源，肾为水之下源"

TCM treatment of asthma follows the fundamental principle of providing symptomatic relief during the acute phase of the disease while focussing on treating underlying cause when the disease is in remission 急则治其标, 缓则治其本. This is re-emphasized by Zhu Zengheng in that Qi should be reinforced during remission but counteracting the effects of pathogenic factors is paramount during an asthmatic onset.

《丹溪心法》: "未发以扶正气为主，既发以攻邪气为急"

Treatment during the acute phase should emphasize on the elimination of phlegm to ease labored respiration. It is also necessary to differentiate between cold or heat-related asthmatic sub-types so that cold be expelled or heat be cleared from the lungs. During the remission phase, the priority should turn toward tonifying and boosting the weakened Qi and normalizing the organ functions.

Allergic conditions such as asthma are associated with a deficiency in the immune system that harbors latent phlegm 伏痰. A weakened or over-sensitive immune system is invariably more susceptible to external pathogenic factors or allergens. In TCM, strengthening the immune system requires a rebalancing of organ Yin-Yang. It, therefore, becomes imperative to identify the deficiencies in the lung, spleen, and kidney or the combination thereof to normalize relative organ functions.

Gua Sha Protocol for Adjuvant Treatment and Symptomatic Relief

a. Occipital-Cervical Sweep
b. Shoulder Sweep
c. Trapezius Sweep
d. Superior Bladder Meridian Dredge
e. Clavicular Sweep
f. Sternal Sweep
g. Ventral Intercostal Space Sweep
h. Sacral V Dredge
i. Lung Meridian Dredge (LU5-LU10) with emphasis on LU5 尺泽, LU6 孔最, LU7 列缺, LU10 鱼际 using acupoint 'press-and-hold' technique

j. Acupoint 'press-and-hold' for PC6 内关 on both hands
k. Acupoint 'press-and-hold' for ST36 足三里, ST40 丰隆 on both legs

Execution — Unless TCM diagnosis suggests otherwise, moderation press-stroke recommended. Acupoints marked for application of 'press-and-hold' technique in each prescription form a set, each set to be repeated three times. 'Press-and-hold' maneuver should be attempted 10 times for each prescribed acupoint within each set. Use of skin lubricant that invigorates Qi and dispels blood stasis preferred. Observation of Sha appearance not mandatory.

Supplementary Notes — Bronchitis

Acute bronchitis is an inflammation of the trachea and major bronchi generally caused by an acute viral infection.[3] The infecting viruses could be air-borne or acquired through direct contact. Major risk factors include exposure to tobacco smoke, dust, and other air pollution.

However, unlike asthma, the inflammation is transient and will usually resolve itself when the infection clears up. As such, the disease is self-limiting and is diagnosed on the premise of clinical presentation of productive cough, malaise and bronchial obstruction such as dyspnoea and wheeze on exertion.

During acute bronchitis, the bronchial-lining tissue is irritated and the mucous membrane becomes inflamed, hyperemic and edematous that compromise bronchial mucociliary function. This set off a vicious cycle of progressive irritation as the airways become increasingly clogged with debris that is not cleared. The airways respond by increasing mucus secretion to flush out debris, causing the characteristic productive cough. Phlegm is clear or yellowish and occasionally purulent. The onset of bronchitis may be preceded by upper respiratory tract infection with symptoms of runny nose, sore throat, low-grade fever, and malaise. Complications of acute bronchitis include bacteria super-infection, pneumonia, and chronic bronchitis.

Chronic bronchitis is associated with excessive tracheobronchial mucus production sufficient to cause cough with expectoration for at least 3 months a year for at least 2 consecutive years. The disease is caused by an interaction between noxious inhaled agents (e.g. cigarette smoke, industrial and other environmental pollutants) and host factors (e.g. genetic and respiratory infections) that results in chronic inflammation in the walls and lumen of the airways. As the disease advances, progressive airflow limitation occurs with pathologic changes associated with emphysema (COPD).

In TCM, the lung is recognized as a delicate organ 肺为娇脏 vulnerable to opportunistic infection and bronchitis is categorized under the broad umbrella of cough 咳嗽, phlegm retention 痰饮 and occasionally asthmatic cough 咳喘. Like asthma, the etiology is due to the invasion of exogenous pathogens in the light of lung, spleen and/or kidney deficiencies.

A dip in the level of defensive Qi creates a window in which exogenous pathogens enter the body through the various orifices. Due to its anatomical position that is superior relative to other organs in the body, the lungs are vulnerable to wind-borne exogenous pathogens which are associated with cold or heat, giving rise to wind-cold 风寒表证 or wind-heat 风热表证 type of superficial syndrome. A wind-cold superficial syndrome may, however, be transformed into internal heat 风寒入里化热 when the pathogens become rampant and penetrated the protective shield of defensive Qi. This is synonymous the observation of 'developing an infection' in contemporary medicine when the symptoms are low-grade fever and yellow to greenish colored phlegm appear.

Gua Sha Protocol for Adjuvant Treatment and Symptomatic Relief

a. Shoulder Sweep
b. Trapezius Sweep
c. Superior Bladder Meridian Dredge (T1-T7) with emphasis on BL23 肾俞 using acupoint 'press-and-hold' technique
d. Sternal Sweep
e. Ventral Intercostal Space Sweep with emphasis on LU1 中府 using acupoint 'press-and-hold' technique

f. Lung Meridian Dredge (LU5-LU10) with emphasis on LU5 尺泽, LU6 孔最, LU7 列缺, LU10 鱼际 using acupoint 'press-and-hold' technique
g. Acupoint 'press-and-hold' for LI11 曲池, LI4 合谷 on both hands
h. Acupoint 'press-and-hold' for ST36 足三里, ST40 丰隆 on both legs

Execution — Unless TCM diagnosis suggests otherwise, moderation press-stroke recommended. Acupoints marked for application of 'press-and-hold' technique in each prescription form a set, each set to be repeated three times. 'Press-and-hold' maneuver should be attempted 10 times for each prescribed acupoint within each set. Use of skin lubricant that invigorates Qi and dispels blood stasis preferred. Observation of Sha appearance not mandatory.

Glossary

Phenotype, as applied in clinical medicine, would be any observable characteristic or trait of a disease, such as morphology, development, biochemical or physiological properties or behavior, without any implication of a mechanism.

Atopic individuals are typically predisposed to a heightened immune response to common allergens, especially inhaled and food allergens. Atopy refers to the genetic tendency to develop allergic diseases such as allergic rhinitis, asthma and atopic dermatitis (eczema).

Hyperemia is an active process where blood volume and flow to specific tissues are increased by active dilatation of arterioles supplying the tissue (increase blood flow) as well as dilatation of venules (expand blood volume).

References

1. Horak F, Doberer D, Eber E, *et al.* Diagnosis and management of asthma — Statement on the 2015 GINA Guidelines. *Wien Klin. Wochenschr.* **128**: 541–554 (2016).
2. National Asthma Education and Prevention Program, Third Expert Panel on the Diagnosis and Management of Asthma. Expert Panel Report 3: Guidelines for the Diagnosis and Management of Asthma. Bethesda (MD), USA: National Heart, Lung, and Blood Institute (2007).
3. Braman SS. Chronic cough due to chronic bronchitis: ACCP evidence-based clinical practice guidelines. *CHEST* **129**: 104S–115S (2006).

Topic 68

Emphysema

Emphysema is a matter of breath or death; an insidious, progressive and irreversible lung damage that causes shortness of breath. The disease tends to manifest no early signs and symptoms until 50% of lung function is lost, due to airway obstruction that begins at the terminal airways (alveoli). It is one of the two main conditions categorized under Chronic Obstructive Pulmonary Disorder (COPD). The other is chronic bronchitis. There is no cure for emphysema. The only available option is symptomatic relief and control of disease progression.

Respiration is fundamentally a mechanical process with the lungs akin to a bellow. The inflow to and outflow from the bellow (lungs) of air depend on the patency of nozzle tube (airways), the rigidity of the air bladder (alveoli) and the functioning of the air bladder's one-way value (condition of alveoli).

A reduction in the effectiveness of the respiratory system may be due to obstruction of the airways at any juncture from trachea to the bronchioles due to airway inflammation or excessive mucus, the loss of elasticity of airways and alveoli and the loss of gas permeability/perfusion or even rupture of the alveoli preventing air to be accessible to the body.

Chronic bronchitis, as previously discussed, is due to the inflammation of and an increase in mucus production in the airways. This causes a reduction of the airway lumen patency, making breathing more laborious.

Pathologically, emphysema is a structural condition defined as an abnormal permanent enlargement of air spaces distal to the terminal bronchioles, accompanied by the destruction of alveolar walls, a reduction in the pulmonary capillary bed and without obvious gross fibrosis.[1] The walls between many of the air sacs are damaged, causing them to lose shape and elasticity, resulting in air being trapped in the alveoli instead. Air trapping in the alveoli causes hyperinflation in the lungs, making it more arduous to exhale and thus shortness of breath.

The exact cause of emphysema is still not well understood. Research, however, suggests a close association between emphysema and smoking,[2] air pollutions and, in some cases, occupation. Another observation is that individuals affected by emphysema showed a deficiency in alpha-1 antitrypsin, a glycoprotein enzyme that protects the alveoli from collateral damage by neutrophils. Alpha-1 antitrypsin deficiency (AATD) is a genetic disorder.

Arising from the deficiency, an imbalance between protease and antiprotease activity in the lung that resulted in increased alveolar wall destruction and/or failure in alveolar wall maintenance is postulated as the major mechanism causing emphysema. The imbalance could be initiated by an increased presence of alveolar macrophages and neutrophils at the lungs due to irritation, chronic inflammation or increased oxidative stress.[3–5]

From a TCM perspective …

The pathogenesis of emphysema is the deterioration of lung disease that progressed to implicate the kidney function 久病及肾, leading to the kidney's failure to retain inhaled air 肾不纳气. Emphysema is classified in TCM under the category of deficiency-related dyspnea 虚喘 or retrograde cough 咳逆上气.

TCM treatment for emphysema is predicated on attempting to strengthen the lung function along with those of the spleen and kidneys. By tonifying the kidney, the kidney would be in better stead to 'hold' inhalation; also improved excretion of the body fluids shall favorably rebalance fluid distribution and thus having less mucus obstructing the air passages.

As a delicate organ 肺为娇脏, the lung is not only vulnerable to injury but also less receptive to treatment directly. The spleen (Earth), by virtue of the Five Element 五行 Theory, is the mother of the lungs (Metal). The spleen, therefore, provides a viable therapeutic proxy for treatment of the lung. In this regard, the deficiency of the lung may be normalized by reinforcing the function of the spleen.

Gua Sha Protocol for Adjuvant Treatment and Symptomatic Relief

a. Sternal Sweep
b. Ventral Intercostal Space Sweep
c. Clavicular Sweep
d. Trapezius Sweep
e. Superior Bladder Meridian Dredge (T1-L2) with emphasis on BL13 肺俞, BL23 肾俞 bilaterally using acupoint 'press-and-hold' technique
f. Para-Vertebral Dredge (T1-T12)
g. Epigastric-Umbilicus Sweep
h. Back Rejuvenation Dredge
i. Epigastric-Umbilicus Sweep
j. Lung Meridian Dredge (LU1-LU10) with emphasis on LU1 中府, LU5 尺泽, LU7 列缺, LU9 太渊, LU10 鱼际 using acupoint 'press-and-hold' technique
k. Acupoint 'press-and-hold' on PC6 内关, LI11 曲池 on both hands
l. Acupoint 'press-and-hold' on ST40 丰隆, KI3 太溪 on both legs

Execution — Unless TCM diagnosis suggests otherwise, moderation press-stroke recommended. Acupoints marked for application of 'press-and-hold' technique in each prescription form a set, each set to be repeated three times. 'Press-and-hold' maneuver should be attempted 10 times for each prescribed acupoint within each set. Use of skin lubricant that invigorates Qi and dispels blood stasis preferred. Observation of Sha appearance not mandatory.

Glossary

Alveoli are tiny air sacs of the lungs which allow for rapid gaseous exchange.

Alpha-1 anti-trypsin (AAT) is a protein produced mainly by the liver. Its primary function is to protect the lungs from neutrophil elastase. Neutrophil elastase is an enzyme in the lung tissue that normally serves to digest damaged or aging cells and bacteria to promote healing.

Protease is an enzyme that breaks down protein into its building blocks, amino acids. The three main proteases are pepsin, trypsin, and chymotrypsin.

References

1. Snider GL, Kleinerman J, Thurlbeck WM, Bengali ZH. The definition of emphysema: report of a National Heart, Lung, and Blood Institute Division of Lung Diseases workshop. *Am. Rev. Respir. Dis.* **132**(1): 182–185 (1985).
2. Sharafkhaneh A, Hanania NA, Kim V. Pathogenesis of emphysema: from the bench to the bedside. *Proc. Am. Thorac. Soc.* **5**: 475–477 (2008).
3. Goldklang M, Stockley R. Pathophysiology of emphysema and implications. *Chronic Obstr. Pulm. Dis.* **3**(1): 454–458 (2016).
4. Morris D, Sheppard D. Pulmonary emphysema: when more is less. *Physiology* **21**: 396–403 (2006).
5. Berg K, Wright JL. The pathology of chronic obstructive pulmonary disease. *Arch. Pathol. Lab. Med.* **140**: 1423–1428 (2016).

TOPIC 69

Influenza

Influenza virus, one of the most common causes of human respiratory infections, is a highly contagious airborne pathogen associated with high morbidity and mortality. The virus, belonging to the orthomyxovirus group, exists in four forms: A, B, C, and D.[1]

Influenza type A is generally responsible for pandemics and epidemics can infect humans, birds, pigs, horses, and other animals. The ability to mutate and cross species-barrier makes Type A virus the most virulent of the influenza virus. Aquatic birds including ducks, geese, and swans are considered to be the host or natural reservoir of type A virus.

Influenza type B and C virus are found only in humans. Type B virus may be less virulent than type A but can still be extremely harmful occasionally. Type B virus does not cause pandemics but localized community-level outbreaks of milder nature whereas type C infections generally cause mild respiratory illness.

Influenza D viruses primarily affect cattle and are not known to infect or cause illness in humans.

Influenza A viruses are divided into subtypes based on two proteins on the surface of the virus: the hemagglutinin (H) and the neuraminidase (N).[2] There are 18 different hemagglutinin subtypes and 11 different neuraminidase sub-types, giving a mathematical combination 198 possible sub-types for Influenza A. Hemagglutinin binds to sialic acid found on respiratory epithelial cell surface glycoproteins and provides for the attachment and fusion of viral and epithelial cell membranes. Neuraminidase digests sialic acid (neuraminic acid) on the surface of target cells, promoting entry of the virus into the cell. Neuraminidase also facilitates penetration of the mucus layer in the respiratory tract. Neuraminidase is the target of the antiviral drugs Relenza and Tamiflu. Subtypes can be broken down further into different strains. Other influenza viruses are not divided into subtypes.

Antigens are molecular structures on the surface of viruses that are recognized by the immune system and are capable of triggering an immune response (antibody production). On influenza viruses, the major antigens are hemagglutinin (H) and the neuraminidase (N).

Antigenic shift occurs when two or more different strains of a virus, or strains of two or more different viruses, combine to form a new subtype having a mix of surface antigens from the original strains. When this happened, presumably during co-infection of a single host, it provides a larger bandwidth for a major reorganization of surface antigens, giving rise to new H and/or new H and N. The most common form of reassortment is genetic recombination of the human virus with that of an animal orthomyxovirus. When this happened, few people would have immunity to the new or 'novel' flu virus resulting in epidemics and pandemics. Reassortment can only occur between influenza viruses of the same type. It is not understood why influenza A virus never exchange RNA segments with influenza B or C viruses.

Antigenic drift of a known strain results from successive point mutations leading to amino acid changes in the two surface antigens, H and N. Inefficient proofreading by influenza viral RNA polymerase results in a high incidence of transcription errors and amino acid substitutions in hemagglutinin or neuraminidase during replication leading to accumulation of natural mutation over time. A loss of host immunity results when the mutated surface antigen becomes unrecognizable to the pre-existing humoral immunity. Antigenic drift occurs in all types of influenza, including type A to C for humans.

Antigenic shift occurs only in Type A because it has a wider ambit of infection beyond humans whereas Types B and C that principally infect humans only may not have the bandwidth for surface antigen reassortment to cause an antigenic shift.

Influenza is an acute respiratory disease characterized by the sudden onset of high fever, coryza, cough, headache, generalized joint pains, body aches, malaise and inflammation of the upper respiratory tract and trachea. Diarrhea and emesis may occasionally be presented and more often observed in children. Acute symptoms and fever often persist for about 10 days but weakness and fatigue may, however, linger for weeks or months. Incubation period for influenza is usually between one and four days, during which the individual may be asymptomatic but capable of spreading the infection at a late stage. Pneumonic involvement is not clinically prominent in most cases.

As the disease is caused by a viral infection, treatment usually involves containment of viral proliferation and symptomatic relief. Rest and hydration are essential to recovery. Therapeutically, antiviral drugs can alleviate the severity of symptoms, avert flu-related complications and shorten the duration of recovery by 1 or 2 days. Center for Disease Control and Prevention (CDC) recommends prophylactic use of antiviral drugs for individuals at high risk of serious complications including those who are aged, diabetic, cardiopulmonary insufficient, immunocompromised or institutionalized. Antibiotics should be prescribed when bacterial infection developed or in individuals with chronic bronchitis, heart or renal disease. Symptomatic relief involves in the use of antipyretic and analgesic drugs but aspirin and other salicylates should be avoided in patients, especially those below 18 years of age. This is due to an association between the use of aspirin during influenza illness and the development of Reye syndrome, a serious pediatric disorder.[3–7]

Most patients recover fully after a fortnight. However, influenza and influenza-related pneumonia are important causes of morbidity or mortality in high-risk patients. Pneumonia is suggested by an aggravating cough, bloody sputum, dyspnea, and rales. Secondary bacterial pneumonia is suggested by persistence or recurrence of fever and cough after the primary illness appears to be resolving.

From a TCM perspective…

Influenza is a seasonal disorder categorized under the ambit of contagious epidemics and was first mentioned during the Han dynasty as the 'plague from the cold 伤寒 that is widely contagious with high mortality'. During this era, the onset of influenza was regarded as a Greater Yang disorder caused by exogenous pathogens of a combined nature: predominantly cold pathogen with wind or dampness pathogen. Because pathogens are still contained within the superficial layer (innate immunity) 体表, the nutritive and defensive Qi are involved, reflecting a position of strength for both defensive Qi and invasive pathogens 正盛邪实. Clinical presentations include fever, headache, body and joint pains, aversion to cold and chills. The primary meridian affected is Greater Yang Meridian of the Bladder. Unabated pathogenic invasion with declining defensive Qi would permit pathogenic entry into the Rising Yang (Stomach/Large Intestine) or Lesser Yang (Triple Energizer/Gall Bladder) area. This is the TCM pathogenesis for influenza based on the Six Meridian Diagnostic Principle 六经辨证 in which strengthening pathogens linger amid the three Yang Meridians depicting Qi being a viable resistive force. With the fundamental premise that exogenous pathogens are cold-related 寒邪, the disease would progress from superficial cold 表寒 syndrome to internal heat 里热 syndrome.[8,9]

At this stage only the Yang Meridian diagnosis appeared relevant to the prediction of disease development for influenza in a clinical setting. When exogenous pathogens invade further into the three Yin Meridians 阳病入阴 giving rise to scenarios of consolidating pathogens in the light of declining Qi 正衰邪盛, predictive gaps were identified by some scholars.[10]

> At the outbreak of an epidemic, physicians wrongly applied earlier prescribed methods but failed to observe therapeutic improvement… physicians were in despair when the disease progressed into a critical state. The more critical the disease progressed, the more chaotic the treatment. If the patient did not succumb under the disease, the patient would perish from the disorderly treatment;

if not dying in the hands of incompetent, it would be death from oversights in the Medical Classics.

《溫疫論·原序》:"始發之際，時師誤以傷寒法治之，未嘗見其不殆也。……醫者傍徨無措，病者日近危篤。病愈急，投醫愈亂。不死於病，乃死於醫；不死於醫，乃死於聖經之遺忘也"

This limitation was duly addressed by Ye Tianshi who took a perspective that febrile epidemics could be initiated by exogenous heat-related pathogens 温邪 instead of only cold-related ones 寒邪. He developed a system of Four Stratum Syndrome Differentiation 卫气营血辨证 for febrile disease progression of increasing severity. This 4-phase Syndrome Differentiation framework even provided a predictive model for expressed viral infection leading to sepsis and delirium 温邪上受，首先犯肺，逆传心包.[11]

Further discussion on the various diagnostic principles is beyond the scope of this topic and avid readers may refer to the original text listed under Topic References.

Gua Sha Protocol for Treatment and Symptomatic Relief

a. Occipital-Cervical Sweep
b. Governor Vessel Dredge
c. Shoulder Sweep
d. Sternal Sweep
e. Superior Bladder Meridian Dredge (T1-L5)
f. Para-Vertebral Dredge (T1-L5)
g. Lung Meridian Dredge with emphasis on LU1 中府, LU5 尺泽, LU6 孔最, LU10 鱼际, LU11 少商 using acupoint 'press-and-hold' technique
h. Acupoint 'press-and-hold' for LI11 曲池, LI4 合谷, TE5 外关 on both hands
i. Acupoint 'press-and-hold' for ST36 足三里 on both legs

Execution — Unless TCM diagnosis suggests otherwise, moderation press-stroke recommended. Acupoints marked for application of 'press-and-hold' technique in each prescription form a set, each set to be repeated three times. 'Press-and-hold' maneuver should be attempted 10 times for each prescribed acupoint within each set. Use of skin lubricant that invigorates Qi and with antipyretic properties preferred. Observation of Sha appearance preferable.

Glossary

Coryza refers to inflammation of and the discharge from the mucous membranes of the upper respiratory tract, sinuses, and eyes.

Humoral Immunity Explained — Before invading cells, pathogens entering the body first move from cell to cell through the fluid-filled extracellular spaces. Extracellular spaces are protected by the humoral immune response, in which antibodies produced by B cells cause destruction of extracellular microorganisms and prevent the spread of intracellular infections. The presence of antigen in the extracellular space activates B cells to differentiate into antibody-secreting plasma cells. To enter host cells, viruses and bacteria must first bind to specific molecules on the target cell surface. Invoked antibodies, however, bind to these pathogens to thwart them from penetrating the cells, thus neutralizing these pathogens and also preventing bacterial toxins from entering cells. To further prevent bacteria from proliferating within the extracellular space, antibodies facilitate the uptake of pathogens by phagocytic cells that specialize to destroy ingested bacteria; by an IgG antibody or C3b complement-mediated opsonization that coats the surface of a pathogen to enhance phagocytosis. Once the pathogens enter the cells, another immunity mechanism, the cell-mediated immunity, takes over and destroy the infected cells. In this instance, no antibodies are involved but operate on the activation of phagocytes, antigen-specific cytotoxic T-lymphocytes and the release of various cytokines in response to the antigen.

Reye's (Reye) syndrome is a rare but serious condition that causes swelling in the liver and brain. Reye's syndrome most often affects children and teenagers recovering from a viral infection, most commonly the flu or chickenpox. There is however a reported case of adult affliction under the same condition. Asia is not spared of this serious condition with reported cases in Taiwan and Japan. The mean mortality rate of Reye's syndrome is approximately 40% and appears to be higher in males than in females.

References

1. U.S. Department of Health & Human Services. Centre for Disease Control & Prevention. *Influenza*.

2. Taubenberger JK, Morens DM. The pathology of influenza virus infections. *Annu. Rev. Pathol.* **3**: 499–522 (2008).
3. McGovern MC, Glasgow JFT, Stewart MC. Reye's syndrome and aspirin: lest we forget. *BMJ* **322**(7302): 1591–1592 (30 June 2001).
4. Malcolmson CH. Reye's syndrome. *Can. Fam. Physician* **33**: 2615–2617 (Nov 1987).
5. Ninovea L, Daniel L, Gallou J, *et al.* Fatal case of Reye's syndrome associated with H3N2 influenza virus infection and salicylate intake in a 12-year-old patient. *Clin. Microbiol. Infect.* **17**(1): 95–97 (2011).
6. Burle S, Desai V. Managing risk of Reye's syndrome in children on long-term Aspirin treatment. *J. Clin. Case Rep.* **7**(Suppl): 9 (2017).
7. Su EJ, Hsieh JH, *et al.* Reye's syndrome arising from the treatment of Kawasaki disease. *HK J. Paediatr.* **23**: 185–187 (2018).
8. Gao YJ, Wang RB. Progress in the study of traditional Chinese medicine for the treatment of influenza. *Clin. Med. J.* Vol. 16, No. 1 (Jan 2018).
9. Zhang Zhongjing 張仲景. Treatise on Cold Damage Diseases 傷寒論 (219 AD).
10. Wu Youke 吳又可. The Epidemiology of the Epidemic 溫疫論 (1642).
11. Ye Tianshi 葉天士. Treatise on Warm Heat Disease 溫熱論 (1746).

Urological

TOPIC 70

Benign Prostate Hyperplasia/ Lower Urinary Tract Symptoms

The prostate is a walnut-sized gland forming part of the male reproductive system. It secretes an alkaline seminal fluid that nourishes and protects sperms during ejaculation. Located anterior to the rectum and distal to the urinary bladder, the urethra passes through the center of the prostate from the bladder to the penis, allowing urine to flow out of the body. The prostate comprises of the anterior fibromuscular stroma, the peripheral, central and transition zones, and is encapsulated by an outer layer of tissue.

Benign Prostate Hyperplasia (BPH) is the proliferation of prostate stromal cells resulting in an enlarged prostate gland that compresses on the prostatic urethra and restricting the urinary flow from the bladder causing discomfort associated with urinary storage, voiding, and postmicturition. BPH is however not a generalized enlargement of the prostate but nodular hyperplasia akin to fibroadenoma of the breast and affecting mainly the transitional and periurethral zones of the prostate with multiple nodules fusing together to form adenomata. In this regard, it is observed that bladder outlet obstruction is contingent on the site as opposed to the size of the benign growth (adenoma).[1]

BPH is a leading cause of Lower Urinary Tract Symptoms (LUTS) characterized by a range of storage, voiding and postmicturition symptoms. Storage (irritative) symptoms, caused by an overactive bladder, are characterized by an altered bladder sensation, increased daytime frequency, nocturia, urgency or urgency incontinence, dysuria, and suprapubic pain.

Voiding (obstructive) symptoms, caused by prostate or bladder neck stenosis/urethral/meatal stricture, include hesitancy, intermittency, weak stream, split or spray streaming, postmicturition dribble, urinary retention, straining and incomplete emptying.

Factors associated with BPH include aging, genetics, metabolic syndrome, inflammation, hormone, diet, lifestyle, environment, oxidative stress and, more recently, suppression of apoptosis in the prostatic tissue.

Aging males have a higher incidence of BPH due to tissue remodeling of basal cells within the prostate, especially in the transition zone. The nodular enlargement is androgen-dependent and the tissue remodeling involves both the epithelium and fibromuscular stroma. BPH could possibly be an inheritable autosomal dominant disease. Men with inherited forms of BPH tend to have larger prostates and disease onset at a younger age than men with sporadic BPH. Genetic factors may contribute as much as 72% to the risk of high moderate or severe LUTS among older men.[2]

Androgens *per se* do not cause BPH but the development of BPH requires the presence of testicular androgens. Testosterone is converted in the prostate to Dihydrotestosterone (DHT) by type II 5α reductase through DHT/androgen receptor signaling and may influence cell proliferation, differentiation, morphogenesis, and functional maintenance. DHT is ten times more potent than testosterone because of its higher affinity with androgen receptors. Therapeutic use of 5α reductase inhibitors (finasteride) markedly decreases serum DHT concentrations and slows the progression of BPH. Serum androgens, however, did not fully explain BPH occurrence in elderly male and it is suggested that estrogen/estradiol could be implicated since free estradiol levels are kept constant by adipose cells of obese individuals. Though inconclusive, estrogens can cause increased stimulation of the prostatic stroma, resulting in excessive tissue proliferation of the prostate and occurrence of BPH.[3]

Metabolic syndrome is a clinical constellation of conditions including obesity, hypertension, dyslipidemia, and hyperglycemia implicated in the development of cardiovascular diseases. Studies have shown that individuals with metabolic syndrome, in particular, dyslipidemia and central obesity, have enlarged overall prostate size (Total Prostate Volume), predominantly in the transitional zone, putting them at increased risk for BPH.[4]

Inflammation is an essential host immunological defense mechanism by which tissues respond to and contain, neutralize or eliminate an injury or infection and initiate regenerative or healing processes. Chronic inflammation, however, is harmful and may result in disease and conditions like cancer and arthritis. There is a growing body of evidence suggesting inflammation is closely linked to the development of BPH and LUTS. Di Silverio *et al.*, in reviewing clinical and pathologic data of some 4000 related urological surgeries, found evidence of inflammation in 42.5% of the patients. The nature of inflammation was predominantly chronic and low-grade but increase significantly with increased prostate volume.[5] Chronic inflammatory injury may contribute to cytokine production by inflammatory cells driving up the concentration of growth factors such as VEGF, leading to angiogenesis in abnormal proliferation of the prostatic tissue.[6] Men with LUTS are more likely to have higher serum C-reactive protein (CRP), a robust marker of systemic inflammation.[2]

Prostaglandin is an essential part of the body's way of dealing with injury and illness but unlike most hormones, it is not secreted by an endocrine gland and carried by the bloodstream to the site of tissue damage or infection. Instead, they are produced on-site and on-demand by nearly all organs in the body, where they cause inflammation, pain and fever as part of the healing process.

Prostaglandins are inflammatory mediators converted from arachidonic acid and mediated by two cyclooxygenase isoforms, COX-1 and COX-2. Both these pro-inflammatory enzymes are expressed in the prostate gland and increased expression of COX-2 in BPH is postulated to upregulate prostaglandin synthesis, especially of prostaglandin E2, that leads to prostatic hyperplasia.

Oxidative stress refers to an imbalance between the production of ROS/free radicals and its neutralization by antioxidants in favor of ROS/free radicals, thereby causing tissue damage. Reactive nitrogen species (RNS) and reactive oxygen species (ROS) are by-products of normal cellular metabolism and excessive production of ROS and RNS induces oxidative stress, causing a significant decrease in antioxidant defense mechanisms. The activities of antioxidant enzymes and the levels of antioxidants have been found to be significantly depressed in prostatic hyperplasia.[7]

A proinflammatory microenvironment akin to BPH stromal hyperproliferation and tissue remodeling promotes local hypoxia induced by increased oxygen demand by proliferating cells. The ensuing chronic inflammation thus becomes a source of oxidative stress leading to tissue injury in the infiltrating area. Inflammation is also a source of ROS/free radicals in the prostatic tissue. Prostatic inflammation can cause the generation of free radicals such as inducible nitric oxide synthase (iNOS), RNS and ROS. While iNOS is not detected in normal prostate, it is expressed in the prostate of all BPH patients even in the absence of prostatitis or systemic signs of an inflammatory condition.[8]

In the light of inflammation being a significant risk factor, the use of NSAIDs may prevent, delay or retard hyperplastic and/or inflammatory processes in the prostate, resulting in a decreased incidence of BPH.[9]

In an Asian-based study,[10] heavy smoking (>50 pack-year) was found to severely exacerbate the deterioration of LUTS, particularly storage symptoms. Heavy smoking was associated with urgency and frequency symptoms as nicotine increases sympathetic nervous system activity and could contribute to storage symptoms by increasing the tone of the bladder smooth muscle. Alcohol consumption, however, was not a significant risk factor for LUTS.

Exercise was found to be a protective factor against voiding symptoms as study participants who were physically active during leisure time were less likely to experience a deterioration of voiding symptoms. Physical activity was found to reduce the risk of LUTS and this benefit is postulated to result from improvements in cardiovascular health, promotion of weight loss, enhancement of vascular flow, normalization of serum lipid and lipoprotein concentrations. Physical activity was also associated with the improvement of insulin sensitivity and changes in sympathetic nervous system activity. It is possible that physical activity directly influences prostate growth pathways through the alteration of hormone levels (exercise ameliorates prostaglandins).

The total energy intake-adjusted protein consumption was associated with storage symptoms. This is consistent with an earlier finding of modest direct associations between BPH and intakes of total energy, protein, and specific long-chain polyunsaturated fatty acids. Energy-adjusted total and animal intake protein were positively associated with total BPH. Energy-adjusted total fat intake was not associated with risk of total BPH, but intakes of eicosapentaenoic (EPA), docosahexaenoic (DHA) and arachidonic acids were associated with a moderate increase in risk of total BPH probably due to lipid peroxidation, free radical generation and a possible role of oxidative stress in the etiology of BPH.[11] Arachidonic acids are also building blocks for prostaglandins.

Yet another study found that a dietary pattern high in vegetables and protein, moderate in alcohol, and low in fat and red meat may protect men from developing symptomatic BPH. There was no evidence that antioxidant nutrients, from either supplements or food, were associated with reduced BPH risk, nor were there evidence that consumption of long-chain omega-3 fatty acids, zinc or calcium was associated with reduced risk.[12]

Enlargement of the prostate is caused by an increase in cell population within the organ arising from either amplified cell proliferation, decreased cell death or both, resulting in net positive cell growth. Apoptosis or programmed cell death is a control mechanism in the body that ensures a balanced rate of cell regeneration and demise to maintain tissue homeostasis. BPH has been shown to result from smooth muscle and epithelial proliferation primarily within the prostatic transition zone.

Several studies suggested that a down-regulation of apoptotic function might occur in BPH when an over-expression of Bcl-2, an apoptotic suppressor, was found in the basal and luminal epithelial cells in BPH as opposed to healthy prostate tissue;[13] and survivin, an inhibitor of apoptosis that counteracts cell death and controls mitotic progression, was over-expressed in the stromal compartment of patients with BPH.[14] Recent studies also showed increased expression of Inhibitors of Apoptosis Proteins (IAPs) in human prostates with BPH.[15,16]

An investigation into the mechanisms of action of the drugs currently being used in BPH management further suggested possible interactions with apoptotic mechanisms. BPH patients treated with finasteride benefitted from an upregulation of Transforming Growth Factor beta (TGF-beta) that affirmed the pro-apoptotic effect of finasteride on the epithelial cells.[17] In another study of finasteride treatment on BPH tissue, a caspase-dependent apoptotic process that acted restrictively on epithelial cells by increasing the expression of pro-apoptotic proteins (Caspases-3, -6 and -9) was also observed. The action was however transient and did not sustain beyond 32 days after treatment.[18]

BPH symptoms arise through two mechanisms: static, where hyperplastic prostatic tissue or overgrowth of the prostatic epithelium compresses the urethra; and dynamic, due to increased adrenergic nervous activity and prostatic smooth muscle tone. Both mechanisms increase resistance to urinary flow at the level of the bladder outlet. Management for BPH/LUTS is therefore targeted at these two levels and range from medication to surgery, the complexity of which is beyond the scope of this article.

Complications of BPH/LUTS include urinary retention, recurrent urinary tract infection, bladder stones, gross hematuria, renal insufficiency, kidney obstruction, and renal failure.

From a TCM perspective...

BPH/LUTS is categorized as a disorder under the generic class of dysuria and may be sub-divided into excess-related or deficiency-related. Dysuria was believed to be caused by kidney weakness and intrinsic heat of the bladder during the Sui Dynasty (640AD).[19] This diagnosis was expanded in the Yuan dynasty to include Qi deficiency, blood deficiency, phlegm stagnation, wind occlusion 风闭, and heat excess 实热.[20] Lung dysfunction as a cause of dysuria was further included during Qing Dynasty,[21] and in the same period, aging and male menopause 命门火衰 became contributing factors to the disorder.[22]

Etiology of the disease is a deficiency in kidney Qi or blood stasis that prevents the normal function of the Triple Energizer 三焦 which consequently impedes the descent of systemic turbidity 浊阴不降. Specific pathogenesis may be categorized into intrinsic damp-heat 湿热内蕴, unregulated Qi mechanism 气化失司, failure of spleen Qi in ascending 脾气不升, heat stagnation in lung 肺热壅滞 and kidney deficiency 肾元亏虚.

If Qi is obstructed due to heat in the lung, the lung loses its function in distributing and channeling body fluids 通调水道 so that fluids do not descend to the bladder 下输膀胱. When liver Qi is stagnated and the liver loses its regulatory 调达 function, Qi mechanism shall be obstructed, leading to interruption in body fluid transport, latency in excretion and water retention 津停水聚. If the spleen Qi is weak and did not ascend 升清降浊, systemic turbidity will fail to descend. If the kidney is deficient, both the vital essence and kidney Qi lack warmth 精寒气冷 and cannot perform its transformation function to maintain overall fluid balance 气不化水.

TCM holds that exogenous factors may cause no harm when Qi remains robust and intact within the body 正气存内，邪不可干 and conversely pathogens may enter the body only when Qi is deficient 邪之所凑，其气必虚. Male quinquagenarians who lived for more than half a century would generally experience gradual depletion of kidney yin and yang, disruption of Qi mechanism and in longer terms blood stasis and phlegm obstruction — the contributing factors for BPH/LUTS.

Treatment for BPH/LUTS should, therefore, focus on stimulation and strengthening of the Kidney, Bladder, Spleen, Liver, Lung and Triple Energizer.

Gua Sha protocol for adjuvant treatment and symptomatic relief

a. Superior Bladder Meridian Dredge (T1-L5)
b. Governor Vessel Dredge
c. Sacral V Dredge
d. Umbilicus-Pubic Sweep
e. Acupoint 'press-and-hold' for SP6 三阴交, SP9 阴陵泉, ST36 足三里, BL39 委阳, BL40 委中, KI3 太溪, LR3 太冲 on both legs
f. Acupoint 'press-and-hold' for LU5 尺泽 on both arms

Execution — Unless TCM diagnosis suggests otherwise, moderation press-stroke recommended. Acupoints marked for application of 'press-and-hold' technique in each prescription form a set, each set to be repeated three times. 'Press-and-hold' maneuver should be attempted 10 times for each prescribed acupoint within each set. Use of skin lubricant that invigorates Qi and dispels blood stasis preferred. Observation of Sha appearance preferable.

Other Considerations — in event of urine retention, additional manipulations of Four Spirit Extension and Sternal Sweep may be attempted.

References

1. Luo GC, Foo KT, Kuo T, Tan G. Diagnosis of prostate adenoma and the relationship between the site of prostate adenoma and bladder outlet obstruction. *Singapore Med. J.* **54**: 482–486 (2013).
2. Parsons JK. Benign prostatic hyperplasia and male lower urinary tract symptoms: epidemiology and risk factors. *Curr. Bladder Dysfunct. Rep.* **5**: 212–218 (2010).
3. Ho CKM, Habib FK. Estrogen and androgen signaling in the pathogenesis of BPH. *Nat. Rev. Urol.* **8**: 29–41 (2011).
4. Gacci M, Corona G, *et al.* Metabolic syndrome and benign prostatic enlargement: a systematic review and meta-analysis. *BJU Int.* **115**: 24–31 (2015).
5. Di Silverio F, Gentile V, *et al.* Distribution of inflammation, pre-malignant lesions, incidental carcinoma in histologically confirmed benign prostatic hyperplasia: a retrospective analysis. *Eur. Urol.* **43**: 164–175 (2003).
6. Bostanci Y, Kazzazi A, Momtahen S, *et al.* Correlation between benign prostatic hyperplasia and inflammation. *Curr. Opin. Urol.* **23**: 5–10 (2013).

7. Udensi UK, Tchounwou PB. Oxidative stress in prostate hyperplasia and carcinogenesis. *J. Exp. Clin. Cancer Res.* **35**: 139 (2016).
8. Minciullo PL, Inferrera A, *et al.* Oxidative stress in benign prostatic hyperplasia: a systematic review. *Urol. Int.* **94**: 249–254 (2015).
9. St Sauver JL, Jacobson DJ, *et al.* Protective association between nonsteroidal anti-inflammatory drug use and measures of benign prostatic hyperplasia. *Am. J. Epidemiol.* **164**: 760–768 (2006).
10. Choo MS, Han JH, *et al.* Alcohol, smoking, physical activity, protein, and lower urinary tract symptoms: prospective longitudinal cohort. *Int. Neurourol. J.* **19**: 197–206 (2015).
11. Suzuki S, Platz EA, *et al.* Intakes of energy and macronutrients and the risk of benign prostatic hyperplasia. *Am. J. Clin. Nutr.* **75**: 689–697 (2002).
12. Kristal AR, Arnold KB, *et al.* Dietary patterns, supplement use, and the risk of symptomatic benign prostatic hyperplasia: results from the Prostate Cancer Prevention Trial. *Am. J. Epidemiol.* **167**: 925–934 (2008).
13. Kyprianou N, Tu H, Jacobs SC. Apoptotic versus proliferative activities in human benign prostatic hyperplasia. *Hum. Pathol.* **7**: 668–675 (1996).
14. Shariat SF, Ashfaq R, *et al.* Expression of survivin and apoptotic biomarkers in benign prostatic hyperplasia. *J. Urol.* **174**: 2046–2050 (2005).
15. Minutoli L, Altavilla D, *et al.* Inhibitors of apoptosis proteins in experimental benign prostatic hyperplasia: effects of Serenoa repens, selenium and lycopene. *J. Biomed. Sci.* **21**: 19 (2014).
16. Rodriguez-Berriguete G, Fraile B, *et al.* Role of IAPs in prostate cancer progression: immunohistochemical study in normal and pathological (benign hyperplastic, prostatic intraepithelial neoplasia and cancer) human prostate. *BMC Cancer* **10**: 18 (2010).
17. Saez C, Gonzalez-Baena AC, Japon MA. Regressive changes in finasteride-treated human hyperplastic prostates correlate with an upregulation of TGF-b receptor expression. *Prostate* **37**: 84–90 (1998).
18. Bozec A, Ruffion A, *et al.* Activation of caspases-3, -6, and -9 during finasteride treatment of benign prostatic hyperplasia. *J. Clin. Endocrinol. Metab.* **90**(1): 17–25 (Jan 2005).
19. Chao Yuanfang 巢元方. *Treatise on the Pathogenesis and Manifestations of All Diseases* 諸病源候論 (610 AD).
20. Zhu Zhenheng 朱震亨. *Danxi's Experiential Therapy* 丹溪心法 《丹溪心法·小便不通》 (1481).
21. Li Yongcui 李用粹 *Collected Supplement to Pattern/Syndrome Identifications and Treatments* 证治汇补 (1687).
22. Chen Shizhen 陈士铎. *Dialectical Anecdote* 辨证奇闻.

Topic 71

Erectile Dysfunction

Erection is a neurovascular incident, which means an event involving both nerves and blood vessels. Anatomically, the penis consists of three cylindrical erectile cavernous tissue structures: two chambers of corpora cavernosa and a corpus spongiosum enclosed by a fibrous capsule, the tunica albuginea. Blood must flow adequately into the lacunar spaces of the penis and at same time venous outflow be impeded before an erection may occur.

This happens when the blood partial pressure of oxygen (PaO_2) increases from 35mmHg in a flaccid state to about 90 mmHg and intra-cavernous pressure to around 100 mmHg at full erection. At rigid erection, the PaO_2 is many folds higher, raising the arterial blood inflow to the corpora cavernosa by as many as six-fold. This engorgement of the encapsulated corpora cavernosa compresses the venular plexus in the penis and reduces the blood outflow.

This process of penile perfusion involving arterial dilatation and venous compression is collaborated by three systems: the neurologic, circulatory and endocrinologic systems.

The neurologic system accounts for vasodilation and venoconstriction of the corporal blood vessels so that blood is shunted to the erectile tissues. Two neurological pathways are elicited during sexual arousal, one originating in the cerebral cortex and another from the genitals to the sacral segment of the spinal cord and cortex. While the cerebral cortex processes visual, auditory, and psychic stimuli, the lower pathway is stimulated by physical sensations to the genitals.

Psychogenic erection results when impulses from the brain mediate the spinal erection centers (T11-L2 and S2-S4) to induce an erection. Reflexogenic erection is caused by tactile stimuli to the genital organs reaching the spinal erection centers via the lower pathway. Cortico-sacral efferent signals are then transmitted via the spinal cord to the pelvic parasympathetic nerves and dilate the corporal vessels to promote increased blood flow.

From an engineering perspective, an erection is the hydraulic action of increased blood flow into the corpora cavernosa that creates the structural rigidity necessary to prevent the collapse of the penile column during copulation. Erectile dysfunction is, therefore, the collapsing or buckling of the penile column in the presence of an axial force when attempting or following vaginal intromission.[1] As such, the circulatory system plays a central role in acquiring and sustaining a penile erection in that blood flow be adequately supplied to the branches of the internal pudendal arteries that feed the corpora cavernosa to generate the needed hydraulic pressure.

Sometimes blood supply may be adequate to obtain an erection at rest but not sufficient to generate the much-needed hydraulic pressure to maintain an erection during intercourse. This is when the thrusting penis is subject to external pressure arising from the act of penetration as well as the reduction in hydraulic pressure caused by the diversion of blood supply to the pelvic musculature that is being placed under greater physical demand.

In the endocrine system, testosterone appears to have a positive effect on the hemodynamics of erection; though its mechanisms have yet to be fully understood. In animal studies, decreased cavernous tissue volume, decreased arterial flow, induced venous leakage and reduced erectile response to stimulation of the cavernous nerve are observed in castrated (reduced testosterone) rats. Castration is also associated with a rapid reduction in neuronal nitric oxide synthase (nNOS) that is suspected to effect on central regulation of blood pressure, a downgrade of smooth muscle relaxation and vasodilatation via peripheral nitrergic nerves and through the NO-cGMP vasodilation pathway.

It is well-known that testosterone from the endocrine system enhances sexual interest, increases the frequency of sexual acts and correlates to frequency of nocturnal erections. The same study correlating nocturnal erections to testosterone levels identified testosterone normal floor value as 200 ng/dl and demonstrated further that testosterone is lower-end sensitive.[2] This was affirmed clinically by the administration of testosterone therapy to impotent men with borderline low testosterone levels reportedly having little effect on potency.[3]

What is lesser known is testosterone has little effect on fantasy-induced or visually induced erections but testosterone and dihydrotestosterone are responsible for male pelvic thrusting vigor and ejaculation.[4]

Erectile dysfunction (ED), commonly referred to as impotence, is the persistent or recurrent inability to achieve or maintain an erection that is sufficient for satisfactory sexual performance.[5] Impotence can be broadly categorized as organic or psychogenic; organic being the inability to obtain an erection firm enough for vaginal penetration or the inability to sustain an erection until completion of intercourse due to physiological issues, while psychogenic impotence is the failure to achieve satisfactory sexual performance is due to emotional and psychological interference.

Organic ED is characterized by insidious and progressive decline leading to total erectile failure. The manifestation is consistent, non-situational and non-selective, i.e. partner or stimulation independent. Most patients with organic impotence are likely to have an underlying or undiagnosed medical condition.

By contrast, psychogenic ED is typically abrupt in onset and often associated with specific psychological trauma. It is therefore manifested intermittently cued by the imagery of the traumatic experience. Psychogenic ED is situational in that erectile failure may be presented with a specific partner(s) or any partner but not during self-stimulation. Impotent patients with Nocturnal Penile Tumescence are likely to be suffering from psychogenic rather than organic causes.

Stress, depression and heightened anxiety can affect the ability to achieve and sustain an erection before or during sexual activity. Psychogenic ED is also known as norepinephrine-mediated ED. As neurotransmitters, epinephrine impinges more on the heart while norepinephrine has more effect on the blood vessels. In a normal male, penile erection is accompanied by a reduction of norepinephrine in the cavernous blood and a rise in epinephrine levels in the systemic and cavernous blood, meaning that while the heart works harder, the blood vessels are relatively relaxed leading to higher blood flow. In patients with ED, the norepinephrine levels in the cavernous and systemic blood increase during sexual arousal leading to less powerful drive from the heart against constricted blood vessels; a probable cause of impaired erectile function.[6]

Organic ED may be further classified as neurogenic, vasculogenic, endocrinologic and iatrogenic.

As penile erection is a neurovascular event involving nerves and blood vessels, any disease or trauma affecting the efferent and afferent neural pathways between the brain and the genital can induce dysfunction.

Neurogenic ED is caused by a deficit in nerve signaling to the corpora cavernosa. Such deficits can be secondary to spinal cord injury, multiple sclerosis, Parkinson disease, lumbar disc disease, traumatic brain injury, radical pelvic surgery (radical prostatectomy, radical cystectomy, abdominoperineal resection) and diabetes.

Depending on the location, nature, and severity of the spinal injury that hampers transmission of neural signals, ED may be implicated. Upper motor neuron lesions (above spinal nerve T10) may not impair reflexogenic erection and ejaculation but can inhibit the central nervous system (CNS)-mediated control of the erection.

Reflexogenic erections are mediated by spinal erection centers (S2–S4) located in the sacral region. Decreased innervation arising from sacral injuries causes reduced nitric oxide (NO) load available to the smooth muscle that functionally hinders arterial flow to the penis. Structural tissue changes may also result in reduced perfusion and lack of pelvic ganglion activity/infrequent erections. A decrease in penile oxygen tension often leads to a reduction of smooth muscle cells as well as collagenization of the smooth muscle that diminishes penile elasticity and compliance causing veno-occlusive dysfunction or venous leak.[7]

The general principle behind vasculogenic ED is the reduction of blood perfusion pressure and arterial flow to the corpora cavernosa due to atherosclerotic or traumatic occlusion of the inner iliac arterial tree. This leads to increased timing taken to reach maximal erection as well as a reduction in rigidity of the aroused penis due to venous leakage. Common causes of arterial insufficiency resulting in vasculogenic ED include hypertension, hyperlipidemia, diabetes mellitus, tobacco smoking, blunt perineal/pelvic trauma and pelvic irradiation.

Vascular lesions, whether atherosclerotic or fibrotic, will limit flow to the corpora cavernosa. Diabetes and aging increase the incidence of fibrotic lesions of the cavernous artery. The arterial vascular bed of the penis was studied histologically in post-mortem material of aging men and men with diabetes. In males more than 38 years of age or with diabetes, there was fibrous substitution of the longitudinal smooth muscle complemented by intimal proliferation with calcification and luminal stenosis; apparently related to age and in particular diabetes mellitus.[8]

Both ED and cardiovascular disease share similar pathophysiological mechanisms and often coincide. Both disease states involve impaired vascular endothelial function and reduced availability of NO. There is also high coexistence between ED and cardiovascular disease such that ED is often cited as the purveyor of cardiovascular disease. Cigarette smoking is well established as a risk factor for cardiovascular disease and stroke. Smoking contributes to ED in different ways and its effects are dose-dependent and reversible. Nicotine may adversely affect erectile function not only by decreasing arterial flow to the penis (penile vasospasm) but also by blocking corporeal smooth muscle relaxation (NO pathway) and thus preventing normal venous occlusion.[9]

Akin to blunt perineal trauma, long-distance cycling that repeatedly traumatizes the rider's perineum area is also a risk factor for vasculogenic and neurogenic ED. One study on amateur long-distance cyclists revealed penile numbness or hypoesthesia with transient impotence in more than 60% of the respondents after a tour/competition. Both genital numbness and impotence were correlated with weakness in the hands after the ride.[10]

Endocrinologic ED is caused by dysfunction of the hypothalamic-pituitary-gonadal (HPG) axis resulting in hypogonadism.

In healthy males, the hypothalamus initiates the release of gonadotropin-releasing hormone (GnRH) into the hypothalamic-pituitary portal system. The anterior pituitary then secretes follicle-stimulating hormone (FSH) and Luteinizing Hormone (LH) which stimulate an increase in gonadal activity. In completing the feedback loop, the increase in gonadal hormones results in lowered FSH and LH secretion at the pituitary level. Within the testes, LH stimulates Leydig cells to produce testosterone, whereas FSH is necessary for tubular growth.

Hypergonadotropic hypogonadism (primary hypogonadism), a downstream HPG axial dysfunction, results when the gonad does not produce adequate sex steroid to suppress the secretion of LH and FSH at normal levels. Hypogonadotropic hypogonadism, an upstream HPG axial dysfunction, results from a disorder of the hypothalamic GnRH pulse generator or inability of the pituitary to respond with LH and FSH secretions. Whilst both hypogonadism types may be acquired from trauma, disease (mumps orchitis) or injury, only hypogonadotropic hypogonadism can be congenital.[11]

Men with hyperprolactinemia present frequently with pituitary macroadenoma. Hyperprolactinemia causes elevated prolactin levels that suppress GnRH secretion and induces low circulating levels of testosterone. Symptoms, reflective of both reproductive and sexual dysfunction, may include impaired libido, ED, galactorrhea, gynecomastia, diminished ejaculate volume and oligospermia.[12]

Iatrogenic refers to complication induced inadvertently by medical treatment or diagnostic procedure but in this instance, the term is used loosely to include situations that the clinician could have known of the adverse effects but chose to proceed with the procedure on balance of medical rationality.

Radical pelvic surgery appears to be the prevalent cause of iatrogenic ED. In spite of advances in nerve-sparing surgeries, damage to the cavernous nerve may be inevitable (neurogenic ED). Injury to the accessory pudendal artery is another cause (vasculogenic ED).

Anti-hypertensive drugs are closely associated with ED and thiazide diuretics, centrally acting-agents and beta-blockers have been reported to be more detrimental to sexual performance than other antihypertensive agents like calcium channel antagonists and ACE inhibitors.[13] Anti-androgens, psychotherapeutics, anti-ulcer drugs, opiates, and digoxin have also been linked with ED. Notwithstanding, a direct association between these medications and ED has yet to be established as the underlying diseases these medication purport to treat are also risk factors of ED.

In summary, ED is a neurovascular disorder that can be caused by underlying conditions, trauma or medical iatrogenesis. Neurogenic ED is the usual cause for failure to initiate an erection, while the failure of penile engorgement due to arterial insufficiency (filling the corpora) and veno-occlusive dysfunction (blood storage at corpora) is related to vasculogenic ED. Endocrinologic ED provides the backdrop.

From a TCM perspective...

There are 5 types of non-performing male 五不男 and the descriptions from the ancient medical text refer to the five observed sexual disorders namely congenital 天, leakage 漏, bullock 犍, timid 怯 and transformed 变, which in modern-day context represent congenital Hypogonadotropic Hypogonadism (absence of gonads/secondary sexual characteristic) 天阉, premature ejaculation 漏, castration or genital mutilation 犍, Erectile Dysfunction 怯 and hermaphroditism (intersexual) 变 respectively.[14]

ED, as identified above, is associated with heart, liver, spleen and kidney systems. The underlying cause is a deficiency in the liver and kidney; with damp-heat, Qi stagnation and blood stasis as clinical presentations 本虚标实. Risk factors for ED are congenital insufficiency 先天禀赋不足, excessive coitus 房劳过度, emotional trauma 情志失调, and gastronomic indulgence 饮食不节.

ED is more closely associated with the liver system because the liver meridian and its collateral transverse the hypogastric-cavernous region, the testicles and penis 径胫上睾，结于茎. And according to TCM principles [*HuangDi's Internal Classics: Miraculous Pivot*], the liver governs the tendons and the genitals (penis) is the gathering place of the ancestral tendon 宗筋.

《灵枢·经脉》: "厥阴者，肝脉也，肝者筋之合也，筋者聚于阴器"

In another segment of Miraculous Pivot, it was documented that disorder of the liver meridian could render the penis incompetent; flaccid when the meridian is internally injured; withdrawn when injured by cold, and priapism when injured by heat.

《灵枢·经筋》: "足厥阴之筋，其病…阴器不用，伤于内则不起，伤于寒则阴缩入，伤于热则纵挺不收。"

To achieve a meaningful erection, Qi and thus blood must reach and nourish the genitals and the liver is instrumental in this regulatory function. Emotional distress that causes dysfunction of the liver and spleen would disrupt the seamless distribution of Qi. As the flow of Qi and blood is concurrent, stagnation of Qi at the liver would impede the flow of blood to engorge the penis, leading to ED.

Similarly, psychological trauma that imposes on the kidney causing Qi mechanism to retrograde and behave in a disorderly manner shall, on a longer term, cause insufficiency of kidney essence and result in the debilitation of the life-gate fire 命門火衰. This means that the kidney essence fails to be transported into the ancestral tendon (penis), leading to the genital being limp and wilted.

In TCM clinical setting, ED may present in the following sub-types: liver Qi stagnation 肝气郁结, liver Qi retrograde 肝气横逆, damp-heat in Liver Meridian 肝经湿热, obstruction of collateral by blood stasis 瘀血阻络, occlusion of collateral by phlegm 痰湿阻络,

occlusion of Liver Meridian by cold 寒滞肝脉, kidney impairment by psychological trauma 恐惧伤肾, kidney Yin deficiency 肾阴亏虚, liver blood deficiency 肝血虚 and spleen/stomach Qi deficiency 脾胃气虚.

Contemporary medicine appears to acknowledge that TCM may have some role to play in the treatment of ED, especially in deficiency syndrome type. The TCM treatment of ED ties in with the treatment of late-onset hypogonadism (LOH). LOH occurs due to the breakdown in coordination between the heart and the kidneys, deficiencies of the spleen and kidney Yang, deficiencies of the liver and kidney Yin and deficiencies of the kidney essence.[15]

The treatment principle is therefore to smooth the flow of liver qi, tonify liver blood and kidney essence, nourish the spleen and unblock the relevant meridians. Damp-heat, phlegm, and cold if present should be cleared to further regulate blood circulation.

Gua Sha Protocol for Adjuvant Treatment and Symptomatic Relief

a. Occipital-Cervical Sweep
b. Back Rejuvenation Dredge
c. Sacral V dredge
d. Umbilicus-Pubic Sweep
e. Acupoint 'press-and-hold' for SP6 三阴交, SP9 阴陵泉, ST36 足三里, KI3 太溪, KI7 复溜, LR8 曲泉 on both legs

Execution — Unless TCM diagnosis suggests otherwise, moderation press-stroke recommended. Acupoints marked for application of 'press-and-hold' technique in each prescription form a set, each set to be repeated three times. 'Press-and-hold' maneuver should be attempted 10 times for each prescribed acupoint within each set. Use of skin lubricant that invigorates Qi and dispels blood stasis preferred. Observation of Sha appearance not mandatory.

Glossary

Partial pressure of oxygen, also known as PaO2, is a measurement of oxygen in arterial blood. It shows how well oxygen is able to move from the lungs to the blood. It explains why oxygen moves from the alveoli (lung) into the blood and carbon dioxide from the blood into the alveoli. This behavior of gas exchange is explained by the principles of Dalton's law and Henry's law. Air containing 21% oxygen at atmospheric pressure of 760 mmHg (sea level) has PaO2 of $0.21 \times 760 = 160$ mmHg at point of inspiration. As air works its way into the alveoli, water vapor and carbon dioxide are added that reduces the PaO2 to about 104 mmHg in the alveolar gas

Nocturnal Penile Tumescence (abbreviated as NPT) is a spontaneous erection of the penis during sleep or when waking up. Men without physiological erectile dysfunction should experience nocturnal penile tumescence, usually three to five times during the night, typically during REM sleep

Atherosclerotic refers to a condition associated with atherosclerosis, a disease in which plaque builds up inside the arteries and progressively thickening and hardening of the inner walls of arteries until the vessel becomes totally blocked

Galactorrhea is a milky nipple discharge unrelated to the normal milk production of breastfeeding. Galactorrhea itself is not a disease but could be a sign of an underlying problem, usually hormone-related.

Priapism refers to a prolonged usually painful erection of the penis that persists for hours and even days. Priapism may not be caused by sexual stimulation

References

1. Udelson D. Biomechanics of male erectile function. *J. R. Soc. Interface* **4**: 1031–1047 (2007).
2. Granata AR, Rochira V, *et al.* Relationship between sleep-related erections and testosterone levels in men. *J. Androl.* **18**: 522–527 (1997).
3. Graham C, Regan J. Blinded clinical trial of testosterone enanthate in impotent men with low or low normal serum testosterone levels. *Int. J. Impot. Res.* **4**: 144 (1992).
4. Beyer C, Gonzalez-Mariscal G. Effects of sex steroids on sensory and motor spinal mechanisms. *Psychoneuroendocrinology* **19**: 512–517 (1994).
5. NIH Consensus Conference. Impotence. NIH Consensus Development Panel on Impotence. *JAMA* **270**: 83–90 (1993).
6. Becker AJ, Uckert S. Cavernous and systemic plasma levels of norepinephrine and epinephrine during different penile conditions in healthy men and patients with erectile dysfunction. *Urology* **59**(2): 281–286 (Feb 2002).

7. Yafi FA, Jenkins L, *et al.* Erectile dysfunction. *Nat. Rev. Dis. Primers* **2**: 16003 (2017).
8. Ruzbarský V, Michal V. Morphologic changes in the arterial bed of the penis with aging. Relationship to the pathogenesis of impotence. *Invest. Urol.* **15**(3): 194–199 (Nov 1977).
9. Biebel MG, Burnett AL, *et al.* Male sexual function and smoking. *Sex Med. Rev.* **4**(4): 366–375 (Oct 2016).
10. Andersen KV, Bovim G. Impotence and nerve entrapment in long-distance amateur cyclists. *Acta Neurol. Scand.* **95**(4): 233–240 (Apr1997).
11. Fraietta R, Zylberstejn DS, *et al.* Hypogonadotropic hypogonadism revisited. *Clinics* **68**(S1): 81–88 (2013).
12. De Rosa M, Zarrilli S, *et al.* Hyperprolactinemia in men: clinical and biochemical features and response to treatment. *Endocrine* **20**(1–2): 75–82 (Feb-Mar 2003).
13. Fogari R, Zoppi A. Effects of antihypertensive therapy on sexual activity in hypertensive men. *Curr. Hypertens. Rep.* **4**(3): 202–210 (2002).
14. Wan Mi Zhai 万全(密斋). *Critical Success Factors for Procreation — On Mate Selection* 《广嗣纪要·择配篇 (1573).
15. Lee JKC, Tan RBW, Chung E. Erectile dysfunction treatment and traditional medicine — can East and West medicine coexist? *Transl. Androl. Urol.* **6**(1): 91–100 (2017).

Topic 72

Premature Ejaculation

In the primate world, procreation is often preceded with competition and aggression; with the threat of aggression and act of guarding persisting even during breeding. Insemination is a prerequisite for procreation in mammals and for the purpose of species survival, the male genital tract is designed anatomically for *coitus citus*, meaning copulation on the move or performed with haste. From a zoological perspective, this reproductive strategy is indicative of an adaptive behavior when an animal is poised for retaliation or escape even during coitus when insemination is accomplished with despatch and security. Intromission and rapid ejaculation, therefore, become essential for 'proliferation in the wild' and spread of genetic material via rapid procreation with multiple partners. This is observed in chimpanzees when the entire process of approach, penetration, and ejaculation lasts merely 6 seconds.[1]

By contrast, the evolved man who holds intellectual development above the highest order of primates ascribes functions beyond mere procreation to coitus. In fact, when he associates the quality of his life and that of his partner to the due performance of these routine encounters, ejaculation control becomes a critical success factor. In this regard, it becomes arguable that premature ejaculation (PE), technically being the failure to coordinate insemination with sexual satisfaction of one's partner, is a cultural issue rather than a natural issue.

Ejaculation is the final phase of coitus for the mammalian male and consists of two coordinated neurological reflexes: emission and ejection. Emission involves peristaltic smooth muscle contractions of the seminal vesicles and prostate and results in the expulsion of sperm and seminal fluid into the posterior urethra. This is mediated by the sympathetic nervous system (T10–L2). Once emission is completed, the ejaculate is ready to be expelled through the urethra.

Seminal ejection occurs when the semen is rapidly and forcefully advanced forward along the urethra and spring out through the penile meatus. This involves the pulsatile contractions of the bulbocavernosus and pelvic floor muscles with the relaxation of the external urinary sphincter. This is mediated by somatic nerves (S2–S4) and involves the sympathetic nervous system with limited voluntary control. These reflexes are stimulated by sensory input from nerve endings in the glans penis, which are relayed via the sacral spinal cord to the sensory cerebral cortex. In male humans, this perceptual-cognitive and pleasurable event associated with ejaculation, hyperventilation of around 40 breaths/min, tachycardia and elevated blood pressure is termed orgasm. Orgasm is followed by a refractory period of transient erectile inhibition.[2]

The fundamental process of ejaculation further involves the operation of complex pathways of central serotonergic and dopaminergic neurons. As essential neurotransmitters, dopamine promotes seminal emission and ejaculation via D2 receptors, while serotonin is inhibitory via the serotonin receptors (5-HT). This inhibitory effect is likely to occur in the brain, as a 5HT effect on ejaculation in the spine is likely stimulatory. Another neurochemical that has an inhibitory role in the ejaculation process is nitric oxide (NO).

Hormonal regulation is also implicated in PE. Contrary to popular belief, testosterone the key hormone to male sexuality did not demonstrate a consistent association with PE. In one study, it was suggested that low testosterone (hypogonadism) could be a possible cause of delayed ejaculation (DE) while high serum testosterone levels were found in PE patients.[3] In a smaller but later study, no significant difference between the levels of total testosterone and free testosterone was detected in PE patients and control group.[4] Looking at the data groups drawn from both studies, PE vs DE and PE vs normal, one interpretation of the two studies could be that inversed effect of testosterone on ejaculation latency time could be more pronounced at the lower serum levels than the effect above the baseline level.

Oxytocin is produced in the hypothalamus and released by the posterior pituitary; it is also produced locally by the testis as well as the prostate. The role of oxytocin in PE is less obvious and believed to reduce ejaculatory latency times through central and peripheral pathways.

Thyroid status may, however, have direct involvement with the physiology of ejaculation. A high prevalence of PE has been observed in hyperthyroid patients, whereas DE was also frequently reported by patients with hypothyroidism; a finding more pronounced in patients with acquired rather than lifelong PE. When thyroid functions were re-established, both ejaculatory dysfunctions extinguished without treatment for the sexual symptom.[5]

Because PE is strictly not a functional failure but shortfall against subjective expectation, the definition is thwarted with many difficulties and remains a challenge even today. The International Society of Sexual Medicine definition (2014) refers to premature ejaculation as ejaculation that always or nearly always occurs prior to or within about 1 minute of vaginal penetration from first sexual experiences (lifelong/primary PE) or a clinically bothersome reduction in latency time, often to about 3 minutes or less (acquired PE); inability to delay ejaculation on all or nearly all vaginal penetrations; and imposes negative personal consequences such as distress, bother, frustration, and/or the avoidance of sexual intimacy.[6]

The ISSM 2014 definition identifies two distinct classes of PE: primary PE that occurs since inception and acquired PE; it further introduces an objective, quantifiable timing to ejaculation latency, which is referred to as the intravaginal ejaculatory latency time (IELT). IELT refers to the time interval from vaginal penetration to ejaculation.

The demarcation between primary and acquired PE allows for a clearer diagnosis and management of the disorder. Primary or lifelong PE is mainly driven by genetic or neurobiological factors while the etiologies for acquired PE are psycho-relational (anxiety, relational issues), urological (prostatitis), hormonal (hyperthyroidism) and andrological (erectile dysfunction).

In studies of genetic influence on PE, the target of assessment was gene polymorphism for the serotonin transporter protein (5-HTTLPR) and the dopamine active transporter gene (DAT-1) as a modulator of ejaculation latency. The outcome of these studies, however, was controversial and suggests at best that individual genetic polymorphisms may exert a minor influence or create a predisposition towards PE rather than a direct cause-and-effect relationship.[6] Major neurological disorders of genetic origin that may cause PE include multiple sclerosis and spina bifida.

Neurobiological factors affecting PE refers mainly to disturbances of central serotonin (5-HT) neurotransmission and 5-HT receptor functioning (serotonin hyperactivity) and glans penis hypersensitivity. The general assumption is the serotoninergic system acts as a suppressor of the ejaculatory reflex at the hypothalamic level. Low serum levels of 5-HT have been associated with an increase in libido while increased serotonin levels are thought to decrease arousal and thus extends IELT. The therapy of choice is the administration of Selective Serotonin Reuptake Inhibitor (SSRI).

SSRIs block the reabsorption (reuptake) of serotonin in the brain, making serotonin more available to the brain and extending the effect of signals caused by serotonin. By limiting its reabsorption (reuptake) into the presynaptic cell, the extracellular level of serotonin is enhanced, increasing the level of serotonin in the synaptic cleft available to bind to the postsynaptic receptor.

Despite the high efficacy, impressive safety profile and low prevalence of Treatment-Emergent Adverse Events (TEAEs), the discontinuation rate of using of SSRIs were high; 79.1% within 6 months and 90.1% at 2 years. The reasons cited for dropping-out were disappointment that PE was incurable and tablets needed for every sexual encounter, side effects (nausea, headache, and vertigo), perceived poor efficacy, high maintenance cost and search for alternative remedies.[7]

Glans penis hypersensitivity can be effectively managed with topical anesthetic agents containing lignocaine, lignocaine/prilocaine or herbal-derived anesthetic components. Applied to the glans penis ahead of coitus and used in conjunction with condoms to avoid numbness in the partner's genitals, these agents can increase IELT and sexual satisfaction.

In acquired PE (APE), hyperthyroidism appeared to be a single cause that is manifestly treatable with a high degree of permanence. In hyperthyroid patients, the increased adrenergic tone may precipitate both PE and ED, either acting directly on smooth muscle contractility/relaxation or indirectly on anxiety and irritability. Further and in the alternative, with widespread distribution of thyroid hormone nuclear receptors within the brain as well as the testis, it can be postulated that iodothyronines can mediate central serotoninergic pathway, leading to diminished ejaculation control which is observed in animal studies where increased serotonin turnover in the brainstem is consistently reported in experimentally-induced hypothyroid mice.

Prostate inflammation/infections, especially chronic prostatitis, have been empirically correlated with PE as prostatic inflammation was found in 56.5% and chronic bacterial prostatitis in 47.8% of the subjects with PE.[8] One reason could be prostatitis-induced erectile dysfunction mediated the PE. If indeed prostatitis is the cause, successful eradication of causative organisms in patients with PE and chronic prostatitis may lead to a marked improvement in ejaculatory control and therefore IELT. In one study, where infection/inflammation is confirmed by expressed prostatic secretion (EPS) culture and white blood cell (WBC) count, 83.9% patients demonstrated increased IELT and reported good control of their ejaculation with no recurrence of PE upon clearance of the prostatitis.[9] This outcome was confirmed in another study that antimicrobial therapy is effective in the treatment of PE associated with inflammatory prostatitis; the results are most pronounced in men with acquired PE and when there are ≥19 pus cells per high–power field (HPF) in an EPS analysis.[10]

Evidence demonstrates that up to half of men with PE also experience erectile dysfunction (ED), with a third of patients being easily confused between the two conditions. A possible interaction between the two sexual dysfunctions was rationalized by Jannini *et al.*, in the form of an ED-PE vicious circle, that men with ED instinctively raise the levels of arousal to attain an erection or may attempt to rush sexual intercourse prior to a loss of erection; in both situations they will be predisposed to reduced ejaculatory control and possibly PE. Conversely, men with PE may instinctively reduce the level of arousal to control ejaculation which may aggravate the erectile function.[11] It has also been suggested that men may ejaculate prematurely for lack of confidence in maintaining a reliable erection. Sexual dysfunction associated with performance anxiety invariably aggravates erectile function.

Phosphodiesterase-5 inhibitors (PDE5i) are the gold standard first-line treatment for ED. PDE5 is expressed in the prostate, vas deferens, and seminal vesicles and may have a physiological role in ejaculation. 5PDEi should, however, be prescribed for treatment of PE in situations where PE coexists with ED.[12]

PE is generally age-dependent with younger patients showing a higher prevalence of anxiety symptoms. Performance anxiety is often treated with behavioral therapy — a gradated protocol of non-demanding genital stimulation that may proceed to erection but not orgasm (Semans' stop-and-start program and Masters & Johnson's squeeze technique). The objective of the protocol is moderation in genital activity to reduce the "pressure to perform" so that the patients learn to (i) evaluate pre-orgasmic pleasure, (ii) be aware of the "orgasmic point of no return", (iii) prolong the plateau phase, and (iv) distinguish between excitation and orgasm.[13] The confidence of the patient to perform is thus reinforced through a "virtuous circle" and perhaps his psychological and interpersonal issues resolved in the process.

Behavioral therapies, however, have limitations in that they are receptive only to highly motivated couples enjoying a strong relationship, of young age and with recently onset sexual dysfunction. But the derived benefits can also be transient and plateau off quickly. As the therapies are designed on the premise of partners' mutual accommodation, they are not applicable to single males with multiple or occasional partners.

Premature ejaculation is a common yet complex male sexual dysfunction that causes significant psychological, emotional and interpersonal distress for the patient and his partner. Complexities of the disorder come from the fact that the etiology could be multifactorial and for a lack of objective measurement. The introduction of IELT resolved the quantitative issue. The classification of PE in whether the disorder is primary or acquired further improves and guides the management of PE.

From a TCM perspective...

Sexual dysfunctions, PE included, were known to the Chinese since the time between 500 BCE and 200 CE. As a response to these disorders, Taoism and TCM practitioners developed a set of effective yet safe techniques that are quite similar to those employed by contemporary behavioral therapists and psychotherapists. Many of these therapies are supported by TCM theories and may even have therapeutic relevance today. This art of sexuality, distilled from the empirical experience of 700 years, is compiled into two manuals entitled The Plain Damsel's Classics 素女经 and The Art of Bed Chamber 房中术.

The liver has a key role in PE as its meridian loops around the genitals with one of its branches terminating at the penis [*HuangDi's Internal Classics: Miraculous Pivot*].

《灵枢·经脉》："肝足厥阴之脉……过阴器……其别者……结于茎"

In 'Notes from Reading Medicine 读医随笔', it was mentioned that people suffering from stagnated or agitated liver meridian are prone to seek rapid relief whenever they encounter anxiety. When the liver Yang is not duly distributed, it descends upon the kidney; and this can be due to liver Qi 志气 being in a state of flux, agitated by anger. For it is the nature of the liver to regulate Qi and energy, and when this is not achieved in an upward direction, the same shall descend and be dissipated downwards.[14]

《读医随笔》："凡肝经郁勃之人，于欲事每迫不遇，必待一泄，始得舒快。此肝阳不得宣达，下陷于肾，是怒之激其志气，使志气不得静也。肝以疏泄为性，既不得疏于上，而陷于下，遂不得不泄于下"

Accordingly, tactile stimulation generated during copulation and transmitted along the liver meridian would invariably precipitate PE in people with liver meridian disturbance.

The kidney is the innate reserve of and keeper for vital essence and dominates the reproductive function. Production and discharge of semen would be duly regulated when the dynamic equilibrium between yin and yang of the kidney is maintained. Premature ejaculation (PE) occurs when this dynamic equilibrium is lost, resulting in the untimely discharge of semen. This is exhaustively deliberated in Dialectical Records 辨证录·种嗣门（九则）in which the kidney and heart are implicated in PE[15]:

"The most severe of PE occurs when runny semen is involuntarily discharged at the vulva of the partner with any immediate attempt to seek further pleasure being futile; a situation many ascribed as a congenital weakness but in reality, deficiency of the heart and kidney. Those who laid claim in coital endurance are endowed with strong 'Gate of Life' (kidney) fire, the power of which is derived from the heart fire. Now that the fire of heart is the imperial fire and that fire of kidney is the ministerial fire, the strength of the ministerial fire would obviously be in pace with the imperial fire. However, if the imperial fire is weakened, control would be transferred to the ministerial fire that would influence the imperial fire instead. In this regard, the ministerial fire would take lead whenever volatility with the heart fire is detected; such as even when the heart fire desired to restraint emission, the ministerial fire would insidiously evacuate semen through the orifice. For those suffering from PE prior to penetration, the imperial fire may not be fully oppressed; neither would the ministerial fire be in full blaze. The general principle of therapy would be to address the deficiency of heart fire and avoid purging the excesses in the ministerial fire. This is because any attempt to dissipate ministerial fire would cause a further decline in the imperial fire"

《辨证录》：男子有精滑之极，一到妇女之门，即便泄精，欲勉强图欢不可得，且泄精甚薄，人以为天分之弱也，谁知心肾之两虚乎？ 夫入房可以久战者，命门火旺也。然作用虽属于命门之火，而操权实在于心宫之火。盖心火乃君火也，命门之火相火也。心火旺则相火听令于心，君火衰则心火反为相火所移，权操于相火，而不在君火矣。故心君之火一动，相火即操其柄，心即欲谨守其精，相火已暗送精于精门之外。至于望门泄精者，不特君火衰极，相火亦未常盛也。治法补心火之不足，不可泻相火之有余，盖泻相火，则君火益衰耳

As in all deficiency syndrome, dysfunction of the spleen is invariably involved. PE, a disorder with underlying deficiency but clinical presentations of excess nature, is no exception.

From the foregoing, the etiologies of PE are deficiency in kidney Qi leading to lower endurance and therefore a decline in ejaculation control; or deficiency of liver and kidney Yin which failed to prevent the descent of kidney fire (ministerial fire) 相火下注 that in turn causes impulsive discharge of semen 火邪逼精妄泄; or deficiencies of the heart and spleen that cause loss in the general retentive 摄纳 power of Qi; or functional damage of the liver arising from emotional distress; transformation of liver stagnation into heat/fire 肝郁化火; or functional damage to the kidney arising from extreme fear, excessive sexual indulgence or self-stimulation that depleted kidney essence.

These causes give rise to five different sub-types of PE in TCM clinical setting: liver Qi stagnation 肝气郁结 type in which patients are constantly emotionally distressed; excessive ministerial 相火亢进 fire type in which Yin and Yang of the person are in a state of imbalance and having inadequate fluid or blood to cool the over-heated organs which could be systemic or organ-specific; kidney Qi deficiency 肾气不固 type in which Yin (fluid, blood) and Yang (warming life force) are lacking in the reproductive system; heart-spleen deficiency 心脾亏虚 type in which emission control is encumbered by general debility; and damp-heat in Liver meridian 肝经湿热 type in which PE follows swiftly after rapid arousal.

Gua Sha Protocol for Adjuvant Treatment and Symptomatic Relief

a. Occipital-Cervical Sweep
b. Trapezius Sweep
c. Superior Bladder Meridian Dredge
d. Back Rejuvenation Dredge
e. Sacral V dredge
f. Umbilicus-Pubic Sweep
g. Acupoint 'press-and-hold' for SP6 三阴交, ST36 足三里, KI3 太溪, LR1 大敦, LR4 中封 on both legs
h. Acupoint 'press-and-hold' for PC6 内关, HT7 神门 on both hands

Execution — Unless TCM diagnosis suggests otherwise, moderation press-stroke recommended. Acupoints marked for application of 'press-and-hold' technique in each prescription form a set, each set to be repeated three times. 'Press-and-hold' maneuver should be attempted 10 times for each prescribed acupoint within each set. Use of skin lubricant that invigorates Qi and dispels blood stasis preferred. Observation of Sha appearance not mandatory.

Glossary

Serotonin or 5-hydroxytryptamine (5-HT) is a monoamine neurotransmitter known to contribute to feelings of well-being and happiness. Made from the essential amino acid tryptophan, it is found in the digestive system, blood and the throughout the nervous system. Its biological function is complex and multifaceted, involving the modulation of cognition, reward, mood, sexual desire and function, appetite, sleep, memory and learning, temperature regulation, and numerous physiological processes. It is also the driver of nausea. Low serum levels of 5-HT have been associated with depression and an increase in libido. Increased serotonin levels are thought to decrease arousal.

In the TCM theory of organ-fire, the fire of heart is referred to as imperial fire 君火 and fire of the kidney (and fire of the liver by some scholars) are called the ministerial fire 相火. The term imperial fire carries the connotation

(*Continued*)

(*Continued*)

that the heart is in the anatomically superior position and, from the perspective of 5-element theory, the heart system is associated with fire. In that sense, imperial fire is the 'fire of fire' and is sterling Yang. By contrast, kidney fire is 'fire within water', positioned anatomically inferior and should not be at parity with that of the heart. The ministerial fire is also the 'fire of passion'. In reality, all five internal organ-system may have fire, except that those of the heart and kidney (and liver) are more volatile.

Under normal conditions, the imperial/heart fire should be kept ablaze in the Upper Energizer 上焦 and the ministerial/kidney fire maintains warmth at the Lower Energizer 下焦 with the communication between the two fires sustained by the triple Energizer 三焦 thoroughfare. The fire of the heart is therefore synchronized with that of the kidney and vice versa. In the event that intensity of the imperial fire is not coordinated with the ministerial fire, disorder of the heart occurs. The converse also holds. Thus in the treatment of heat-related disorders, it is imperative to pinpoint the exact organ-fire. Excessive heart fire should be controlled by bitter cold 苦寒 herbs but for excess kidney fire, cold salty 咸寒 herbs are more appropriate. If the excess heat is caused by deficiencies of heart and kidney Yin, the obvious prescription would be Yin nourishing herbs.

References

1. Jannini EA, Ciocca G, *et al.* Premature ejaculation: old story, new insights. *Fertil. Steril.* **104**: 1061–1073 (2015).
2. Alwaal A, Breyer BN, Lue TF. Normal male sexual function: emphasis on orgasm and ejaculation. *Fertil. Steril.* **104**(5): 1051–1060 (Nov 2015).
3. Corona G, Jannini EA, *et al.* Different testosterone levels are associated with ejaculatory dysfunction. *J. Sex. Med.* **5**: 1991–8 (2008).
4. Canat L, Erbin A, *et al.* Assessment of hormonal activity in patients with premature ejaculation *Int. Braz. J. Urol.* **43**(2): 311–316 (2017).
5. Carani C, Isidori AM, *et al.* Multicenter study on the prevalence of sexual symptoms in male hypo- and hyperthyroid patients. *J. Clin. Endocrinol. Metab.* **90**: 6472–6479 (2005).
6. Althof SE, McMahon CG, Waldinger MD, *et al.* An update of the International Society of Sexual Medicine's Guidelines for the Diagnosis and Treatment of Premature Ejaculation (PE). *J. Sex. Med.* **2**: 60–90 (2014).
7. Park HJ, Park NC, *et al.* Discontinuation of Dapoxetine treatment in patients with premature ejaculation: a 2-year prospective observational study. *Sex. Med.* **5**: e99–e105 (2017).

8. Screponia E, Carosa E, *et al.* Prevalence of chronic prostatitis in men with premature ejaculation. *Urology* **58**(2): 198–202 (Aug 2001).
9. El-Nashaar A, Shamloul R. Antibiotic treatment can delay ejaculation in patients with premature ejaculation and chronic bacterial prostatitis. *J. Sex. Med.* **4**: 491–496 (2007).
10. Zohdy W. Clinical parameters that predict successful outcome in men with premature ejaculation and inflammatory prostatitis. *J. Sex. Med.* **6**: 3139–3146 (2009).
11. Jannini EA, Lombardo F, *et al.* Correlation between ejaculatory and erectile dysfunction. *Int. J. Androl.* **28**(Suppl 2): 40–45 (2005).
12. McMahon CG, McMahon CN, *et al.* Efficacy of type-5 phosphodiesterase inhibitors in the drug treatment of premature ejaculation: a systematic review. *BJU Int.* **98**(2): 259–272 (2006).
13. Jannini EA, Carosa E, *et al.* Update on pathophysiology of premature ejaculation: the bases for new pharmacological treatments. *Eur. Urol. Suppl.* **4**(4): 141–149 (2006).
14. Zhou Xuehai 周学海. *Reading Medical Essays* 读医随笔 (1644–1911).
15. Chen Shizhen 陈士铎. *Dialectical Record* 《辨证录.》种嗣门（九则）(1644–1911).

Epilogue

We have come to the conclusion of this book.

This book presents *Gua Sha* as a time-honored ancient Chinese therapy that survived the baptism of disapproval in its march of time into modern society. Along the way, many skeptics with formal healthcare training have labeled it as unscientific and consigned it to the realms of quackery. It did not help, for lack of understanding, that the 'bruising' surfaced during treatment was often mistaken by less informed social workers in other cultures to be evidence of physical abuse especially when the patient was a child or an institutionalized elderly. This grave misconception further distanced *Gua Sha* from the medical community.

Having said that, few are aware that since 2005, there have been more than 120 studies on *Gua Sha*, mostly investigating its efficacy in alleviating painful musculoskeletal conditions. On a wider scope, Harvard-led researchers, in 2011, found *Gua Sha* having anti-inflammatory and immunological properties. In yet another 2013 Harvard report, *Gua Sha* demonstrated promise in reducing liver inflammation in chronic active hepatitis B patients.[1]

Gua Sha has come a long way. From a rudimentary therapeutic technique that subsumes acupuncture and popularly adopted for myofascial pain treatment, it has evolved to include non-invasive acupoint stimulation. Needless to say, the ambit of treatment for *Gua Sha* has also expanded to encompass many of the ailments that are addressed by acupuncture.

Gua Sha is known to accord her practitioner a wide latitude of error during execution. Perhaps another but lesser mentioned attribute of *Gua Sha* is it provides her user the same tolerance in therapeutic decision error. *Gua Sha* has a characteristic of acquiescence in that "the administered healing protocol would only demonstrate effect by the presence of a disease 有病则病受之". Coupled with the fact that *Gua Sha* has now become the *de facto* "acupuncture without needles", the technique has evolved into a comprehensive home-based healing system that harbors little iatrogenic permanence. In short, *Gua Sha* is a treatment with little downside risk but high upside reward.

Readers would probably notice a trend in the choice of *Gua Sha* patterns, engagement of meridians and selection of acupoints for disorders related to a specific organ dysfunction are relatively similar. This is deliberately highlighted for readers' attention by organizing illnesses accordingly in the Application Section of this text.

On a different note and interestingly, cupping therapy with the same fundamental principles had its share of disbelief and criticisms too. But when Michael Phelps and fellow Olympians proudly paraded the 2016 Olympics ground at Rio De Janeiro with purple circular tell-tale skin marks on their bodies like badges of honor, their act immediately sparked off a tsunami of interest and acceptance from the world for cupping as a miraculous fatigue recovery modality. Yet another instance of ancient Chinese treasure being first appreciated by the Western world.

This book is dedicated to all readers with the fervent wish that, through the introduction of this ostensibly simple topic of *Gua Sha*, the interest of all in TCM would be ignited.

In the course of writing, the author has been ever mindful that "any third-grade presenter can increase the complexity of things, but it takes someone with profound understanding to make things simple again". The author hopes that he did not inadvertently commit this literary mistake.

Reference

1. Chan ST, Yuen JW, Gohel MD, *et al.* Guasha-induced hepatoprotection in chronic active hepatis B: A case study. *Clin. Chim. Acta* **412**(17–18): 1686–1688 (17 Aug 2011); Chan ST, Yuen JW, Gohel MD, *et al.* Does guasha offer hepatoprotective effect to chronic inactive hepatis B carriers? A built-indesign to control subject expectation. *J. Alterm. Complement. Med.* **19**(9): 772–776 (Sep 2013).

APPENDIX

China Historical Timeline

Pre-historic China	
Dawn of Civilization	Before 2070 BC
Xia Dynasty 夏代	2070–1600 BC
Ancient China	
Shang Dynasty 商朝	1600–1050 BC
Zhou Dynasty 周朝	1066–771 BC
Spring and Autumn Period 春秋时期	771–475 BC
Warring States Period 战国时期	475–221 BC
Qin Dynasty 秦朝	221–206 BC
Han Dynasty 汉朝	206 BC–220 AD
Chinese "Middle Ages"	
Three Kingdoms Period 三国时期	220–265
Jin Dynasty 晋朝	265–420
Southern & Northern Dynasties 南北朝	420–589
Sui Dynasty 隋朝	581–618
Tang Dynasty 唐朝	618–907
Five Dynasties & Ten Kingdoms 五代十国	907–960
Sung Dynasty 宋朝	960–1279
Yuan Dynasty 元朝	1279–1368
Ming Dynasty 明朝	1368–1644
Qing Dynasty 清朝	1644–1912
Republic of China 中華民國	1912–1949
People's Republic of China 中华人民共和国	1949 onwards

www.ingramcontent.com/pod-product-compliance
Ingram Content Group UK Ltd.
Pitfield, Milton Keynes, MK11 3LW, UK
UKHW020352150926
8624IPUK00004B/132